Developmental Paediatrics

POSTGRADUATE PAEDIATRICS SERIES

Under the General Editorship of

JOHN APLEY
C.B.E., M.D., B.S., F.R.C.P.

Emeritus Consultant Paediatrician, United Bristol Hospitals

Developmental Paediatrics

Perspectives and Practice

K. S. Holt

MD (USA)., MD (Manc)., FRCP., DCH

Professor of Developmental Paediatrics, and
Director, The Wolfson Centre, Institute
of Child Health, University of London.
Hon. Consultant. The Hospital for Sick Children,
Great Ormond Street, London.

BUTTERWORTHS
LONDON - BOSTON
Sydney - Wellington - Durban - Toronto

The Butterworth Group

United Kingdom	Butterworth & Co (Publishers) Ltd	London: 88 Kingsway, WC2B 6AB

Australia Butterworths Pty Ltd
Sydney: 586 Pacific Highway, Chatswood, NSW 2067
Also at Melbourne, Brisbane, Adelaide and Perth

Canada Butterworth & Co (Canada) Ltd
Toronto: 2265 Midland Avenue, Scarborough,
Ontario, M1P 4S1

New Zealand Butterworths of New Zealand Ltd
Wellington: T & W Young Building,
77–85 Customhouse Quay, 1, CPO Box 472

South Africa Butterworth & Co (South Africa) (Pty) Ltd
Durban: 152–154 Gale Street

USA Butterworth (Publishers) Inc
Boston: 19 Cummings Park, Woburn, Mass. 01801

First published 1977
Reprinted 1978

ISBN 0 407 00065 8

© Butterworths & Co (Publishers) Ltd 1977

Library of Congress Cataloging in Publication Data

Holt, Kenneth Sunderland.
    Developmental paediatrics.

    (Postgraduate paediatrics series)
    Bibliography: p.
    Includes index.
    1. Child development. 2. Child development--Testing.
I. Title. II. Series. [DNLM: 1. Child development.
WS103 H756d]
RJ131.H64 1975 612.6'5 76-7221
ISBN 0-407-00065-8

Typeset by Butterworths Litho Preparation Department

Printed in England by Billing & Sons Ltd,
Guildford & London

Contents

Preface

Our children inherit the future. Their best equipment to meet the challenges ahead consists of a healthy body, enquiring mind and stable personality. Prominent amongst those helping children to acquire these vital attributes are paediatricians, i.e. those medical specialists who are concerned with child development and care, and the treatment of children's illnesses.

The relatively slow expansion of paediatrics and the preoccupation of many paediatricians with investigative medicine has led to a neglect of child health and rearing just at a time when knowledge of child development is increasing rapidly, and when parents are seeking a high level of fitness and performance from all their children. This situation is being remedied by the establishment of developmental paediatrics.

This book was written in response to demands for information about developmental paediatrics. It is written for paediatricians, especially those just entering the profession. In this book I have tried to show the depth and breadth of child development, and to indicate how an understanding of development enriches clinical work, especially work with handicapped children. I hope that reading this book will help paediatricians to appreciate the contributions of other professions such as psychology, therapy, and education, and that members of these other professions, who are also concerned with the promotion of child health and care, will find the book useful and interesting.

Much of the material in this book is based upon my work in the Department of Child Heath of the University of Sheffield and, during the last ten years, in the Department of Developmental Paediatrics of the Institute of Child Health of the University of London. I am indebted to colleagues, past and present, for ideas, stimulation and help. Dr (psychologist) R.M.C. Huntley and Dr (paediatrician) P. Sonksen helped me by their kind critical reading of the text during preparation. The delightful line drawings were executed by Miss A. Wisbeach, and Mr A. Blakey took some of the photographs. Invaluable assistance was given by my departmental secretaries Miss S. Brown and Miss A. Feist.

I am only too aware of my reliance upon material from many sources which I have tried to acknowledge throughout the book. If there are any omissions these are due to oversight and not to unawareness of my indebtedness to external assistance. I wish to acknowledge the sources of the following illustrations which are reproduced by permission.

Figures 1, 9 (b, c), 10, 11 (a), 12, 17, 20 (a, b), 31 (a, b, c), are reproduced by permission from a tape/slide recording prepared by Dr K. S. Holt for the Medical Information Service of the Royal College of General Practitioners.

Figures 33 (a), 34 (a), 36 (a, b, d), 38 (b, c), 40 (a, b, c, d), 41 (a, b, d), 42, are reproduced by permission from tape/slide recordings prepared by Dr M. D. Sheridan for the Medical Information Service of the Royal College of General Practitioners.

Figures 4, 5, are reproduced from *Gray's Anatomy,* 34th edition, by permission of Messrs. Churchill Livingstone, Edinburgh.

Figure 6 is reproduced from *Human Development,* 1966, by permission of the author, J. C. Larroche, and the publishers W. B. Saunders Company, Philadelphia.

Figure 11 (b) is reproduced from *Baby File* by permission of Glaxo-Farley Foods Ltd, Plymouth.

Figures 13, 14, 16 are reproduced from Prechtl H. F. R. and Beintema, D. J., 1968, A neurological study of newborn infants. *Clinics Dev. Med.* 28, Heinemann, London by permission of the authors, the publishers, and Spastics International Medical Publications.

Figures 28, 60, are reproduced from Klaus, M. H., Kennell, J. H., Plumb, N., and Zuehlke, S. (1970) *Pediatrics* 46, 187 by permission of the authors and the editor.

Figures 27, 81, 82, were published originally in my book, *Assessment of Cerebral Palsy,* Lloyd Luke (Medical Books) Ltd, London (1965) and are reproduced by kind permission of the publishers.

Figure 35 (a) was taken in the nursery of Dr E. Pikler in Budapest, and is reproduced by permission.

Figure 37 is reproduced by permission of Dr G. M. Bryant and the editor of *Developmental Medicine and Child Neurology* (1974), **16**, 475.

Figure 43 (a) is reproduced by permission of the publishers.

Figure 43 (b) is reproduced by courtesy of Dr J. K. Reynell.

Figure 50 is reproduced from Murphy, K. P., (1962). *Panorama,* Dec 3. by permission of the author and Linco Acoustics Ltd., Reading.

Figure 51 is reproduced by permission of the publishers.

Figure 74 is reproduced by permission of Dr M. D. Sheridan and the editor of *Developmental Medicine and Child Neurology,* (1975), **17**, 167.

Figures 86 (a, b) are reproduced by permission of the authors.

The quote on p. 263 from Tinbergen and Tinbergen's *Early Childhood Autism* is reproduced by permission of the authors and publishers.

Finally, the publication of this book would not have occurred without the gentle persuasion of Dr John Apley.

K. S. H.

CHAPTER 1

Developmental Paediatrics: Definitions, Scope and Nature

Developmental paediatrics emphasizes the importance of a developmental approach to the practice of paediatrics.

Paediatrics is defined by the Oxford English Dictionary as: 'the branch of medical science dealing with the study of childhood and the diseases of children'. Much of paediatric practice has to be concerned with seeing children when they are sick on isolated or repeated occasions. This episodic type of practice does not provide a clear picture of child development, nor is it possible to give much attention to children's developmental progress when some acute disturbance takes priority. It is necessary, however, to give attention to the development of all children and particularly to those showing delayed or distorted patterns of development. By studying child development and using this knowledge to help children with these problems it is found that the doctor's understanding of children is enriched and his paediatric practice is given greater continuity. Consequently, a steadily increasing number of doctors are actively practising developmental paediatrics. The nature of developmental paediatrics and the forces leading to its emergence are described in this chapter.

Over the years in different countries several paediatricians have been especially interested in the problems and deviations of child development and their contributions have made them internationally renowned. Arnold Gesell was the American pioneer of developmental paediatrics and Hilda Knobloch continues this type of practice in the USA. In the UK the names of Ronald Illingworth and Mary Sheridan are well known. Dr Mary Sheridan's definition of developmental paediatrics is as follows:

'Developmental paediatrics is concerned with maturational processes (from fetal viability to full growth) in structure and function, of normal and abnormal children, for three purposes; first, to promote optimal physical and mental health for all children; second, to ensure early diagnosis and effective treatment of handicapping conditions of body, mind and personality; third, to discover the cause and means of preventing such handicapping conditions.' (Sheridan, 1962).

Developmental paediatrics has evolved from both advances in medical science and changes in the pattern of child health and illness. There have been three major influences. Firstly, medical scientific advances have occurred so rapidly that individual paediatricians have had to concentrate upon certain sections in order to be able to encompass the available knowledge and to be able to continue to make progress. Thus, specialist groups have appeared within paediatrics concerned with cardiology, neurology, nephrology and so on. These changes have occurred so rapidly that at times it has seemed that preoccupation with the technicalities of the particular speciality is so great that the paediatric aspects are overlooked. To some extent this is an inevitable accompaniment of such rapid change, but it need be neither serious nor prolonged so long as a compensatory balance is maintained by greater interest in developmental paediatrics.

Secondly, the decline of acute illness, and the more frequent survival of congenitally deformed and weak babies has resulted in an increase in the numbers of chronically disabled children who are developmentally handicapped. Their opportunities for development are stunted and consequently they need much help to make educational progress and acceptable social adaptations. Many aspects of their development must be studied and understood in order to plan and provide effective assistance for them.

Thirdly, the advances in medicine in recent years have greatly enhanced the prospects of survival, especially in childhood. The infant mortality is only a tenth of what it was a century ago. In the past families were larger than at present, and it was not uncommon for children to die in their early years. Nowadays the majority of babies survive to enjoy a long adult life. As a result of medical and social advances, we now unquestionably expect survival for all our children and we are becoming more and more concerned with the quality of their survival (Holt, 1972). Consequently, there is an increased demand by parents to know that their child is normal, or if not, the reasons and remedies for the situation. So it is important to detect deviations from normal development, and whenever possible to correct them.

This demand for high quality survival and an intolerance to accept anything less is stimulating the expansion of developmental paediatrics. This new emphasis in paediatric practice is clearly stated in the following paragraph which was introduced into the 9th edition of one of the major international textbooks of paediatrics (Nelson, Vaughan and McKay, 1969).

'No appraisal of the child is complete which does not assess his developmental status, not any program of management complete which does not continuously evaluate how illness or treatment may change or distort his pattern of growth or behaviour. The thoughtful physician must be concerned also with ways in which assets or liabilities in the child's family, neighbourhood, school or community may facilitate or impede his progress towards healthy and productive childhood.'

Developmental paediatrics is not a sub-speciality or branch of paediatrics but is an essential part of clinical practice with children. It requires an understanding of all the features of normal child development and the underlying mechanisms, and the utilization of this knowledge to detect deviations of development and then to plan treatment, training and care for the children in need. It is closely allied to developmental neurology, developmental psychology and child psychiatry.

A thorough knowledge of normal development makes clinicians more sensitive to the presence and significance of deviations. This is soon apparent whenever developmental paediatrics is practised. For example, whilst working in Sheffield with Professor R. S. Illingworth, I learnt that by using a developmental approach it was possible to detect cerebral palsy in the early months of life, often a year or more earlier than in the case of children referred from areas where this experience and approach were not available. Rogers (1968), working in Reading, found that the increased alertness of medical officers to developmental problems which followed the introduction of the 'At Risk' register resulted in a considerably earlier detection of deviant development in all babies,—and in the 'not at risk' group just as much as in the 'at risk' group.

A developmental basis for treatment and management programmes for children is both rational and effective, and discourages many of the harmful practices which unfortunately exist. For example, therapists sometimes exhort handicapped children to walk before they are developmentally ready to do so; and children are sometimes admitted to hospitals and nurseries in ways which show that there is no appreciation of the impact of these events upon them. Perhaps Robertson's (1967) dramatic illustration of the effects of fostering would not have been necessary, or even possible, if everyone concerned with children had been aware of their developmental needs. Aids and appliances made on developmental lines are more effective and so save time and money. Wheelchairs for handicapped children are often unsatisfactory because they are designed on the assumption that children are miniature adults. When account is taken of children's growth and developmental characteristics they are more satisfactory. (Holt, 1966)

Although one of the reasons for the emergence of developmental paediatrics was the need to compensate for excessive preoccupation with 'scientific paediatrics', it should not be assumed that scientific methods are not applied in developmental work. Developmental paediatricians in fact do use the scientific advances made by other specialists, and apply them to the needs of developing children. The fact that many children with developmental problems have in the past been treated with compassion and sympathy, but with little scientific study, has contributed to ineffectual treatment and their limited progress. It is not only in the biochemical and electronic laboratories that a scientific approach can be pursued—later chapters give examples of the scientific analysis of many developmental problems, some of which are carried out not in a laboratory, but in the nursery, classroom and home.

In order to appreciate the scope of developmental paediatrics several terms must be understood. These are defined and discussed below.

Defect, Deformity, Disability and Handicap

These terms are all too often used loosely and interchangeably (Mitchell, 1973).

Defect: any abnormality of structure.
Deformity: any deviation from the normal shape and form.
Disability: any failure of function or skill.
Handicap: any condition which impedes an individual's development, opportunities, expectations and activities.

The adjectival form of defect, 'defective', is often used loosely to describe impairment of function and not just abnormality of structure. Thus, 'a defective ear drum', meaning one which is abnormal and perforated, is an appropriate use of the word, whereas 'defective hearing', meaning impairment of hearing without necessarily any structural abnormality, may be misleading and 'hearing disability' or 'impairment' are preferable terms.

Deformity is applied particularly to acquired abnormalities which arise during the course of an illness, e.g. equinus deformity in cerebral palsy.

Defects and deformities may give rise to disability, but need not necessarily do so. Many who see children with defects and deformities assume that they will be disabled and so underestimate their capabilities. This tendency has to be guarded against in all rehabilitation work. During the course of a long-term disorder such as cerebral palsy the degrees of deformity and disability may change in opposite directions with one improving whilst the other becomes worse. For example, a child with cerebral palsy may increase his speed and distance of walking and so considerably reduce his disability, but the muscular effort required to achieve this improvement may result in an increase in deformity. This situation produces very considerable therapeutic dilemmas (Holt, 1963). Clear distinctions between defect, deformity and disability need to be kept constantly in mind.

A disabled child may be handicapped, but there is neither a direct nor a close relationship between the extent of disability and associated handicap. The extent to which a child is handicapped depends not only upon the nature and extent of the disability, but also upon the significance of the disability to the child and the success or otherwise with which the child can by-pass or compensate for the disability. For example, the extent to which a child with disability of the hands is handicapped depends, amongst other things, upon his drive to overcome his limitations and the amount he is required to do with his hands. Literature contains many examples of individuals with considerable defects, deformities, and disabilities who were able, nevertheless, to lead very full, productive and satisfying lives. Far from handicapping them, their difficulties seemed to spur them to ever greater achievements. It should not be assumed that a disabled child will be handicapped. One should never adopt a negative and pessimistic outlook towards such children.

The qualifying word 'multiple' or 'multiply-' is often associated with the terms defect, deformity, disability and handicap. A child may have several of these problems so it is quite appropriate for the word 'multiple' to be added. But the addition of 'multiple' to one of these terms should not be transferred automatically to the other terms. For example, a child with multiple defects may suffer only a single disability. Thus a child with defects in various parts of the body, such as malformed ears, congenital heart defect and lower limb deficiency, may be disabled only with respect to walking. And another example: a child with a single disability such as severe hearing impairment may be multiply handicapped, e.g. educationally, emotionally, and socially.

Handicapped, Disadvantaged, Deprived (Sheridan, 1962; 1969)

The unwary may use these terms interchangeably, but they have quite distinct meanings which often have legal significance.

'A handicapped child is one who suffers from any continuing disability of body, intellect, or personality which is likely to interfere with his normal growth and development or capacity to learn.'

'A disadvantaged child is one who suffers from a continuing inadequacy of material, affectional, educational or social provisions, or who is subject to detrimental environmental stresses which are likely to interfere with the growth and development of his body, intellect, or personality, and thus prevent him from achieving his inherent potential.'

Sheridan makes this clear distinction between handicapped and disadvantaged. The former arises from a disturbance primarily affecting the child, the latter indicates a potentially normal and healthy child whose development is stultified by unfavourable environmental conditions. Whilst the distinction is a valuable contribution to clear thinking and discussion, it should not be followed too rigidly, because in practice the situations sometimes overlap. Thus, the extent to which a disabled child is handicapped is determined by the demands of his environment. Likewise the exposure of a normal healthy child to unfavourable circumstances of sufficient severity for long enough may produce permanent disability which will persist even when the environmental stresses are corrected.

'A deprived child is one who, for any reason, is deprived of a normal home life and who in consequence needs the temporary or permanent care or protection of a recognised child care agency.'

According to Sheridan this definition, in contrast to the others, is official and legal.

Normal, Average

Normal: usual, typical, regular, healthy, free of abnormality.
Average: the calculated point around which other values are dispersed.

Both these terms are in everyday use. Confusion arises when they are used loosely and interchangeably. 'Normal' is a descriptive term which can be applied to any child who shows typical characteristics for his age. The term 'average' is derived from statistics and implies that measurements have been taken of some particular feature. A normal child can be in a group with a lot of other normal children. The average child in such a group with respect to some measured characteristic such as height, weight or intelligence will have other above-and below-average children around him. These terms must be used carefully in discussions with parents in order to avoid unnecessary confusion and distress. Parents may describe their child as 'average' when they mean that he appears to them to be normal and typical of their family. Children with widely differing abilities from families in different social classes may all be described in this way as 'average'. If parents are told that their child is average intellectually, meaning that his scores on intellectual tests correspond to the 'average' figure for the population, they may think that their child is 'normal and acceptable', when in fact he may be considerably above or below the normal pattern for that particular family.

Development and Maturation

Development: the process of unfolding or revealing, of becoming fuller and more complete.

This term is usually used to describe what is observed and recorded without any implications about the underlying mechanisms.

Maturation: the process of ripening and reaching maturity.

Although this term may be, and sometimes is, used synonymously with development, it is usually taken to refer more directly to the basic mechanisms. Thus, in connection with human development, maturation is often meant to be the gradual elaboration of the structure and function of the nervous system which underlies the process of development.

In the chapters which follow the observable pattern of child development will be described and the underlying mechanisms, including maturation, will be discussed. This will lead on to a description of the nature and practice of developmental paediatrics.

REFERENCES

Holt, K. S. (1963). Deformity and disability in cerebral palsy. *Devl Med. Child Neurol.,* **5,** 629
– (1966). Principles of child health as seen in the care of handicapped children. *Proc. R. Soc. Med.,* **59,** 135
– (1972). The Quality of Survival. *Occasional Papers, No. 2,* Institute for Research into Mental Retardation. London: Butterworths
Mitchell, R. (1973). Defining medical terms. *Devl Med. Child Neurol.,* **15,** 279
Nelson, W. E., Vaughan III, V. C. and McKay, R. J. (1969). Prologue to the section on Developmental Paediatrics. *Textbook of Pediatrics,* 9th edn. Philadelphia:Saunders

Robertson, J. (1967). *Foster Care for 27 Days*. (Guide to film). London: Tavistock Institute of Human Relations

Rogers, M. G. H. (1968). Risk registers and early detection of handicaps. *Devl Med. Child Neurol.*, **10**, 5, 651

Sheridan, M. D. (1962). Infants at risk of handicapping conditions. *Mon. Bull. Minist. Hlth.* **21**, 238

− (1969). Definitions relating to developmental paediatrics. *Health Trends* (Dept. of Health and Social Security), **1**, 2, 4

CHAPTER 2

The Basis of Development

GROWTH OF THE BRAIN

It is axiomatic that many of the features of human development are dependent upon and occur as a result of development of the brain. The brief synopsis of brain development which follows cannot possibly do justice to all that takes place as the brain grows, differentiates, and matures, but it will perhaps convey an impression of the magnitude and complexity of the processes involved.

The easily observed increase of head size clearly demonstrates the growth of the brain. On those occasions when the brain itself is inspected the increasing complexity of its structure with advancing age is readily apparent. These, however, are crude manifestations of the brain's growth, and all the vital changes occur at cellular level. The study and investigation of brain mechanisms at cellular level are increasing as a result of technical advances. Consequently, our knowledge of brain growth and development is expanding as a result of careful studies of the histological, chemical, and electrical features of the brain, and considerable advances can be anticipated in the coming years.

Gross Structural Development

The growth of the brain is reflected in the increase of head size with age. The clinician's most useful guide to this growth is measurement of the head circumference. The measurement is made with an accurately marked, non-stretchable, narrow tape passed firmly around the head just above the base of the nose and over the occipital prominence, as shown in *Figure 1*.

9

The measurements are used in two ways:

(a)   They are compared with standard data to determine whether the head circumference deviates markedly from that expected for the age of the child. For this purpose it is useful to know the source of the

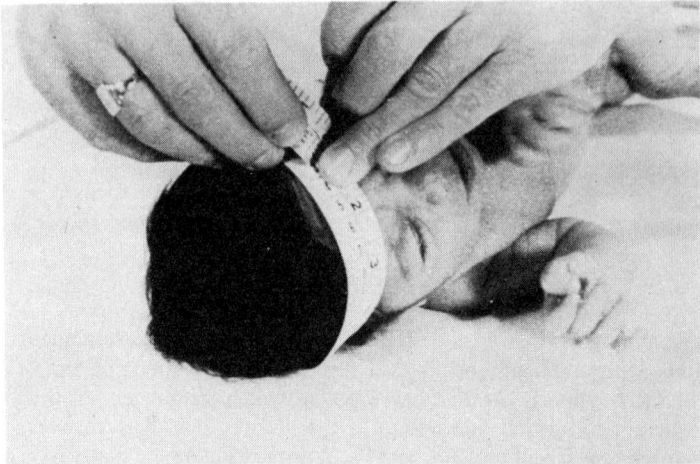

Figure 1. Measurement of the head circumference of a baby

standard data, so as to be satisfied that it was collected from an appropriate and adequate non-selected population. This data should be expressed either in centiles or as mean and standard deviations.

(b)   Serial measurements are plotted on a graph to show the changes with age. Various graphs exist for this purpose. Some are more satisfactory and reliable than others. It is almost impossible to devise a practical graph which covers the whole period of the child's growth. At least two graphs are usually needed, one covering the period from mid-fetal life to about two years of age, and the other covering the period from about three years to adulthood.

Figures 2 and *3* are based on head circumference/age charts which have been found to be satisfactory for general use (Nellhaus, 1968). Four sets of measurements are shown to illustrate the following.

(a)   Initial and subsequent measurements all within the expected range—a normal child with normal brain growth.

(b)   Initial measurement considerably below expectation—an abnormally small head.

(c)   Initial measurement greater than expectation and subsequent measurements showing an excessively high rate of growth—a child suffering from hydrocephalus.

(d)   Initial measurement within the expected range, but subsequent measurements fall below expectation—slowing of brain growth in a moderately retarded child.

Some variation of head circumference occurs between different ethnic groups, but this is not very large, and certainly is not great enough to justify the almost impossible task of producing separate charts for each ethnic group.

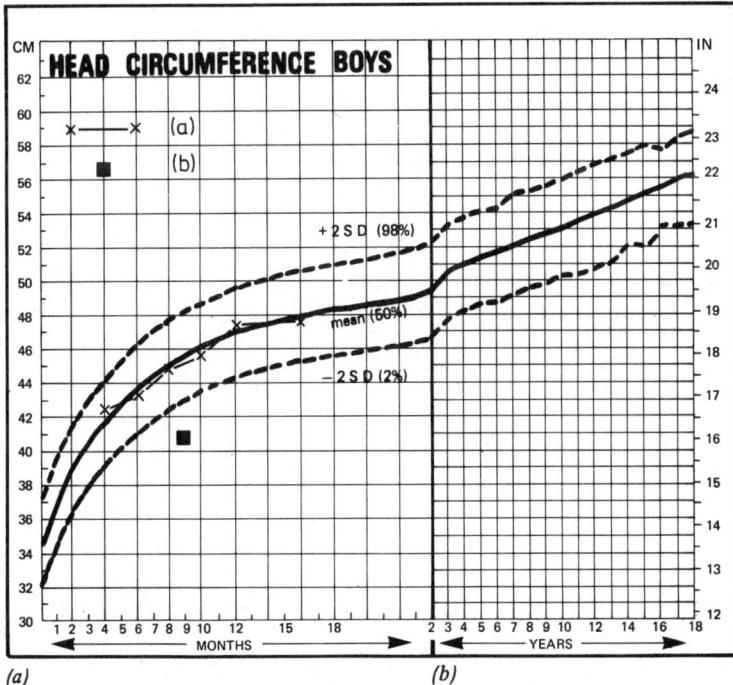

Figure 2. Head circumference/age chart for boys: (a) in a normal child; (b) an abnormally small head

More significant variations of head circumference occur with body weight, so allowances should be made if the infant is much bigger or smaller than expected for his age (Illingworth and Lutz, 1965). The following is a useful working rule.

Babies under 6 months of age:
    Allow 1.3 cm in the head circumference for each kg deviation of body weight from the mean.

Babies aged 6–12 months:
    Allow 1.0 cm in the head circumference for each kg deviation of body weight from the mean.

The brain volume and brain weight increase at comparable rates as growth takes place. At birth the human brain is about half its adults size. It increases rapidly and is about three-quarters its adult size by 18 months of age and 90 per cent by 4 years of age. By this latter age the rate of growth has slowed considerably and the remaining 10 per cent of growth occurs gradually throughout childhood.

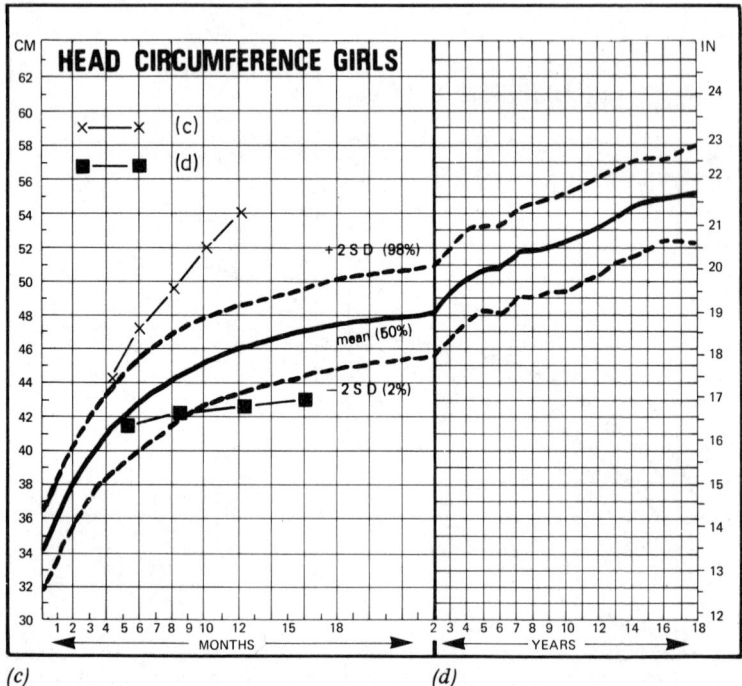

(c)   *(d)*

Figure 3. Head circumference/age chart for girls: (c) hydrocephalus; (b) slowing of brain growth in retarded child

In the early stages of growth of the brain it is possible to identify five major parts. These are the forebrain, mid-brain and hind-brain, and the cerebral hemispheres and cerebellum. The fore-, mid-and hind-brains appear as distinct bulbar swellings of the initial tubular cell mass which constitutes the primitive brain. These then become overlaid by the mantle of the cerebral hemispheres, and the cerebellum appears as a mid-line posterior structure (*Figures 4, 5*). This essential basic structural differentiation of the brain occurs during the first trimester of pregnancy. As early as 10 weeks the five major parts of the primitive brain can be identified despite the fact that it is still quite small—little more than 1.5 cm in length and weighing only 20–30 g. Any interference with the growth of the brain in this early stage is likely to produce serious malformations such as anencephaly.

During the second trimester the brain increases rapidly in size. Most noticeable upon inspection is the increase of the cerebral hemispheres which appear to be appreciably larger each week. Throughout most of this period, however, the hemispheres remain smooth. In contrast, the

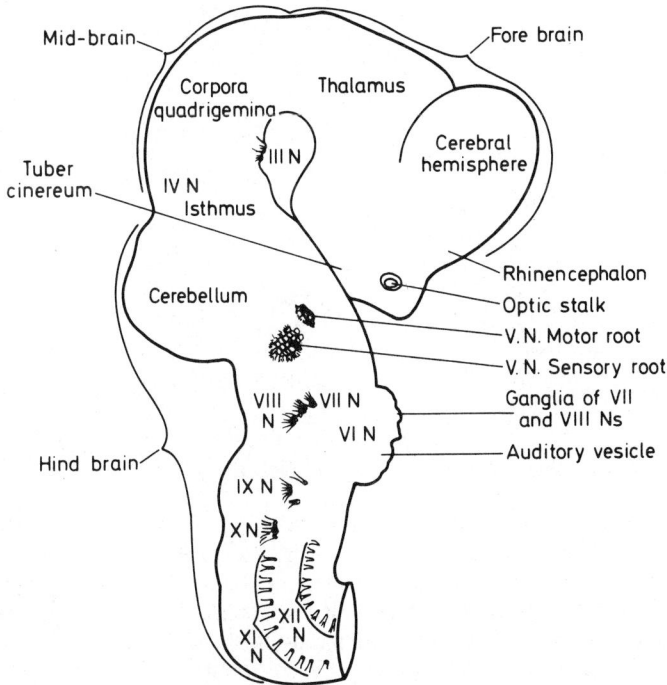

Figure 4. Right lateral surface of brain of human embryo about 10.2 mm long

third trimester is characterized by the appearance of indentations and convolutions of the cerebral cortex. *Figure 6* shows the typical appearance of the developing brain at successive stages of fetal life.

Cellular Development

The formation of the basic structure of the brain during the first trimester of pregnancy is followed by a rapid growth spurt due to development at a cellular level. The cellular development follows an

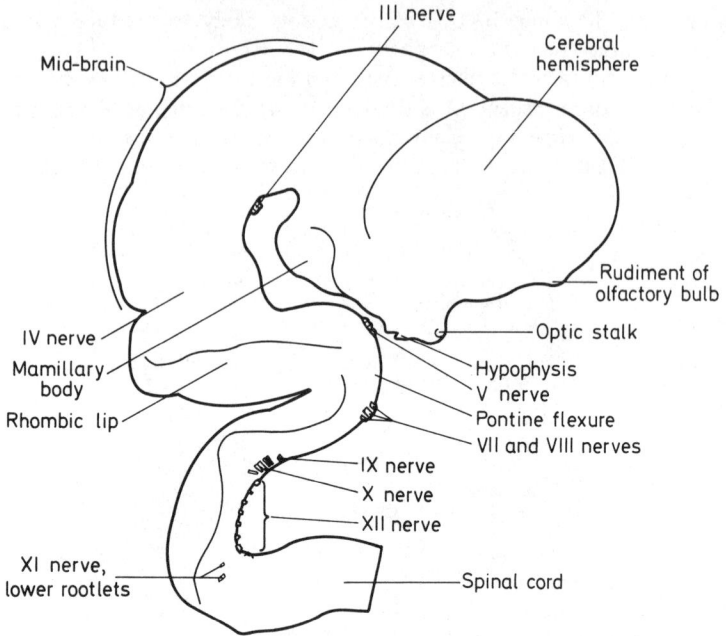

Figure 5. Right side of brain of human embryo about 13.6 mm long

orderly sequence. First of all masses of neuroblasts proliferate in several germinative zones such as the subependymal and sub-pia-arachnoid and the periventricular areas. McIlwain (1966) reported that in the rat brain 97 per cent of the brain cells appear in the fetal period. The fact that in the same period the brain achieves only 15 per cent of the adult weight shows how much the subsequent dendritic elaboration and myelination contribute to the size of the mature brain.

Proliferation of the cells is followed by migration and functional differentiation. Cellular migration is one of the most remarkable features of brain development. It appears to be a self-organizing process which is guided by the characteristics of the cell membranes (Herschkowitz and Rossi, 1972). A variety of enzymes which are genetically regulated control the cell membrane characteristics (Paigen, 1971) and their appearance and disappearance at certain developmental stages (Baurlacher, 1973). The cells migrate from their origin in successive concentric layers or in long thin chains, or in clusters until they reach their destination when they assume the distinctive features and functions of the cells in that particular area. In this way distinctive cell agglomerations appear as nuclei and bands. The rapidity with which these changes

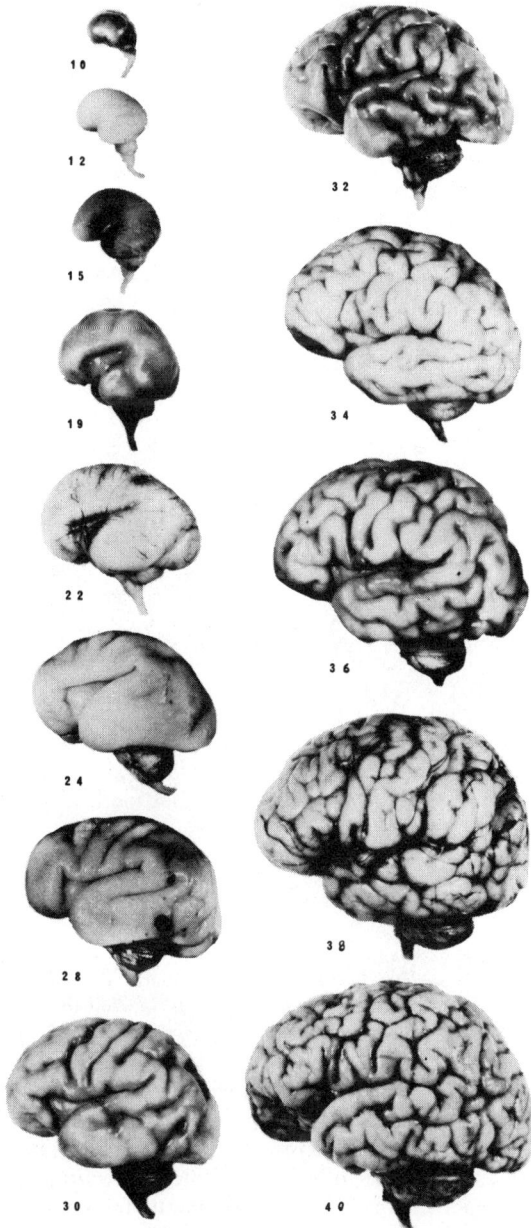

*Figure 6. Appearance of brain at successive fetal ages
(age in weeks shown by figures)*

occur may be judged from the fact that in human fetuses the cerebral cortex is just identifiable at 10 weeks, yet by 26 weeks the cortex is well developed and all six cellular layers are evident. The extent of migration is illustrated by the anatomy of the seventh nerve, the cells which form the nucleus of the seventh (facial) nerve follow an exceptionally long, winding migratory path (*Figure 7*). Initially the nucleus of the facial nerve forms under the floor of the fourth ventricle slightly proximal and dorsal to the nucleus of the sixth (abducens) nerve. Then, in relation to the sixth nucleus it migrates dorsally, medially and caudally, and then sweeps ventrolaterally. As a result the tract of the facial nerve follows a long arc-like course around the sixth nerve nucleus before emerging from the ventral surface of the pons.

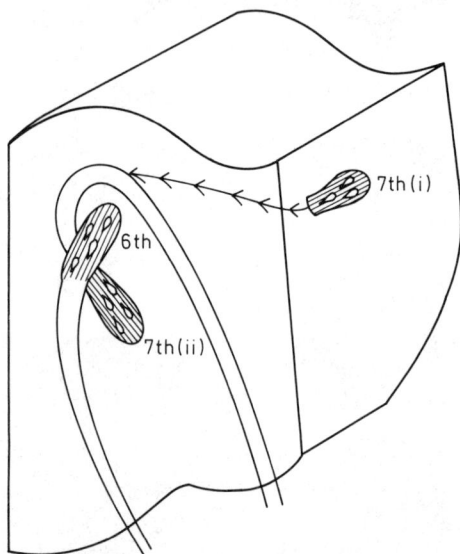

Figure 7. The migration of the facial (7th) cranial nerve. The diagram shows a portion of the pons indicating the initial position of the 7th nerve nucleus (i), and the final tracts of the 6th and 7th nerves (ii)

The proliferation, migration and differentiation of neurones in the developing human brain occur during the second and third trimesters. Although some glial cells are formed during fetal life it is in the months immediately following birth when these cells proliferate. Dendritic elaboration occurs very actively at the same time. Myelination begins early (about 22 weeks) in the spinal cord roots, and by birth there is some evidence of myelination in almost all parts of the central nervous system. The peak period of myelination, however, occurs postnatally, after the peak activity of glial formation. The rapidly developing brain requires an abundant supply of energy and nutrients. Although knowledge about the metabolism of the growing brain is still rudimentary it is clear that there are many biological features and adjustments which enable the rapidly growing brain to obtain the energy it requires and which help to protect it during this vulnerable period. For example, there may be qualitative as well as quantitative differences between the proteins and enzymes of the growing brain as compared with the mature brain (Sterman, McGinty and Adinolfi, 1971); the blood-brain barrier matures at different times for different substances (Myers and Bito, 1973); and ketones may play an exceptionally important role in the metabolism of the growing brain (Wilkinson and Buckley, 1973).

The developing brain is susceptible to the effects of nutritional deprivation. Dobbing and colleagues (1973, 1974) hypothesize that such deprivation would be expected to have greatest impact upon the most rapidly growing tissues at that particular time. For example, intra-uterine nutritional deprivation might be expected to have greatest effect upon the neurones, whereas postnatal deprivation would affect glial cells, myelination, and dendritic processes.

There is much still to be learnt about brain growth and development and many can make some contribution. The developmental paediatrician may feel that his clinical observations cannot match the sophisticated investigative methods of the cellular physiologist and biochemist. He must realize however that there are limits to both the understanding of human brain development from studies upon other species and the opportunities for investigations upon humans. In these circumstances careful developmental observations and clinical analysis may provide occasional clues to improve our understanding of brain function. For the present it is as well to remember how far we have still to go and to be aware of our present limitations.

'There is, however, a considerable discrepancy between the amount of structural data and the sparse observations on the functional properties of the neocortex, particularly during the early phases of development.' (Bernhard and Meyerson, 1973).

Electrical Changes

One of the few ways of exploring the activity of the functioning human brain is by recording and analysing the electrical potentials which come from it. Considerable skill is required to overcome the many technical problems, and much experience is needed to interpret the findings when this technique is used to study the developing brain. The problems which have to be overcome include devising ways of making intra-uterine recordings from the fetus; increasing the effectiveness of trans-abdominal recordings; and trying to ensure that anything recorded represents true brain activity and is not due to brain damage or anoxia. Because of these difficulties relatively few reports have been published and there is still much to be learnt. Dreyfuss-Brisac (1966) has de-scribed what is known of the appearance of electrical activity in the brain. She considers that the electroencephalogram (EEG) correlates closely with the stage of maturation of the brain. In support she quotes the rapid changes of the EEG which parallel the rapid growth of the young brain, and the fact that the EEG patterns correspond well with the conceptual age. The characteristic patterns are as follows:

Conceptual age	*Characteristic pattern*
24–28 weeks:	discontinuous tracing with polymorphic rhythms, but without organized features. Bursts of very slow waves (0.3–1.0 H_z) of 3–20 seconds duration with amplitudes up to 300 microvolts, and shorter (1–2 seconds) bursts of alpha activity of 8–14 H_z and 5–6 H_z. Occasional spikes.
28–32 weeks:	a simpler pattern than earlier with long quiet periods and 1–2 second bursts of regular theta activity of 4–6 H_z and amplitudes of 25–100 microvolts.
32–37 weeks:	the record now shows more continuous activity, especially in the occipital areas. Delta waves of 10–14 H_z are present.
37–41 weeks:	differences between the sleeping and awake records are present for the first time. The awake records show a continuous pattern. In light sleep the pattern resembles that of the earlier stage, whilst with deep sleep the pattern becomes discontinuous, paroxysmal and asynergic.

A visually evoked response can be obtained from 50 per cent of newborns. It shows a longer latency and higher potential than a typical adult record. When the response is obtained from prematures the initial phase is usually absent and the latency is even longer. It is said that the length of the latent period correlates with the conceptual age.

The auditorily evoked response is more variable.

The structural and cellular development of the brain and the changes of electrical activity provide a useful perspective for understanding reflex activity in infancy.

REFLEX ACTIVITY IN INFANCY

The nervous system of a newly born baby is well developed and capable of complex activities. This is shown, for example, by the facts that the neurological control of such a vital function as breathing is well established, and that there are many reflex responses which can be obtained by appropriate stimulation. But this is not the final state and further development of the nervous system occurs rapidly during the early years. Understanding the nature and mechanisms of the neurological reflex activities and their evolution provides a sound basis for a full appreciation of human development.

A reflex action consists of a prompt, stereotyped and often very considerable response to a specific and often quite minor stimulus. There is no opportunity for variation or choice of action. The promptness, consistency and predictability of the neonatal reflex responses show that neurological pathways are already established and defined.

As the nervous system develops many of the early reflexes are inhibited, and others are modified and incorporated into more complex actions. These developmental changes are necessary because the continued activity of the early reflexes would interfere with the development of other actions, an effect which is seen in some neurologically disabled children.

The pattern of reflexes shown by young infants reflects the phylogenetic evolution of the nervous system. Many of the reflexes are evident in other species. For example, the trunk righting reflexes which appear for a time during early human development are also shown by quadrupeds. Some reflexes are considered to be the persisting remnants of vitally important reflexes in the past. For example, the grasp reflex would serve an essential survival function when it was necessary for the animal infant to be able to cling to the mother's fur. Other reflexes are unique to man, especially those concerned with the attainment and maintenance of the upright posture.

Our understanding of reflex activity in the infant comes from several sources, including neurophysiological experimental studies and observations of the evolution of reflex activity in both normal and abnormal babies. The neurophysiological studies of Magnus (1924),

Magnus and de Kleijn (1930), Rademaker (1931), Sherrington (1898) and others have provided information about the mechanisms of many of the reflexes. They were concerned with identifying the areas and pathways within the brain used by the various reflexes and, amongst many other things, showed the important role of the labyrinth for the maintenance of the upright posture and balance. Peiper (1961) was convinced of the importance of the neurophysiological approach in understanding cerebral function in infancy and childhood and reference to his work is recommended to all who seek to understand reflex activity in early life. Other useful references in this connection are to Thomas, Chesni and Dargassies (1960), Paine and Opie (1966), and Milani Comparetti and Gidoni (1967).

Clinical and Developmental Significance

Some of the many reflexes which have been described are of only passing interest and curiosity, whereas others are more important because they provide useful diagnostic signs; they influence the child's development; and they can be made use of therapeutically.

Those reflexes which are of diagnostic value indicate abnormality by such variations as weakness, absence, excessive strength or undue persistence to an inappropriate age. For example, the Moro reflex is a particularly useful diagnostic reflex. It is present so consistently and is so easily elicitable in the newborn period that any variation from the fully normal response at this time is a reliable indication of probable abnormality, and its persistence after 6 months of age also indicates cerebral abnormality.

The most interesting reflexes are those which influence development. For example, the asymmetrical tonic neck reflex is normally most evident at 2–3 months of age when it appears to prepare the way for the integration of head turning, visual fixation and reaching, and so is probably fundamental to the establishment of visually directed reaching and eye-hand co-ordination. That reflex affects development favourably. An example of a reflex which impedes development as a result of its abnormal persistence is seen with respect to the grasp reflex. Manipulative skill is one of man's great assets which requires individual finger action and release, but these become possible only as the grasp reflex wanes. Its persistence delays the acquisition of such skill.

Some reflexes are utilized in therapeutic programmes for children with cerebral palsy. For example, tactile stimulation in certain areas is used to promote reflex muscle contractions and movements.

Qualifying Definitions

The simplest reflex consists of a prompt, but brief stereotyped response to an appropriate stimulus. Many of the reflexes elicited in a clinical examination are of this nature. Others are more complex. Some show a persistence of the response as long as the stimulus lasts—this is called a *tonic* effect. Some reflexes, especially those concerned with posture and movement, trigger off a series of *chain* responses which may lead to some form of effective action. Very forceful reflexes which cannot be resisted and overcome are said to be *obligatory*. An obligatory response is usually abnormal.

Changes with Age

The pattern of reflex activity changes with age. Some activity can be seen quite early in fetal life. Thereafter it increases rapidly in both intensity and complexity. The study of the appearance and evolution of reflex activity from fetal life and infancy onwards is a fascinating exercise which provides much insight into the elaboration of the nervous system. The reflexes fade after serving their purpose or as they are superseded by others, but they seldom disappear entirely. Normally they persist throughout life without our being aware of them. For example, the continued maintenance of our posture and movement against gravity is possible only as a result of the continued action of the reflex postural mechanisms, and we only become aware of this when control is lost. Reflexes sometimes reappear following cerebral catastrophe in later life.

Production by Several Stimuli

In a pure reflex a specific stimulus is followed by a stereotyped and predictable response. The afferent stimulus may be auditory, visual, tactile (especially touch, pressure and pain), labyrinthine or kin-aesthetic. Sometimes different stimuli give rise to similar responses. This phenomenon is valuable biologically because in the case of important actions it ensures that if one method of elicitation fails others will still produce the appropriate responses. For example, head-righting upon the body may occur as the result of kinaesthetic stimulation from the neck, optic stimulation and labyrinthine stimulation. When several different stimuli can produce a particular reflex response their relative importance varies, and each may predominate at different stages of development.

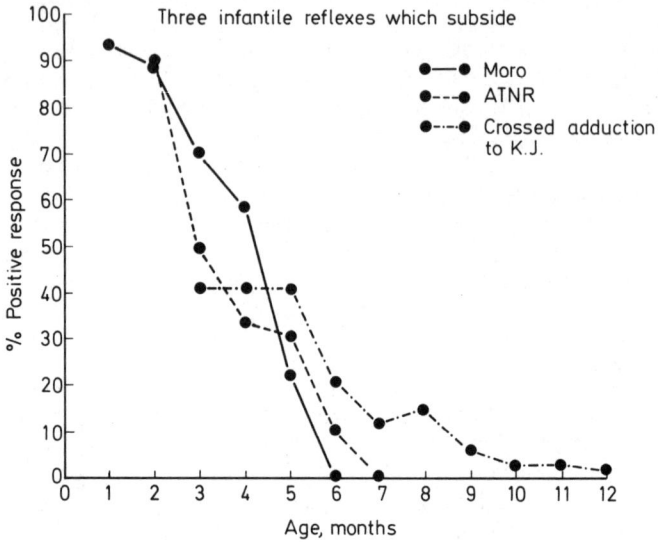

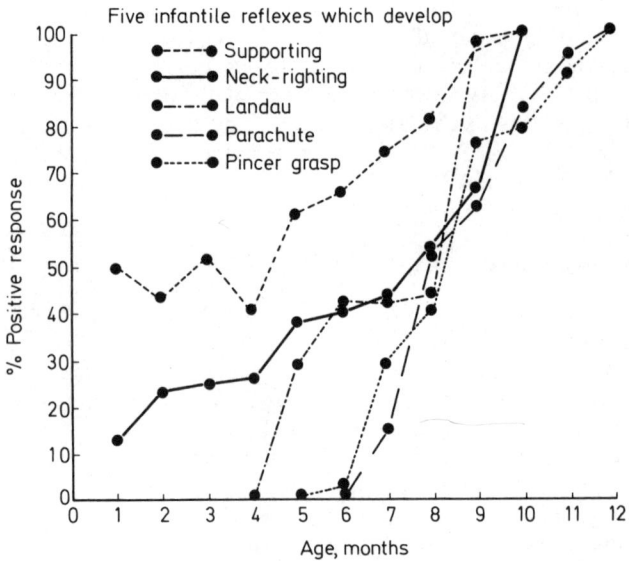

Figure 8. Some primary reflexes which (a) disappear, and some secondary reflexes which (b) appear, during the first year (prepared from data of Paine and Opie, 1966)

Terminology Confusion

Unnecessary confusion is produced when the same reflex response is described as different reflexes according to the way it is produced. For example, pressure upon the sole of an infant's foot causes the leg to extend. The essential stimulus comes from the sole of the foot and the response consists of extension of the leg. When this reflex is elicited by holding the infant upright and allowing the sole of the foot to contact a flat surface the response constitutes a useful anti-gravity supporting reaction and it is often given this name. The reflex can also be demonstrated with the child lying down. The sole of the foot is touched by the examiner's hand and as this hand is withdrawn the leg extends as if following the stimulating hand. This is called the magnet reflex for obvious reasons. These are not different reflexes. The magnet reflex is basically identical with the supporting reaction.

Classification

Reflexes may be grouped according to their function. Some are protective and have a survival value for the infant; others promote appropriate orientation, as for feeding (e.g. rooting reflex) and use of the sensory organs; and others promote postural support and balance. Reflexes may be grouped according to their time of appearance—the primary reflexes are present at birth and then fade to be replaced by secondary reflexes. *Figure 8* shows several primary reflexes which disappear during the first year and other secondary reflexes which appear in the second 6 months of the first year. They may also be grouped according to the method of elicitation, or by the part of the body taking part in the reflex.

The better known and more important reflexes are described below. They are grouped according to the type of stimulus required for their initiation.

REFLEX RESPONSES TO LIGHT TOUCH

Light touch produces a variety of reflex responses depending upon the area stimulated and the age of the individual. The motor responses are most marked in the early months of life.

The grasp reflex: palmar and plantar

Light touch of the palm or sole produces reflex flexion of the fingers or toes. The most effective way to elicit the reflex is to slide the stimulating

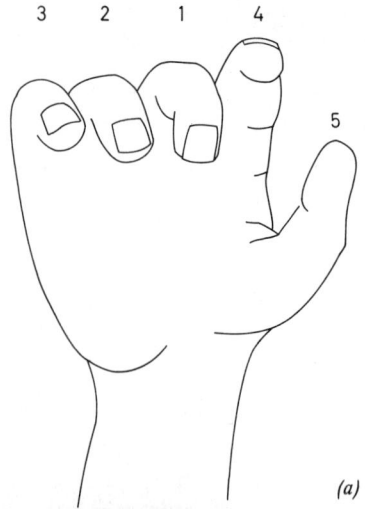

(a)

Figure 9. The grasp reflex: (a) the sequence of finger flexion; (b) the tonic component of the palmar grasp reflex; (c) the plantar grasp reflex

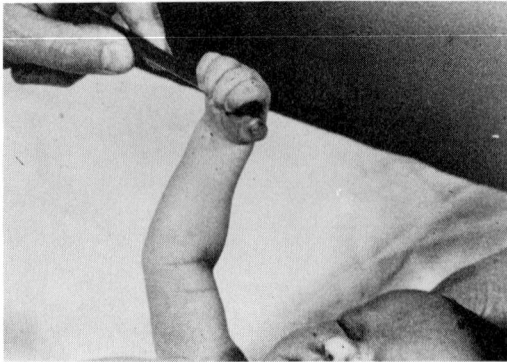

(b)

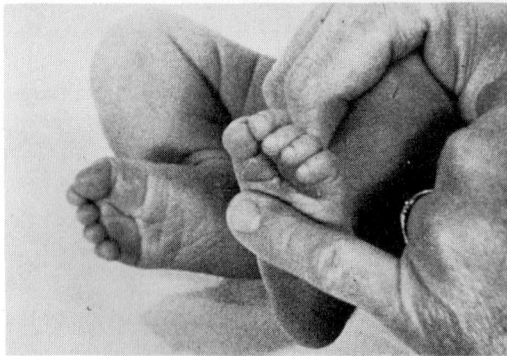

(c)

object such as a finger or pencil across the palm or sole from the
lateral border. Prechtl (1953) described the beautiful neurological
organization of the palmar grasp reflex in which finger flexion follows
a definite sequence: mid–ring–little–index–thumb (*Figure 9 (a)*).

Chain responses follow the initial reflex producing two further stages
which are seen best in the palmar reflex. The first follows initial flexion
of the digits and consists of tensing of the flexed muscles to produce a
strong grasp. A strong tonic component at this stage of the reflex
ensures maintenance of the grasp as long as the stimulus persists. The
second stage occurs when traction is exerted by the stimulating finger
or pencil. This is followed by progressive contraction of the arm muscles
which is sometimes so strong that the baby can be lifted from the
examination couch (*Figure 9(b)*). The palmar and plantar (*Figure 9(c)*)
grasp reflexes are easily demonstrable in the neonate, but then fade
rapidly and are seldom seen after 4 or 5 months of age.

Phylogenetically the reflex is suggested to have had survival value by
enabling the infant to cling to the mother's fur.

Clinically the reflex is of value diagnostically as follows:

(a)   determination of maturity of the neonate (the tonic grasp and
traction reinforcement phases are less evident in the less mature babies)
(Holt, 1965);

(b)   detection of abnormality of the neonate (absence, weakness,
extensive strength or persisting asymmetry of the reflex indicating
abnormality):

(c)   early diagnosis of cerebral lesions (persistence of the reflex after
4–5 months of age indicating abnormality).

The placing reflex (Figure 10)

Stimulation of the dorsum of the foot of the neonate produces flexion
of the same leg. Probably the easiest way to show this, and the method
used in clinical examination, is to hold the infant upright and to let
the dorsum of the foot touch the lower side of the edge of the table.
The infant flexes the leg and appears to do so in order to place the foot
on the table. This reflex is readily demonstrable in the newborn and
persistent failure to elicit it at this stage is thought to indicate neurological abnormality. It fades rapidly in the early months.

The rooting reflex

Light touch of the cheek or stimulation of the edge of the mouth
results in turning of the head in the direction of the stimulus and

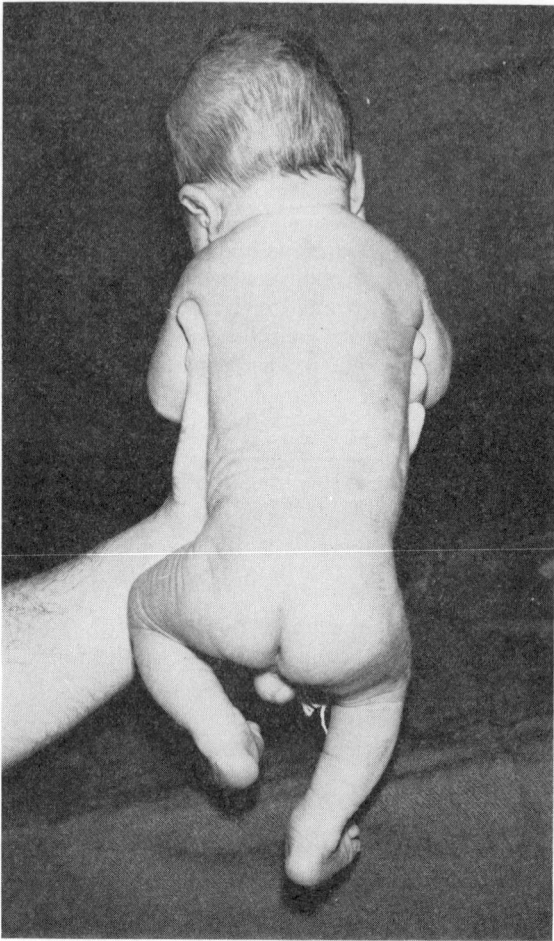

Figure 10. The placing reflex (the left leg is flexed after the dorsum of the foot touched the table edge—the right leg is about to be stimulated in the same way)

simultaneous opening of the mouth and extension of the tongue (*Figure 11 (a)*). It is sometimes called the cardinal points reflex because it is elicited by stimulation of cardinal points in all four quadrants around the mouth. The reflex, which is seen at its best during breast feeding, appears to have an adaptive and survival function. Utilization of the reflex during feeding ensures that the infant takes the nipple well into its widely opened mouth and so avoids painful pressure

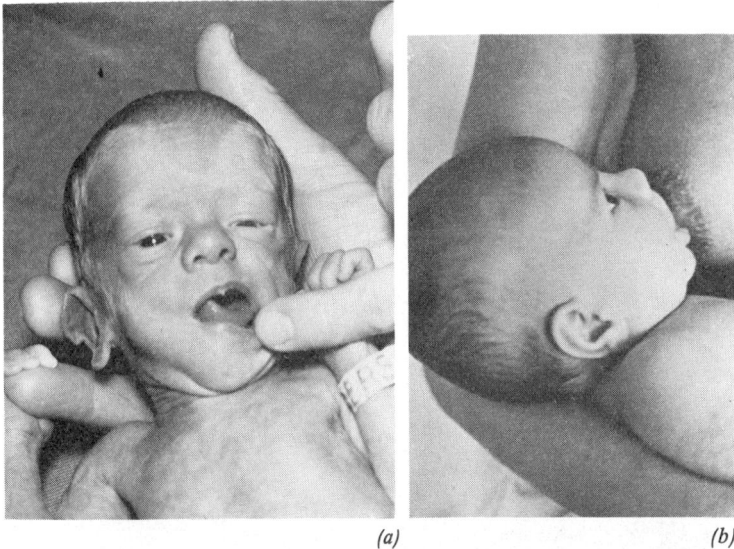

(a)   (b)

Figure 11. The rooting (cardinal points) reflex: (a) elicitation of the reflex; (b) utilization of reflex in breast feeding

upon the end of the nipple (*Figure 11(b)*). Undue haste over breast feeding or other faulty techniques which prevent use of this reflex lead to incomplete acceptance of the nipple into the infant's mouth and cause the nursing mother discomfort. The reflex is demonstrable in the newborn period and then fades during the early months. I have found it valuable to use this reflex to obtain an indication of the infant's alertness by noting its ease of elicitation (Holt, 1972).

REFLEX RESPONSES TO PRESSURE AND PAIN

Although some of the responses to pressure serve a constructive and functional role (such as the support reaction), the majority have a protective and survival value (for example, the withdrawal response). Many of these responses are so well ingrained that only the most profound cerebral depression inhibits them. The persistent absence of, say, Galant's response in the neonatal period is a sign of a poor prognosis.

Galant's reflex (*Figure 12*)

Firm sharp stimulation alongside the spine with the finger nails or a pin produces contraction of the underlying muscles. This causes curving of

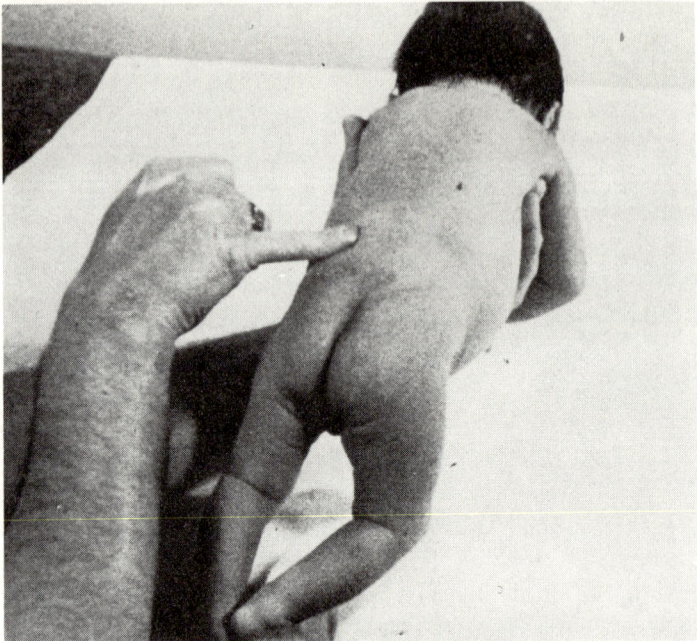

Figure 12. Galant's reflex (trunk incurvation). Following stimulation the back is arched concave to the stimulating finger

the back convexly on the side of the stimulus. This response is readily seen when the infant is held upright and the trunk movement is unrestricted whilst the stimuli are applied. It is best seen in the neonatal period and thereafter gradually fades.

Withdrawal reflex (Figure 13)

A pinprick or other sharp painful stimulus results in flexion and withdrawal of the stimulated limb. This is best seen in the leg when the sole of the foot is stimulated in this way. The protective value of the reflex is obvious.

Crossed extension reflex (Figure 14)

If the leg is kept extended at the knee whilst the sole of the foot is repeatedly stimulated by firm strokes with a finger or other firm object, the opposite leg flexes and then extends. Because the extension phase is associated with some adduction at the hip, an impression is obtained of the moving leg crossing the stimulated one as if to push away the

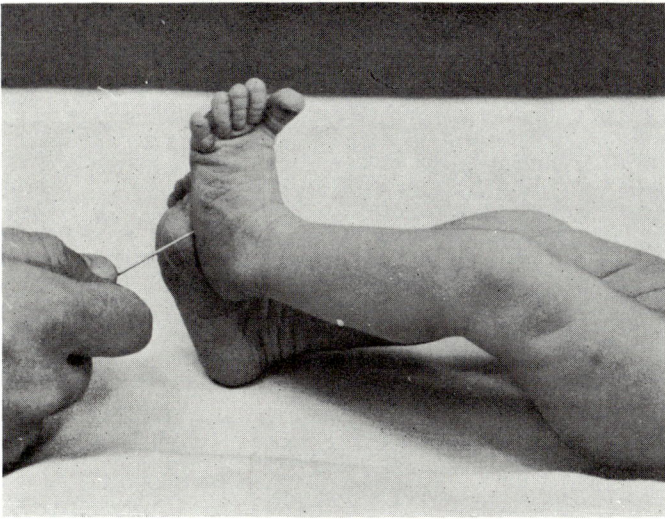

(a)

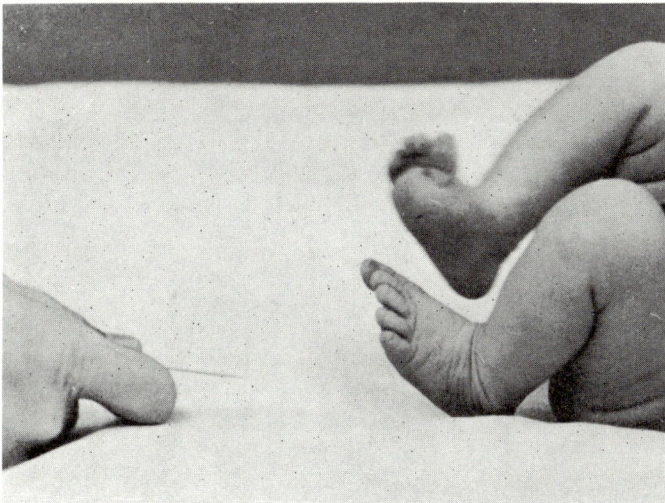

(b)

Figure 13. The withdrawal reflex: (a) stimulation; (b) response

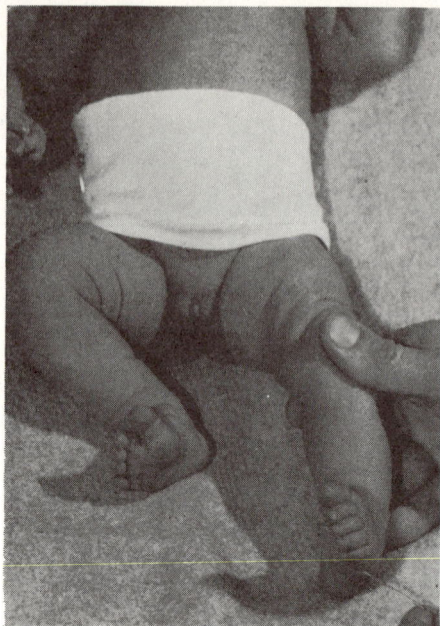

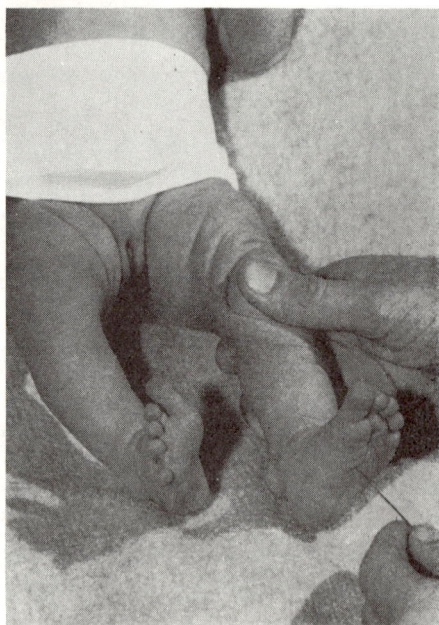

Figure 14. The crossed extension reflex: (a) stimulation; (b) response

stimulating hand. This reflex is present in the neonate and even in the premature baby. Brett (1965) uses this reflex when determining the maturity of the newborn. This reflex gradually fades during the first year, but it is difficult to ascribe a precise time after which it is no longer seen. I have been impressed by the diagnostic value of this reflex, having found it to be present at a year of age as the only clue to diagnosis in several babies who later showed a well developed picture of cerebral palsy.

Babinski (Plantar) reflex (Holt, 1961) (Figure 15)

This reflex is one of the fundamental signs of classical neurology. The stimulus consists of a firm, almost painful stroke along the lateral border of the sole from heel to toe. The response consists of movement (flexion or extension) of the big toe and sometimes movement (fanning) of the other toes as well. Techniques have been described to elicit the response by stimulating other areas (e.g. stroking the lateral border of the dorsum of the foot, squeezing the calf, or running the fingers along the anterior border of the tibia). These manoeuvres are most effective when the reflex is pathologically exaggerated. The reflex is present throughout life. In the first year or two the surface area from which stimuli are effective is quite extensive. Thereafter it shrinks until the lateral side of the sole is the principal area from which a response can be obtained. The motor response is similarly widespread at first so that movement of all the toes is noticeable, and extension of the big toe usually predominates over the weaker flexion movement. After this age, however, the motor response becomes more controlled and restricted. The extensors of the big toe do not appear to be stimulated so flexion of the big toe is the normal response. It is probable that progressive reduction of both the area of effective stimulation and the motor response reflects increasing neurological maturation. After two or three years of age extension of the big toe is probably abnormal and usually indicates a lesion of the pyramidal tract. This reflex is most useful diagnostically, and great reliance is placed upon it in neurological examinations.

The magnet (traction) reflexes (Figure 16)

Steady firm pressure is applied to the sole of the foot or to the palm of the hand with the limb flexed, and is then gently withdrawn to be followed by extension of the limb as if being drawn forwards by a magnet. This reflex is demonstrable in the early months.

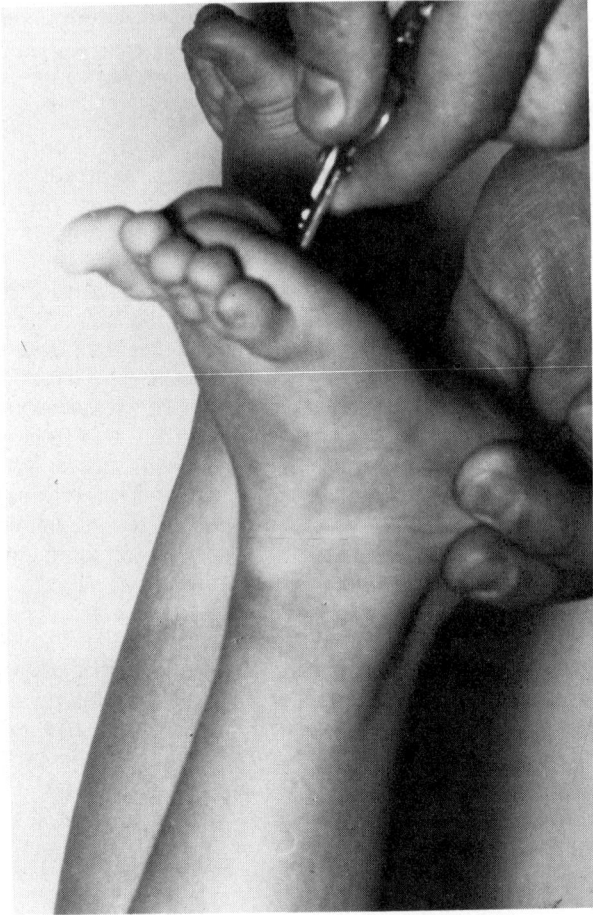

Figure 15. The Babinski (Plantar) reflex

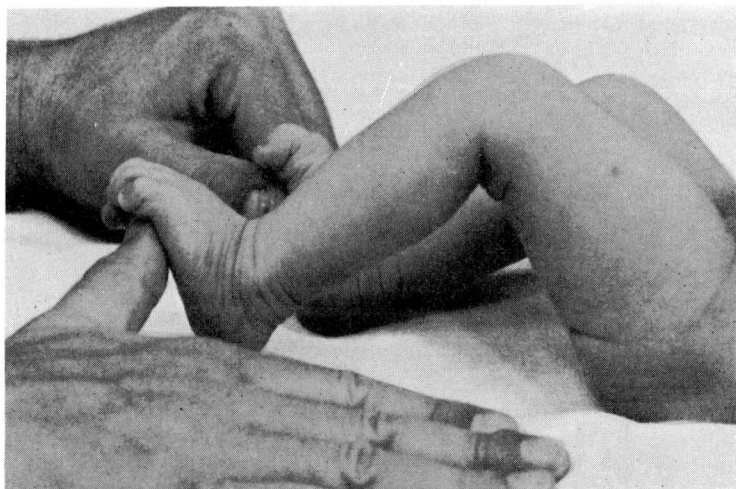

(a)

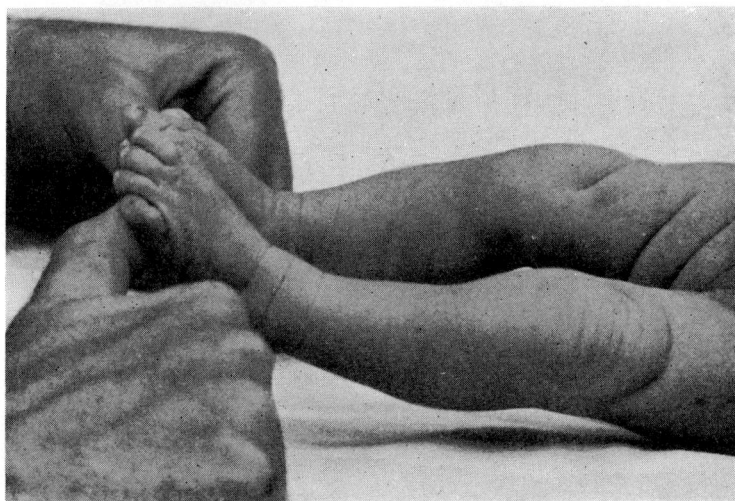

(b)

Figure 16. The magnet reflex: (a) stimulation; (b) response

Babkin reflex

The stimulus for this reflex consists of deep pressure applied simultaneously to the palms of both hands whilst the infant is in an appropriate position, ideally supine. The stimulus is followed by flexion or forward bowing of the head, opening of the mouth and closing of the eyes. The reflex can be demonstrated in the newborn, thus showing a hand-mouth neurological link even at that early stage. It fades rapidly and normally cannot be elicited after 4 months of age. Elicitation of the reflex after this age indicates a cerebral lesion.

Stepping reflex (Figure 17)

Pressure upon the sole of the foot of the neonate causes first flexion then extension of the leg. As this occurs on alternate sides, an

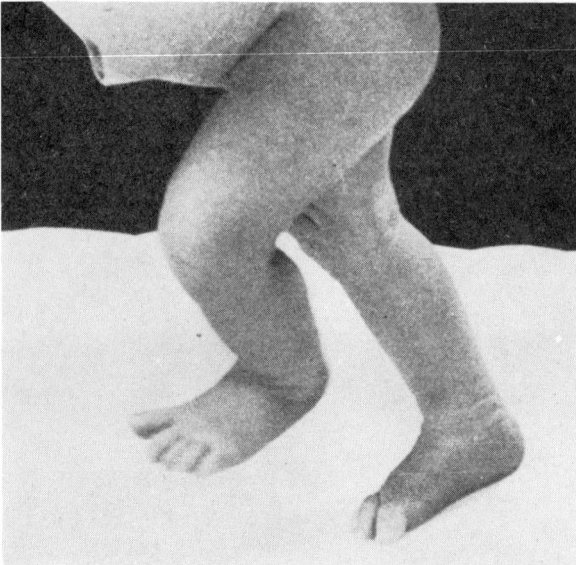

Figure 17. The stepping reflex (contact of the sole with the table top produces flexion of the leg and alternate stepping)

impression is created of automatic stepping. It is not true walking, however, because there is no pelvic stability—this is acquired through the support reflex which develops later. MacKeith (1964) showed very neatly that head position affected the ease of elicitation, strength

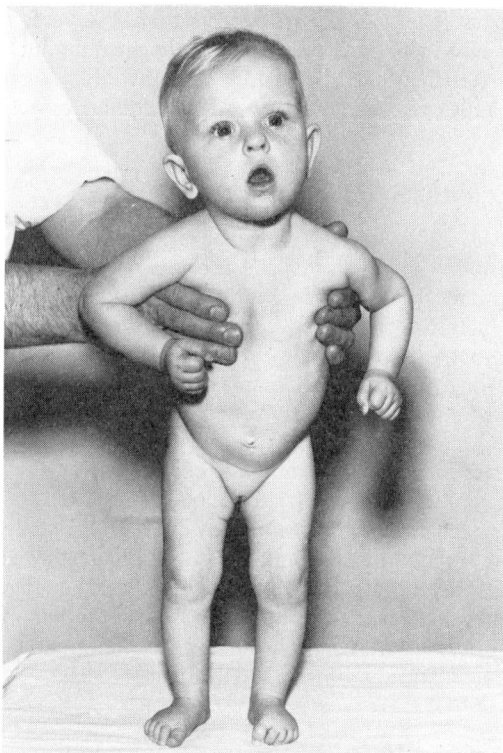

(a)

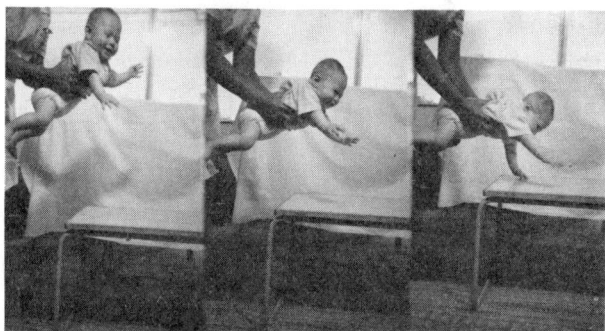

(b)

Figure 18. The support reflex: (a) lower limbs; (b) upper limbs

and duration of this reflex. The stepping reflex should disappear by six months. This reflex sometimes persists for many years in children with cerebral palsy, and parents think that their child must be near to walking, little realizing that he is merely demonstrating the persistence of a primitive reflex.

Support reflex (legs) (Figure 18(a))

The similarity of this reflex to the magnet reflex was mentioned earlier. When an infant is held vertically and the soles of the feet allowed to come into contact with a table or floor, the pressure on the soles causes reflex extension of the legs. A chain response producing secondary stiffening of the legs follows the initial reaction and makes the legs strong supporting pillars. This complex reflex is important for the development of the upright posture and locomotion. The secondary part of the reflex at least occurs in response to kinaesthetic stimuli in addition to deep pressure. The reflex is elicited with difficulty in the early months and even when it is obtained it lasts only a few brief moments. It gradually becomes more evident as the stepping reflex fades, and by six months it should be obtained readily and should persists for several minutes. Failure of this reflex to appear at the right time delays locomotor development. Persistence long after it has served its purpose is a sign of neurological abnormality, and also produces characteristic abnormal gait patterns.

Support reflex (arms) (Figure 18(b))

A support reflex appears in the arms several months later than the similar reflex in the legs. Preparation occurs by extension of the arms as the body is tilted forwards or sideways. Contact of the palms of the open hands with a firm surface then provides the stimulus for tensing of the arm muscles. Visual and labyrinthine righting reflexes are responsible for the early part of the reflex but the supporting part follows pressure stimulus on the palms.

REFLEX RESPONSES TO KINAESTHETIC STIMULI

Many reflex responses originate from stimuli from the tendons, muscles and joints. Most of them are important in the maintenance of posture and orientation of the body in space. Some of these reflexes are as follows.

Tendon reflexes

These are simple monosynaptic spinal reflexes which are elicited by a
sudden stretch of a muscle tendon such as occurs when the tendon is
tapped. They are present throughout life and are most useful diagnostically for the detection of upper motor neurone lesions (exaggerated
response); myopathic conditions, (depressed or absent response); and
localization of segmental lesions of the cord. The cord levels served by
the various tendon reflexes are shown in Table 1.

TABLE 1

The Spinal Cord Levels of the Tendon Reflexes

Reflex	Cord level
Biceps (elbow)	C 5.6
Brachioradialis	C 5.6
Triceps	C 6.8
Long finger flexors	C 6–T 1
Adductors	L 2.4
Quadriceps (knee)	L 2.4
Gastrocnemius-Soleus (ankle)	S 1.2

C, cervical; T, thoracic; L, lumbar; S, sacral

Eye righting (doll's eye) reflex (Figure 19)

Passive turning of the head of the newborn leaves the eyes 'behind' and
a distinct time lag occurs before the eyes move to a new position in
keeping with the head position. Within a week or two of birth, this
doll's eye phenomenon has disappeared as a result of an eye righting
reflex which ensures rapid adjustment of the eye position when the
head is turned. Failure of this reflex to appear, i.e. persistence of the
doll's eye phenomenon, indicates a cerebral lesion. Although listed
here with the reflex responses to kinaesthetic stimuli it is probable that
the labyrinths also have a major influence on this reflex (Kestenbaum,
1930).

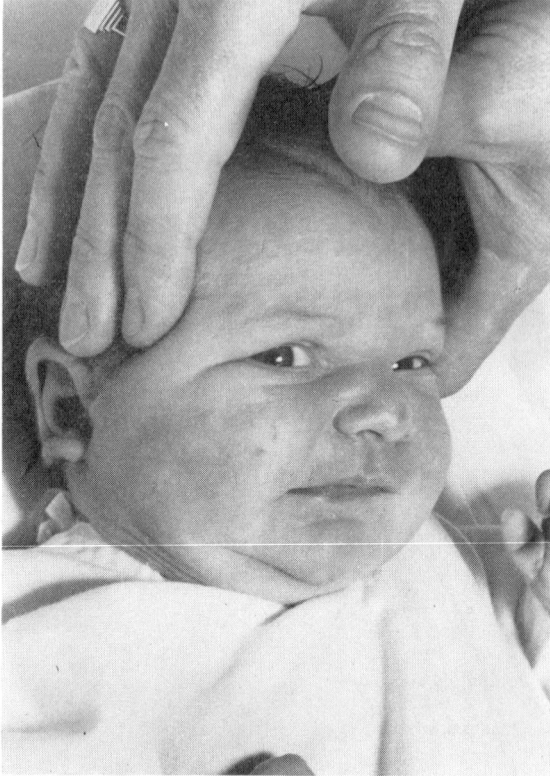

Figure 19. The doll's eye reflex (the eyes lag behind as the head rotates)

Moro reflex (Figures 20(a, b and c))

This is one of the best known and most useful clinically of all the neonatal reflexes. The afferent stimulus is produced by a sudden movement of the head on the shoulders. It can be produced in several ways. One way is to allow the head to drop about one inch into the palm of the hand (*Figure 20(a)*); another way is to raise the supine baby a short way from the couch by pulling upon the hands and then to release them suddenly. The response consists of wide abduction of the arms and opening of the hands. Within moments the arms come together again simulating an embrace (*Figure 20(b)*). The response often includes tensing of the back muscles, flexion of the legs and crying. The response should be symmetrical; asymmetry indicates a central or peripheral nervous system lesion, or injury to the bones or

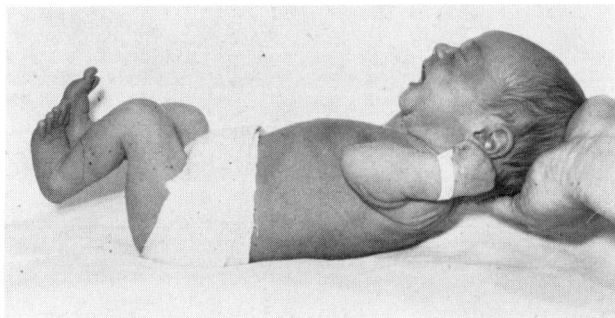

Figure 20 (a)

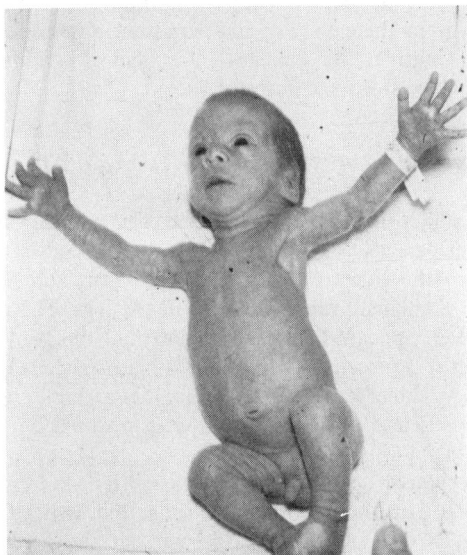

Figure 20 (b)

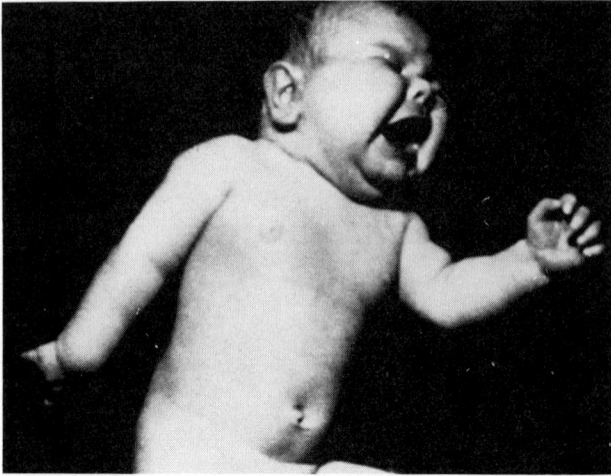

(c)

Figure 20. The Moro reflex: (a) one method of elicitation; (b) normal response; (c) asymmetrical response due to Erb's palsy

muscles of the defective arm (*Figure 20(c)*). Failure of the arms to move freely and of the hands to open fully indicates hypertonia, and feebleness of response occurs with hypotonia and prematurity. The reflex is present in the newborn (its persistent absence or asymmetry should cause considerable concern), but fades rapidly and is not normally elicitable after six months of age.

The asymmetrical tonic neck reflex (ATNR) (Figure 21)

The stimulus which initiates this reflex consists of sideways turning of the head, either passively or actively. The response consists of extension of the arm on the side to which the head turns and flexion of the opposite arm. Similar movements occur in the legs. The precise age at which this reflex appears continues to be the subject of controversy; some deny that it is present in the neonatal period, whereas others think that it can be produced at that early stage. It is certainly not frequently seen nor easily elicited at that time, and it is most evident between two and four months of age.

This reflex would seem to play an important role in visuomotor development. It is present during the time that visual fixation upon nearby objects is developing and it seems that the nervous system is making sure that the appropriate arm stretches out towards visualized

objects. As the hand touches the object the seeds are sown of awareness of distance ('at arm's length') and hand-eye co-ordination.
The reflex fades rapidly and is not normally seen after six to seven
months of age. Persistence of the ATNR is the most frequently
observed abnormality of the infantile reflexes in infants with neurological lesions (Paine, 1964). Its persistence, usually in an exaggeratedly
strong form, is a clear indication of abnormality of the nervous system
and greatly disrupts development.

The symmetrical tonic neck reflex

Experimental observations of animals have shown that flexion and
extension of the head can profoundly influence the posture of the
animal. The response has been linked with the feeding needs and habits
of the animals. When this reflex is strong in an experimental dog, for
example, flexion of the head causes flexion of the forelimbs and extension of the hind limbs, just as if the animal was bending the head
forward in order to take food; whereas extension of the head produces
extension of the forelimbs and flexion of the hind limbs just as if the
animal was preparing to take a tasty morsel held above him. This
reflex is not normally easily seen or elicited in normal infants, but may
be seen in exaggerated form in some children with cerebral palsy.

Head-body and body-head righting reflexes (Figures 22, 23)

As mentioned earlier, various stimuli may produce the same response.
Orientation of the head in relation to the body and *vice versa* is so
important that it is not surprising that it is produced by several
righting reflexes. Some of them arise from kinaesthetic stimulation of
the muscles and joints of the neck. As the head is turned the trunk
realigns itself so as to remain in the normal relationship to the head.
Similarly turning of the trunk is followed by reorientation of head
position. These righting reflexes are present early in life, and during
the second half of the first year of life they reinforce the action of the
visual and labyrinthine righting reflexes. A clear understanding of the
righting reflexes is necessary for the treatment of young children with
central neurological disorders. For example, in the case of a child who
cannot roll sideways it is necessary to study these reflexes to know
whether it is therapeutically better to rotate the head and have the
trunk follow or *vice versa*.

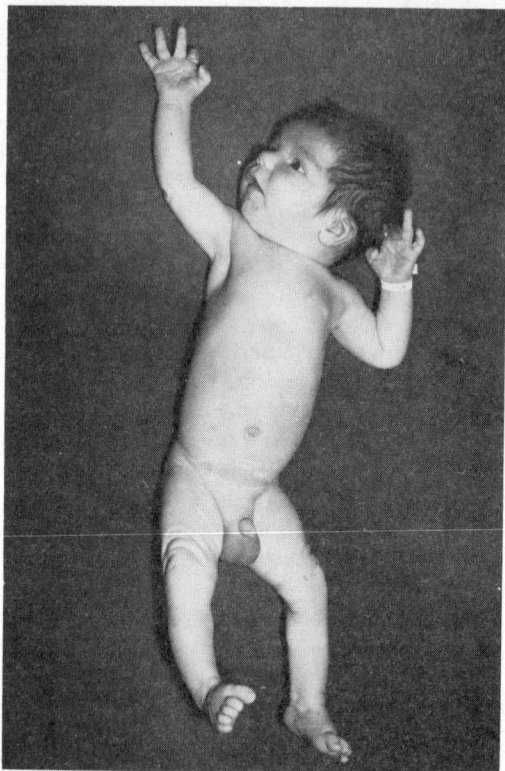

Figure 21. The asymmetrical tonic neck reflex

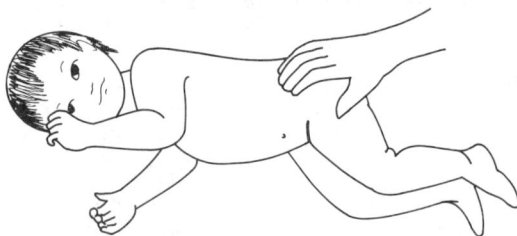

Figure 22. Head righting reflex (rotation of the trunk is followed by righting of the head)

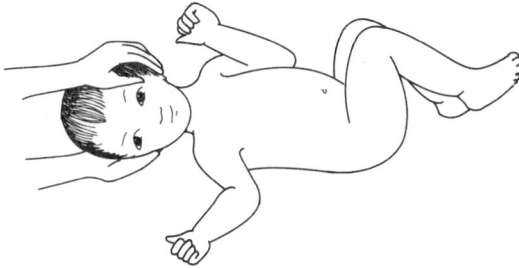

*Figure 23. Body righting reflex (rotation of the head is
followed by righting of the trunk)*   flink - neonate →

REFLEX RESPONSES TO VISUAL AND AUDITORY STIMULI

As our visual and auditory senses are able to receive stimuli from a
distance, they are well equipped to act as warning mechanisms. Consequently many of the reflexes produced by visual and auditory stimuli
have a protective and survival value.

The blink reflex

A bright light suddenly shone into the eyes, a puff of air upon the
sensitive cornea, or a sudden loud noise produce an almost immediate
response of blinking of the eyes. This may be associated with tensing
of the neck muscles and turning of the head away from the stimulus,
and may be followed by grimacing and crying. These reflexes are
easily seen in the neonate in whom the responses are well marked and
widespread. They continue to be present throughout life.

The visual righting reflex (Figure 24)

Once some visual awareness of orientation has developed, infants do
not readily tolerate distorted views and reflexly attempt to right their
head position in order to correct the view. This visual righting reflex
develops in close association with the labyrinthine righting reflexes.

The auditory orientating reflexes (Figure 25)

A sudden noise, especially if it is loud and unpleasant, may produce the
blink reflex as described above, or the infant may remain still and show

44

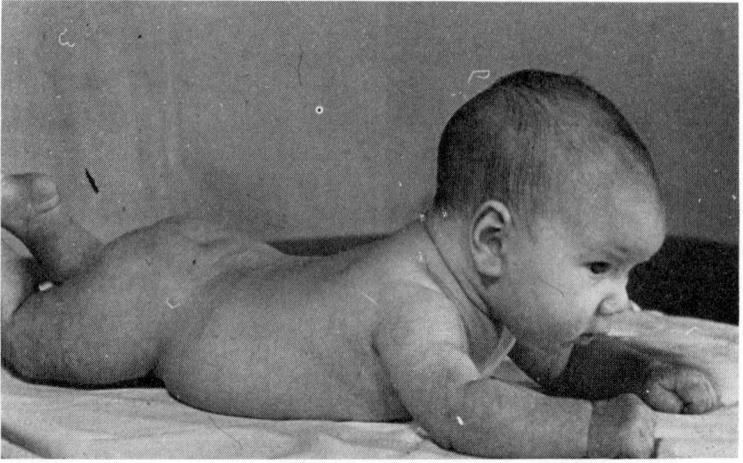

Figure 24. Head extension due to labyrinthine head righting reflex reinforced by visual righting reflex

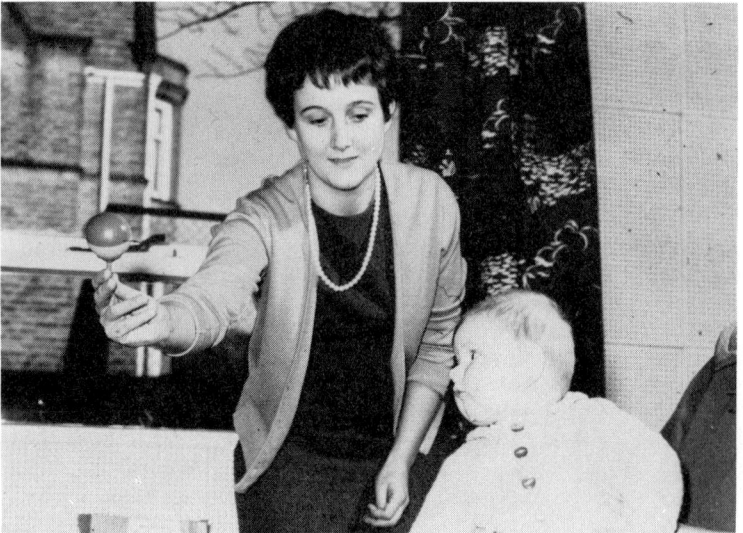

Figure 25. Head turning to auditory stimulus (see also Figure 52)

increased alertness. Quieter sounds usually cause reflex eye and head turning to the side of the sound, as if to locate it. This auditory orientation reflex is seen first clearly about four months of age. Thereafter head turning towards sound stimuli becomes more complex, and the accuracy of localization increases rapidly until by nine to ten months the sound source is located directly and promptly within about five degrees (Murphy, 1962). These reflex responses are made use of in screening tests of infants for hearing loss as will be described in later chapters. The pattern of the localization responses also indicates the level of neurological maturity.

REFLEX RESPONSE TO LABYRINTHINE STIMULI

The attainment and maintenance of upright postures against gravity are essential requirements for the successful motor development of the human infant. The labyrinths are the most important organs concerned with the development of anti-gravity postures and balance. Movement of the head in any dimension stimulates some part of the labyrinths and, after the early weeks, produces appropriate responses.

Labyrinthine head righting

Once this reflex has developed, the infant's head is always moved into a position in which the vertex is uppermost and the mouth horizontal whatsoever the position of the child. Thus, if the infant is held by the feet with the trunk and head downwards, the head will be extended backwards in order to get it upright against gravity. Similarly, if the infant is held in ventral suspension, i.e. horizontally with a hand supporting the trunk, the head will be extended to achieve an upright posture. The response elicited in this latter position has been described as the Landau reflex.

Labyrinthine head righting is not present at birth (*Figure 26(a)*), but develops during the early months. Its influence is clearly seen in the progressive ease with which the infant raises his head in the prone position (*Figure 26(b)*). In humans head righting responses also occur in response to visual stimuli, so that when observing the motor development of infants it is difficult to know the relative contributions made by these two head righting mechanisms. Those children who fail to develop any head righting ability at all, such as some children with cerebral palsy, are very disabled in consequence (*Figure 27*).

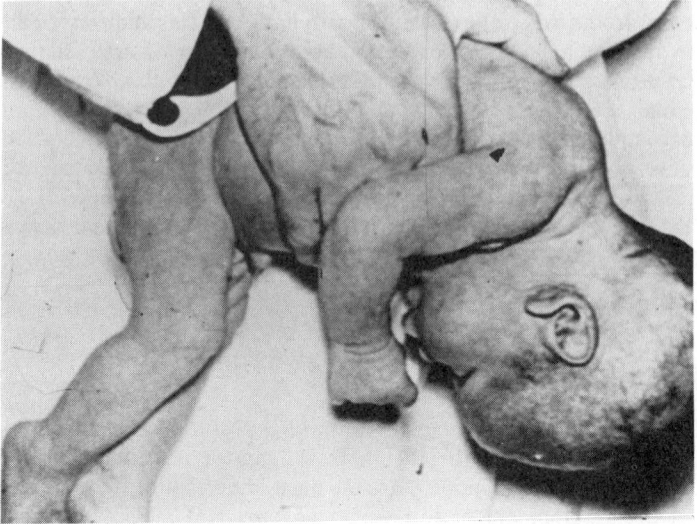

(a)

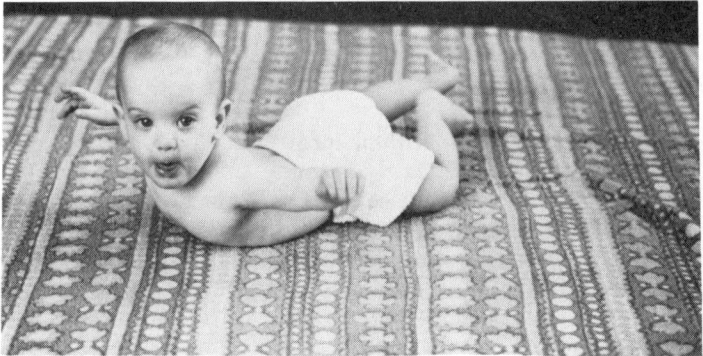

(b)

Figure 26. (a) Absence of head righting in neonate; (b) Ease of raising head in prone position

The development of head righting and of the ability to control the head position irrespective of gravity opens up great possibilities for further motor development. A series of chain reactions ensue as various reflexes influence the body position and the attitudes and movements of the limbs. For example, once an infant can raise his head in the prone position the way is open for him to get to crawling. The sequence is as follows:

Head righting—increases in strength and extent until shoulders are raised—this facilitates forward movement of arms—support reflex of arms then enables chest to be raised—this facilitates raising of pelvis—leads to drawing up of knees and then support reflex enables pelvis to

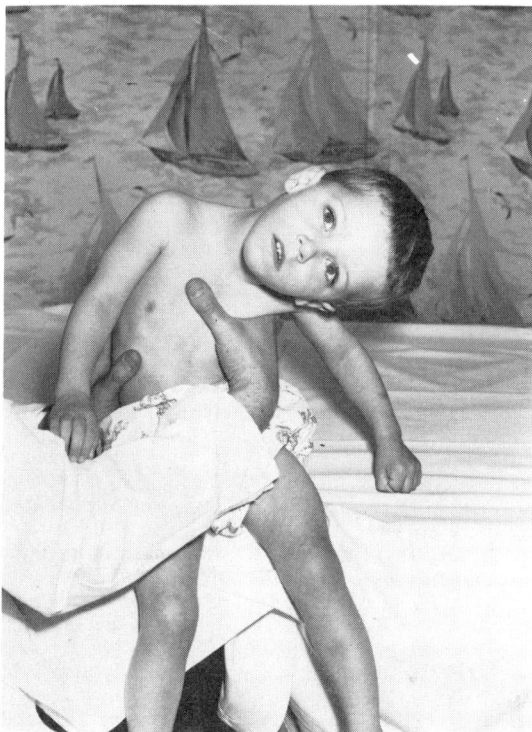

Figure 27. Absence of head righting in child with cerebral palsy

be raised—as security of support increases limbs can be freed in succession to develop an alternating reciprocal movement—crawling is achieved.

Tonic labyrinthine reflexes

The labyrinths are thought to exert a tonic influence upon the distribution of muscle tone throughout the body, and to control the balance between the extensor and flexor muscles. It is very difficult to isolate and study these effects in normal infants, but the effects of disturbances of these tonic reflexes are very obvious in neurologically damaged infants, many of whom exhibit dystonic syndromes.

FURTHER DEVELOPMENT

The growth and development of the brain are essential for an infant's progress. In the early stages the infant is controlled by the many reflexes which are preparing the way for his motor development. Once this basis is established further progress ensues as can be observed, stage by stage, whilst the child grows older.

REFERENCES

Amiel-Tison, C. (1968). Neurological evaluation of the maturity of newborn infants. *Archs Dis. Childh.,* 43, 89

Baurlacher, K. E. (1973). Developmental aspects of amino acid transport. In *Inborn Errors of Metabolism*, ed. Hommes, F. A., and van den Berg, C. J. London: Academic Press

Bernhard, C. G. and Meyerson, B. A. (1973). Morphological and physiological aspects of the development of recipient functions in the cerebral cortex. In *Fetal and Neonatal Physiology*, Barcroft Centenary Symposium. Cambridge: Cambridge University Press

Brett, E. M. (1965). The estimation of foetal maturity by the neurological examination of the neonate. *Clinics Dev. Med.,* 19, 105

Dobbing, J. (1974). The later development of the brain and its vulnerability. In *Scientific Foundations of Paediatrics*, ed. Davis, J. A., and Dobbing, J. London: Heinemann

— and Sands, J. (1973). Quantitative growth and development of human brain. *Archs Dis. Childh.,* 48, 757

— and Smart, J. L. (1974). Vulnerability of developing brain and behaviour. *Brit. Med. Bull.,* 30, 2, 164

Dreyfuss-Brisac, C. (1966). The bioelectrical development of the central nervous system during early life. In *Human Development,* ed. Falkner, F. Philadelphia: Saunders

Dubowitz, V. and Goldberg, C. (1970). Clinical assessment of gestational age in the newborn infant, *J. Pediat.,* 77, 1

Farr, V., Mitchell, R. G., Neligan, G. A. and Parkin, J. M. (1966). The definition of some external characteristics used in the assessment of gestational age in the newborn infant, *Devl Med. Child Neurol.,* 8, 507

Herschkowitz, N. and Rossi, E. (1972). Critical periods of brain development. In *Lipids, Malnutrition and the Developing Brain,* Ciba Foundation Symposium. London: Associated Science Publications

Holt, K. S., (1961). The plantar response in infants and children. *Cerebr. Palsy Bull.* 3, 449

— (1963). In *The Development of the Infant and Young Child Normal and Abnormal,* ed. Illingworth, R. S., 2nd edn. Edinburgh: Livingstone

– (1965). Age, growth, and maturity of the neonate. *Clinics Dev. Med.*, **19**, 100
– (1972). Neurological examination of the newborn. *Hosp. Med. N.Y.* **8**, 86
Illingworth, R. S. and Lutz, W. (1965). Head circumference of infants related to body weight. *Archs Dis. Childh.*, **40**, 672
Kestenbaum, A. (1930). Zur Entwickling der Angenbewagungen und des Optokinetishen Nystagmus. *Archs Ophth.* **124**, 113
McIlwain, H. (1966). *Biochemistry of the Central Nervous System.* London: Churchill
MacKeith, R. C. (1964). The primary walking response and its facilitation by passive extension of the head. *Acta Paediat.* **17**, suppl. 6
Magnus, R. (1924). *Körperstellung.* Berlin.
– and de Kleijn, A. (1930). Körperstellung, Gleichgewicht und Bewegung bei Säugern. Haltung und Stellung bei Säugern. *Handb. Physiol* **15**, 1, 29 and 55
Milani Comparetti, A. and Gidoni, E. A. (1967). Routine developmental examination in normal and retarded children. *Devl Med. Child Neurol.* **9**, 631
Murphy, K. P. (1962). Ascertainment of deafness in children. *Panorama*, December
Myers, R. E. and Bito, L. Z. (1973). Ontogenesis of blood-brain barrier function in primate : CSF cation regulations. In *Fetal and Neonatal Physiology*, Barcroft Centenary Symposium. Cambridge: Cambridge University Press
Nellhaus, G. (1968). Composite international and inter racial graphs. *Pediatrics*, **41**, 106
Paigen, K. (1971). Enzyme systems and degradation. In *Mammalian Systems*, ed. Recheigl, M. Washington, D. C. :Karger, Basel
Paine, R. (1964). The evolution of infantile postural reflexes in the presence of chronic brain syndromes. *Devl. Med. Child Neurol.*, **6**, 345
Paine, R. S. and Opie, T. E. (1966). Neurological Examination of Children. *Clinics Dev. Med.* 20/21. Heinemann : London
Peiper, A. (1961). *Cerebral Function in Infancy and Childhood*. London : Pitman Medical
Prechtl, H. F. R. (1953). *Umschau*, **53**, 656
Rademaker, G. G. J. (1931). *Das Stehen.* Berlin
Robinson, R. J. (1966). Assessment of gestational age by neurological examination, *Archs Dis. Childh.*, **41**, 437
Sherrington, C. S. (1898). Decerebrate rigidity and reflex coordination of movements. *J. Physiol.* **22**, 319
Sterman, M. B., McGinty D. J. and Adinolfi, A. M. (1971). *Brain Development and Behaviour*. London : Academic Press
Thomas, A., Chesni, J. and Dargassies, S. Saint Anne. (1960). The neurological examination of the infant. Little Club Clinics 1. London: Heinemann
Wilkinson, D. H. and Buckley, B. M. (1973). Role of ketone bodies in brain development. In *Inborn Errors of Metabolism*, ed. Hommes, F. A. and van den Berg, C. J. London : Academic Press

CHAPTER 3

Observable Development :
Pattern, Range and Variations –
The Neonate and Infant

THE FEATURES OF HUMAN DEVELOPMENT

Living beings are constantly changing. This is one of the most characteristic properties of life. As they increase in size and ability we say they are developing, and when they decrease in size and cease to function as well as they did in the past we say they are regressing and dying. Development is an integral feature of life, and it follows a definite pattern for each species.

As the tissues multiply and differentiate, the organism develops more functions and abilities which then are seen as outward signs of development. Behind each visible aspect of development lies much activity—the preparation and integration of the various functions which make it all possible. To understand development fully it is necessary to look behind the observable actions and to try to understand what is happening that makes them possible.

Many organisms exhibit a stereotyped pattern of development, but human beings show variations of the common pattern. This is because their highly elaborate central nervous system enables them to select and to reinforce the sensory stimuli they receive and to modify the responses they make. They are able to train and to teach themselves, and also others, and in this way to modify their behaviour and development.

Human development requires many years to reach completion. Life begins with the union of two minute cells which then quickly multiply and differentiate so that at birth some 40 weeks later the baby already weighs about 3½ kg (7½ lb) and is a complex organism (*Figure 28*).

Even so the baby is dependent and immature. During the succeeding years the child acquires the ability to take up various postures such as sitting, squatting, lying and standing, and to move about in different ways such as crawling, walking, running and climbing. The child develops the ability to use his hands in innumerable ways as in reaching, fingering, screwing, carrying and shaping. On the receptive side the child becomes able to identify, differentiate and select a wide range of rapidly changing visual, auditory and other sensory stimuli, and on the responsive side learns to make a variety of responses according to circumstances.

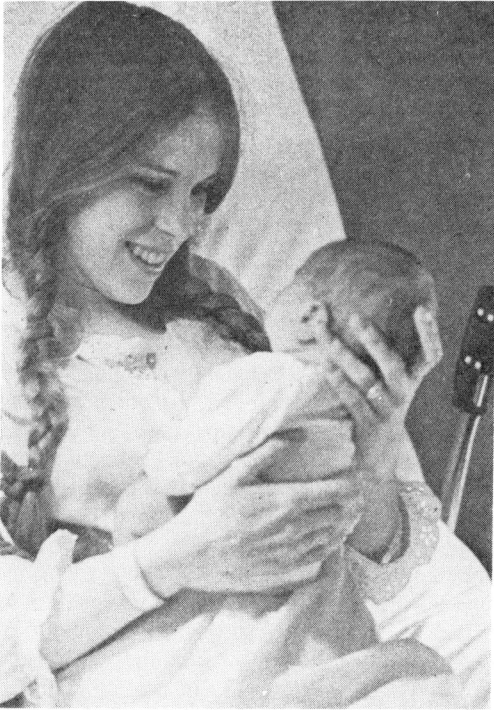

Figure 28. A new baby—little more than a twentieth of the size of the mother

Nor is this all. As development proceeds the child develops a range of emotional feelings and he acquires an awareness of these feelings and a sensitivity towards them in both himself and in others.

Remarkable as it is, human development does not lead to the greatest skills in all abilities. There are many species who can move more quickly, see and hear more acutely, and react more completely than man. But man's achievement is to utilize his great brain capacity to devise ways to extend his basic skills. Thus he devises means to move more quickly and to fly, to perceive sensations of which he would not otherwise be aware such as radio waves, and to communicate and share his knowledge and understanding with his fellows.

Although the basic pattern of human development is similar in all, and is genetically determined, it requires environmental stimulation and opportunities to reach its full manifestation. Both maturational forces and environmental experiences are essential and interdependent. To reach their full potential humans require teaching and training linked with their own drives to achieve even more.

In this and the following two chapters the outward manifestations of human development from birth to 15 years are described. Later chapters contain discussions about the underlying mechanisms. The descriptions are arranged to illustrate development as an interplay between maturational forces which equip a child to be receptive and responsive to environmental stimuli, and the environmental influences and experiences which he receives.

THE NEONATE

In one respect the neonate is reasonably well equipped biologically for survival outside the uterus. Basic bodily functions such as circulation, respiration, digestion, elimination, homeostasis and temperature regulation are well developed. In other respects the neonate is quite immature. Sensory perception is poorly developed and it takes a long time for him to acquire mobility and manipulative skills and to learn to utilize all his potential abilities.

Flexion dominates the neonate's postures. When he is picked up and laid in a prone position, the head turns sideways as a result of a protective reflex which prevents suffocation, the arms are flexed, and the legs are flexed and drawn up under the abdomen so that the pelvis is raised (*Figure 29(a)*). Some movements of the limbs and trunk occur in this position, but they occur more freely in the supine position, because the limbs are less restricted. There is very little head control at this stage and the head flops downwards when the baby is lifted into ventral suspension (*Figure 29 (b)*), (i.e. supported in the prone position with just a hand under the abdomen), or into an upright posture.

The neonate shows awareness of both auditory and visual stimuli by quietening if the stimuli are tolerable, or by blinking, grimacing, startling and crying if they are stronger.

The neonate exhibits a number of reflexes in which a relatively minor stimulus suffices to trigger off an almost instantaneous stereotyped response. These primary reflexes demonstrate the activity of the neonate's central nervous system and they provide the basis for motor development. The nature and purpose of these reflexes is described more fully in Chapter 2 and their evaluation as part of the clinical examination of the neonate is described below.

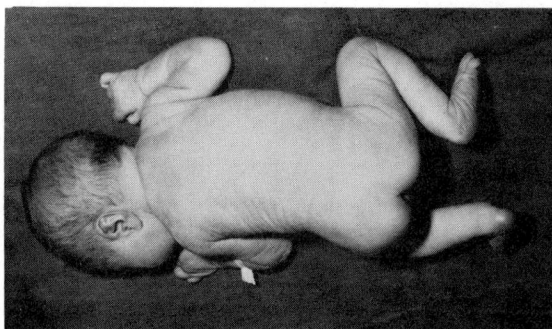

(a)

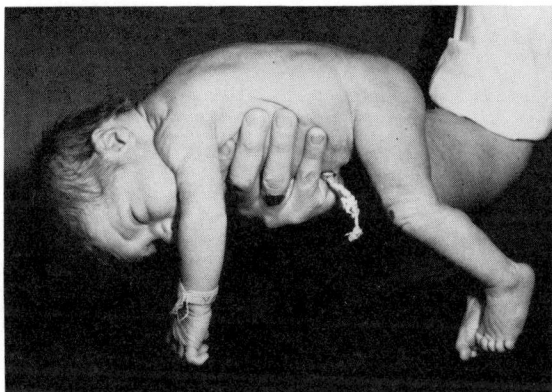

(b)

Figure 29. The neonate: (a) prone; (b) ventral suspension (see also Figures 26 and 32)

Clinical Examination of the Neonate

Birth provides the first opportunity for a clinical examination of a baby. Information is obtained at this first examination about the current state of the baby especially the adjustment to extra-uterine existence, the presence of malformations, the effects of previous antenatal and natal events, the degree of maturity, and to some extent the future prospects of the baby.

There are three principal types of examination.

(a)   An immediate examination at delivery to assess the physiological status of the baby and its preparedness for extra-uterine existence, and to note any gross malformations.

(b)   A general clinical examination to determine the intactness of the baby and freedom from malformations.

(c)   An appraisal of the baby's neurodevelopmental status.

A technique for the first type of examination described by Apgar (1953) is now practised in most places. In this method a score of 0, 1 or 2 is given to each of 5 important physiological parameters (Table 2). The lower the total score the greater the physiological derangement of the baby. According to the original description the Apgar score should be calculated one minute after birth, but this is not at all easy because of all the other things which have to be given attention. It is useful to calculate it at a later time, say 3, 4 or 5 minutes after birth, or even to record it serially at 1-minute intervals and to write down when it was done.

TABLE 2

The Apgar Score

Sign	Score		
	0	1	2
Heart rate	Absent	Below 100	Over 100
Respiratory effort	Absent	Weak, irregular	Good, crying
Muscle tone	Flaccid	Some flexion of extremities	Well flexed
Reflex irritability (Catheter in nose)	No response	Grimace	Cough or sneeze
Colour	Blue, pale	Body pink Extremities blue	Completely pink

A score of 7 or more at one minute indicates a good prognosis for the baby with respect to mortality and subsequent neurological abnormality. Low scores at 1 minute are associated with a high mortality (8 per cent for scores of 2–3 and 23 per cent for scores of 0–1) and a high risk of neurological abnormality at 1 year in the survivors (3.6 per cent for scores of 0–3). Low scores persisting to the 5th minute are even more ominous, scores of 2–3, mortality 30 per cent; 0–1, mortality 49 per cent; and 0–3, neurological abnormality at 1 year 7.4 per cent (Drage and Berendes, 1966).

The methods of general clinical examination have been described many times elsewhere (e.g. Dargassies, 1954; Thomas, Chesni & Dargassies, 1960; Paine, 1961; Prechtl and Beintema, 1968; Braselton, 1973). The main features of such an examination are summarized below.

(a) Measurement of weight, and head circumference (the maximum circumference passing through occiput and just above the bridge of the nose). As the head circumference is measured the opportunity is taken to palpate the fontanelles and sutures. Whilst measurement of length is useful it is not recommended by some because of the difficulty in getting a reliable measurement which requires at least two people, and the risk of damage to the hips by over-strenuous attempts to obtain full extension of the legs.

(b) Confirmation of the intactness and normal function of the body systems especially respiration and circulation, including palpation of the peripheral pulses.

(c) Detection of any congenital malformations, searching particularly for those which are often overlooked, namely;
(i) the hips for undue laxity;
(ii) the eyes for cataract;
(iii) the genitalia and anus for malformation;
(iv) the spine for irregularities and dermal sinuses;
(v) the various minor malformations which when several are present together indicate the likely presence of a major malformation (Smith, 1970).

Table 3 gives a list of the minor malformations to be looked for.

Examination of the neonate's eyes is often best done during feeding when the eyes may open. It should not be necessary to force the lids apart nor to use mydriatics. Ophthalmoscopic examination is not part of a routine examination of the neonate, but if it is decided to perform such an examination it is usually possible and even easy to do so whilst the baby is sucking at a bottle.

The hips are examined by Barlow's (1962) modification of the Ortolani test in the following way. The baby lies supine. The examiner

TABLE 3

Minor Malformations of Clinical Significance (Smith, 1970)

Eyes

Prominent epicanthic folds
Widely spaced eyes (inter-canthal
distance > 3 cm between 1–2 years
and > 3.5 cm between 2–10 years)
Slanting palpebral fissure
Irregularities of iris, including
Brushfields spots
Anomalies of eyebrows

Hands

Single, or atypical palmar creases
Short, inturned little fingers
Syndactyly and polydactyly
Anomalies of nails
Dermal ridge abnormalities

Miscellaneous

Deep dimples at bony points, e.g. elbows
Hirsutism not otherwise explained
Low hair line
Multiple hair whorls
Malformations of genitalia
Malformations of sternum

Ears

Undue prominence
Incomplete development
Pre-auricular tags and fistula
Low set (cranial attachment of
helix lies below horizontal line
through lateral angle of orbit
with head set erect)

Feet

Variations in length of toes
Syndactyly and polydactyly
Wide separation of hallux
Anomalies of nails
Rocker-bottom feet

stands at the feet, facing the baby. He places each hand on the corresponding shin causing full flexion of the knees and flexion of the hips to a right angle. In this position he can place the middle fingers of each hand firmly over the greater trochanters and the thumbs over the lesser trochanters (*Figure 30*). Each leg is held steady in turn whilst the opposite leg is abducted. At or just beyond mid-abduction inward pressure is exerted by the middle finger. If the hip is dislocated the femoral head will be felt to slip over the aectabular lip when this manoeuvre is performed.

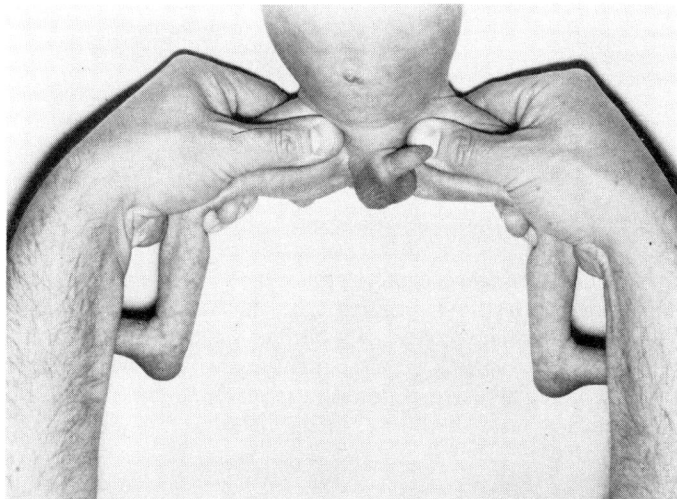

Figure 30. Examination of hips for instability and dislocation

Appraisal of the neurodevelopmental status of the neonate is particularly interesting to paediatricians because of the wealth of neurological activity which can be seen, and the clues which it provides to later development. It is an exacting type of examination which enables the paediatrician to estimate the maturity of the baby and to detect discrepancies which might lead to later difficulties and delays in development. Many of the responses observed during the examination are affected by the state of the baby and by external circumstances (e.g. time after feeding, temperature, draughts), and the examination should be done at the most appropriate stage of alertness of the baby. Beintema and Prechtl (1968) described an exceptionally careful technique. Their criteria and classification of the baby's state are shown in Table 4.

TABLE 4

Classification of State of Neonates (Prechtl and Beintema, 1968)

State of neonate	Criteria considered			
	Eyes	Respiration	Movements	Crying
1	Closed	Regular	None	–
2	Closed	Irregular	No gross movements	–
3	Open	–	No gross movements	–
4	Open	–	Gross movements	No crying
5	Open or closed	–	–	Crying
6	Any state not classifiable as 1–5			

In a clinical setting it is not always possible to carry out such thorough examinations. Nevertheless paediatricians should have opportunities to do so in their training so that they become familiar with all that they reveal and are also able to judge the limitations of abbreviated examinations, which they may have to resort to in practice.

The principal features of the examination are as follows:

(1) Alertness of the baby

This is determined by noting the general responsiveness, spontaneous movements, respiratory pattern, feeding behaviour, and the strength and promptness of the rooting reflex. This information is used both to judge the state of the baby and as a background against which to evaluate the observations of the rest of the examination. Persistently reduced alertness indicates abnormality.

(2) Symmetry of responses

This is noted with regard to the range of joint movement, reactions of muscles, and pattern of reflexes, having first made sure that the baby is in a symmetrical position at the beginning and throughout the examination. Persisting asymmetry indicates probable abnormality.

THE NEONATE 59

(3) Range of movement

This is estimated at certain joints—especially the following:

Movement	Normal response
Rotation of head on shoulders (*Figure 31 (a)*)	chin to acromial tip
Movement of arm across chest (*Figure 31 (b)*) (scarf sign)	fingers to opposite acromial tip
Extension of arm at elbow	180°
Flexion of wrist (*Figure 31(c)*)	150°
Abduction of flexed hips	approx. 75° each side
Extension of leg at knee when flexed to 90° at hips	approx. 150°
Dorsiflexion of foot	approx. 120°

Persisting definite variations indicate possible abnormalities. Reduced range of movement is usually due to increased muscle resistance. Increased range of movement may be due to hypotonia, or to immaturity. Sometimes variations occur as a result of the position *in utero*. For example, the findings on examination in the first few days of a baby born by breech with extended legs are different from those on a baby born by vertex.

(4) Muscle responsiveness to stretch

This is examined with respect to both slow and fast movements. Slow stretch should not produce resistance. If this occurs it is probably abnormal. Rapid repeated stretching of a muscle does produce resistance normally so that after three or four beats the movement tends to be arrested. This is the basis of the French test for 'passivité'. Reduced resistance to rapid stretch which permits the hand or leg to continue to swing freely in the test usually indicates immaturity or abnormality.

(5) Neonatal reflexes

Some of the more easily elicited and useful ones are examined. Abnormality might be indicated by their absence or exaggeration or asymmetry, as summarized below.

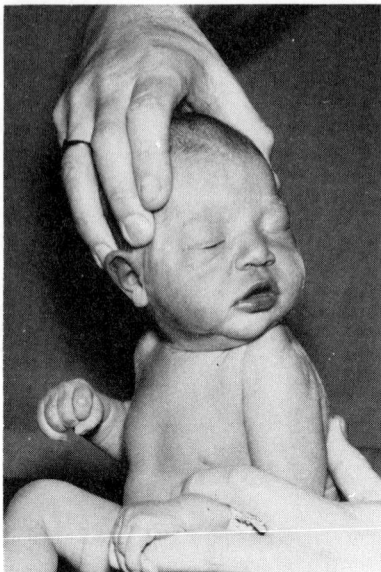

Figure 31. Range of joint movement in neonates: (a) head rotation; (b) scarf sign; (c) wrist flexion (this shows that in a premature baby flexion is limited to 90° producing a window effect)

(a)

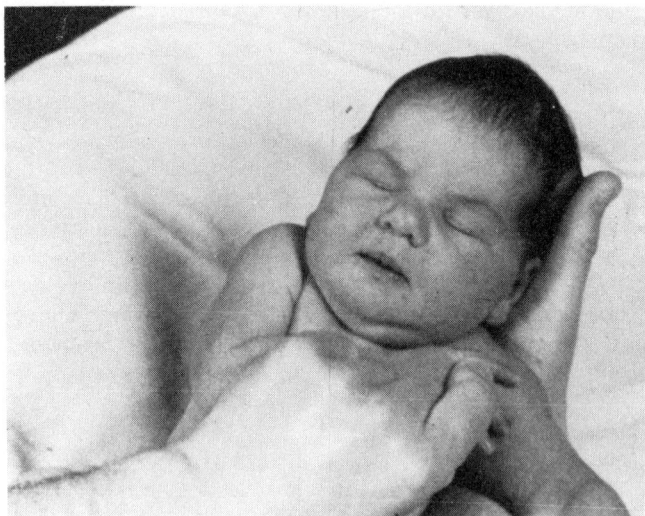

(b)

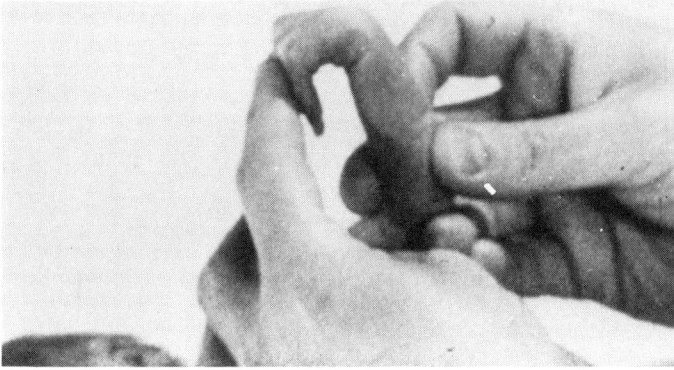

(c)

Reflex: Moro (*Figures 20 (a–c)*)

Method of elicitation   A sudden movement of the head on the shoulders brought about by allowing the head to drop an inch or so into the palm of the hand, or by raising the shoulders a little by drawing up the arm and then suddenly releasing them. Both these manoeuvres are done with the baby supine and symmetrical.

Normal response   Both arms abduct and extend and the hand opens, and then the arms come together as if in an embrace. The legs may be drawn up and the baby may grimace or even cry at the same time.

Abnormal response   Excessive sensitivity so that the reflex is precipitated with the slightest of movements; exaggeration of the response so that when it occurs there are quivering movements of the extended arms. Diminution, sluggishness, or asymmetry of the response may all be due to cerebral lesions. Marked asymmetry is usually due to obstetric damage of the humerus or brachial plexus.

Reflex: Rooting (Mouthing) (*Figures 11 (a, b)*)

Elicitation: Gentle stimulation is applied with a finger to one angle of the mouth.

Normal response   Opening of the mouth, turning of the head towards the stimulated side, and protrusion of the tongue towards the side stimulated.

Abnormal response   Persisting sluggishness or diminution of this reflex may indicate cerebral depression.

Reflex: Crossed Extension (*Figure 14*)

Elicitation   One leg is held extended at the knee, and the sole on that side is stimulated with a finger.

Normal response   The opposite leg flexes, adducts and then extends as if to push away the stimulating hand.

Abnormal response   This reflex is inhibited usually only when there are severe degrees of neurological disturbance.

Reflex: Grasp (*Figures 9a—c*)

Elicitation   A stimulating finger or rod is slid across the palm from the ulnar side.

Normal response   The fingers close upon the stimulating object. If the object is now raised, there is progressive tensing of the forearm and arm muscles, sometimes enabling the baby to be raised up. A similar response of flexion of the toes can be obtained by stimulating the sole.

Abnormal response   Feebleness, especially failure of the second part of the reflex, may indicate immaturity or abnormality. Persisting asymmetry indicates abnormality.

Reflex: Stepping and Placing (*Figures 10, 17*)

Elicitation   The baby is held first so that the sole touches the table (stepping), and second so that the dorsum of the foot touches the edge of the table (placing).

Normal response The first action initiates a stepping reflex in which the leg flexes and then extends, and the second action causes flexion of the leg as if the foot were being lifted to be placed on the table.

Abnormal response Marked suppression indicates a cerebral lesion.

Reflex: Trunk Incurvation (Galant's) (*Figure 12*)

Elicitation The side of the spine is stimulated with a moderately sharp object, e.g. finger nail.

Normal response Contraction of the musculature on that side causing curving of the spine concave to the stimulated side.

Abnormal response This reflex is usually only diminished when there is marked cerebral disturbance.

Reflex: Response to Diffuse Light (Photo-Tropism)

Elicitation The baby is held upright in the examiner's arms near a source of diffuse light, e.g. a window. The examiner then slowly rotates.

Normal response The baby adjusts his head position as rotation occurs so as to continue to face the diffuse light.

Abnormal response Diminution or absence may indicate cerebral disturbance.

Interpretation of the Neurodevelopmental Examinations

It is unwise to make any interpretation on the basis of finding a single abnormal item. This situation seldom occurs, however, and usually the findings fall into one of three patterns—normal, immature and abnormal.

The criteria for judging neonatal maturity are summarized in Tables 5 and 5(a).

TABLE 5

Some Criteria of Neonatal Maturity

(Amiel-Tison, 1968; Brett, 1965; Dubowitz & Goldberg, 1970; Farr, Mitchell, Neligan & Parkin, 1966; Holt, 1963, 1965; Robinson, 1966)

Criteria	Gestational age			
	28 weeks	32 weeks	36 weeks	40 weeks
Posture				
Arms	Limp, abducted, extended	Extended	Flexed weekly	Flexed strongly
Legs	Limp, abducted, extended	Abducted and flexed	Flexed and less 'frog like'	Flexed strongly
Head	Lateral	Lateral	Maybe control	Control
Spontaneous activity				
General	Always	Always	Sometimes	Sometimes
Persists with other activity	Yes	Sometimes	No	No
Individual limbs	Never	No	Sometimes	Yes
Feeding behaviour				
Ease of stimulation	Very difficult	Difficult	Fairly easy	Easy
Response	Feeble	Slow	Fairly brisk	Brisk
Persistence	None	Slight	Fairly good	Good

Range of movement

Head rotation	Well past acromion	Rather less	Rather less	To acromion
Scarf sign	Well past acromion	Rather less	Rather less	To acromion
Hips	Foot to ear	Rather less	Leg vertical	Leg vertical
Knees (popliteal angle)	140–150°	About 110°	About 100°	90° or less
Feet (dorsiflexion)	About 120°	Rather more	Rather more	On to front of shin
Wrist (flexion)	About 100° (window)	Rather less	Rather less	Acute angle
Reflexes				
Sucking	Weak	Stronger	Strong	Strong
Rooting	Weak and slow	Stronger	Strong and quick	Strong and quick
Grasp				
a) response	Feeble	Slow	Easier to obtain	Brisk
b) reinforcement	None	Little or none	Incomplete	Good
Crossed extension				
a) flexion	Weak	Present	Present	Present
b) extension	Absent	Weak	Present	Present
c) adduction	Absent	Absent	Absent	Present
Moro	Weak	Feeble	Stronger	Strong
Pupillary	Absent	Present	Present	Present
Head turning	Absent	Present	Present	Present
Traction	Absent	Feeble	Feeble	Present
Glabellar tap	Absent	Present	Present	Present
Neck righting	Absent	Absent	Present	Present

TABLE 5 (a)

Some Other Neonatal Criteria Scored for Maturity
(Farr, Mitchell, Neligan and Parkin, 1966)

Body feature	Grade of maturity				
	0	1	2	3	4
Skin texture	Very thin, gelatinous feel	Thin smooth	Medium thick, smooth	Thickening stiff feel, cracking and peeling	Thick parchment-like, cracking
Skin colour	Dark red	Uniformly pink	Pale pink, variable	Pale, only extremities pink	—
Skin opacity	Numerous veins seen	Veins seen	A few large vessels clear	A few large vessels indistinct	No vessels seen
Oedema	Obvious	Not obvious tibial pitting	None	—	—
Lanugo	None	Abundant	Thinning	Area of baldness	Over half back bald

Skull hardness	Soft	Springy	Some hard, some springy	Hard but displaceable	Hard, not displaceable
Ear form	Flat, shapeless	Some incurving	More incurving	Incurving of all upper pinna	—
Ear firmness	Soft, easily folded	Soft, easily folded slowly returns	Cartilage palpable, springs back after folding	Firm, definite cartilage	—
Breast size	Nothing	Tissue palpable up to 0.5 cm	0.5–1.0 cm	> 1.0 cm	—
Nipple	Barely seen, no areola	Well defined + areola	Well defined + areola raised	—	—
Plantar skin	No creases	Faint creases	Creases indent < 1/3 sole	Creases indent > 1/3 sole	Definite deep creases
Genitalia	No testis in scrotum; labia maj widely separated, labia min large	One testis in scrotum; labia maj almost cover labia min	One testis at least well down; labia maj cover labia min completely	—	—

Table 5 lists various characteristics at four-week intervals between the ages of 28 and 40 weeks. Table 5 (a) (Farr, Mitchell, Neligan and Parkin, 1966) lists other characteristics each of which is given a score of 0—4 according to maturity. The higher the scores for each individual item and for all items together the greater the maturity of the infant (Farr, Kerridge, and Mitchell, 1966). A total score of 10 or less usually indicates a gestational age of 32 weeks or less; a score of 21 or over usually indicates a gestational age of 38 weeks or more; and scores between 11 and 20 usually indicate gestational ages of 32—38 weeks.

The finding of abnormalities alerts the paediatrician to the need for continued observation and, possibly, treatment, and to the risk of persisting disability. Despair is never justified at this stage because even the neonate with the most markedly abnormal examination may make surprisingly good progress. The observations of Dargassies (1971) are interesting in this connection. She followed up 130 babies who had very abnormal findings on neonatal examination and found that at 2 years of age 82 were still abnormal but the other 48 appeared to be normal.

The abbreviated and modified neurodevelopmental examinations which have to be used by most clinicians do not detect all abnormalities, and indeed it is probable that, however detailed and painstaking are the examinations, not all abnormalities could be detected in this way. To quote Dargassies again, out of a group of 150 babies with normal neonatal examinations, 2 showed abnormalities at 2 years of age. Nor does the usual clinical examination detect the minor changes which Prechtl and his colleagues (Prechtl, 1965; Beintema and Prechtl, 1968) were able to find with their painstaking technique.

Prechtl and his colleagues found variations from normal which fell into three groups—the apathetic, hemi-syndrome, and hyperexcitable groups—and in these groups there was a higher incidence of neurological abnormalities at 2—4 years to which subsequent problems such as restlessness, epilepsy and learning disorders were thought to be related.

The neonates in the apathetic group spent long periods in state 3, and showed marked depression of motility, resistance to passive movements, and intensity of reflex responses. The hyperexcitable group of neonates showed a tremor when making gross movements. The tremor was of low frequency (6 beats per second) and high amplitude (3 cm). The neonates also showed increased tendon reflexes and a low threshold of excitability of the Moro reflex. Neonates showing the hemi-syndrome had three or more persisting asymmetries. The frequency and significance of these syndromes according to Prechtl and his colleagues are shown in Tables 6 and 7. Although it is desirable to identify children with such problems as early as possible in order to

TABLE 6

Frequency of Apathetic, Hyperexcitability and Hemi-Syndromes in Neonates

Pre-& Perinatal conditions	Number and percentage showing syndrome		
	Apathetic	Hyperexcitability	Hemi
252 babies with obstetric complications	31 (12.5%)	101 (40.1%)	49 (19.4%)
116 babies with uneventful history	4 (3.4%)	16 (13.8%)	0 (0%)

TABLE 7

The Frequency of Neurological Abnormalities at 2–4 Years in Relation to
Presence of Prechtl Syndromes in Neonatal Period

Neonatal state and numbers of babies	Number and percentage with neurological abnormalities at 2–4 years
150 with syndromes	110 (73%)
102 without syndromes	14 (14%)

begin remedial work, the general feeling at present appears to be that
it is seldom possible to translate Prechtl's technique from the research
laboratory to the clinical field, and also that harm may result from too
early labelling of children.

REVIEW OF DEVELOPMENT IN THE FIRST YEAR (Table 8)

The changes occurring in the 12 months after birth are so well known
that their magnitude and remarkable nature are frequently overlooked.
The weight trebles, the length doubles, and the head circumference
increases by a third. There are also great changes in behaviour and
abilities. From being a predominantly flexed and dependent individual,
the infant acquires the ability to alter his position and to move about;
he actively and increasingly seeks to learn about his near surroundings
with all his senses; and he selects and modifies his responses by choice
and according to circumstances.

TABLE 8

Summary of Development in the First Year

Age (months)	Gross Motor	Vision and Manipulation
1	Gradual development of head control. Movements coarse and jerky.	Begins to fixate on nearby familiar objects. Watches mother's face.
2	Dominance of primary reflexes on posture and movements.	Following with eyes. Visually takes 'hold' of objects.
3	Head lag, when pulled from supine to sitting, disappearing.	Holds objects placed in hands momentarily.
4	In prone head and chest raised. Later, support taken on forearms.	Visually associated reaching develops.
5	Feet to mouth, plays with toes.	Recognizes everyday objects, e.g. cup.
	Rolls front to back, and usually later back to front.	Watches hands.
6	Held upright takes weight on legs.	Mature visual following and convergence. Eyes used together, no squint.
7	In sitting head steady and back straight.	Transfers objects, e.g. cubes, hand to hand.
8	Reciprocates with legs. Protective support reflexes of limbs appearing.	Looks for dropped objects.
9	Stable in sitting position. Sideways and forward support with arms.	Moves cover in order to see object. Index finger use appearing.
10	Attempts to move—creep, crawl, squirm, shuffle. Pulls to stand.	Visually very alert. Pincer grip for small objects.
11	Plays standing holding on. Cruises around furniture.	Glances around, makes quick visual appraisals. Beginning to look at pictures and may point with index finger.
12	May take first steps.	

TABLE 8 (contd)

Hearing and Vocalization	Social
Cries when hungry or uncomfortable. Freezes or quietens to sounds.	Sleeps and feeds. Evokes much affection and accepts this passively.
Response to sounds varies, e.g. dislikes loud harsh sounds, may excite to familiar sounds.	Quiets in response to cooing and rocking. Regards nearby face. Smiles in response. Reacts to familiar pleasant situations, e.g. feeding, bathing.
Cry pattern more mature. Vocalizes in response to overtures.	Likes handling. Feeding now a social activity.
Turns to sounds. Wider range of vocalization. Chuckles.	Spontaneously responsive and smiling.
Beginning to imitate rhythms of sounds.	
Practises vocalization.	Beginning to be aware of strangers and to modify responsiveness.
Babbles, uses voice purposefully. Vocal imitation.	Responds to adults; plays imitative games.
Mature localization of sounds.	Reacts to encouragement and discouragement.
Beginning to understand words and single simple commands. Beginning to vocalize recognizable words.	Shows affections. Plays pat-a-cake; waves bye-bye.

Stabilization of the head on the shoulders occurs early and is especially noticeable because of the considerable benefits it brings to the child, such as greater ease in feeding and opportunities to use the eyes and ears from a steady position of the head. Such activities in turn stimulate further head control and movement.

Progress in the supine position is towards sitting, which is a useful position once the head is steady. Support is necessary at first when the back is rounded and the legs drawn up. Gradually a straighter back is acquired, the legs extend and come closer together to reduce the area of the sitting base, and the arms are used for support. Some infants spend many happy hours sitting on the floor playing with toys around them. Some pull to standing from this position and some will roll over to a crawl position. An occasional infant will shuffle in this position.

Development during the year in the prone position leads to the *creep* (abdomen flat to ground) and *crawl* (abdomen raised) positions from which the infant may move about actively and effectively. Reciprocal crawling can be very fast and enables the infant to explore his surroundings, but it has the disadvantage that the useful hands are engaged, and in order to use them for play and exploration the infant will often sit back. Left to his own devices, the infant would not spontaneously get to the upright position until nearly the end of this first year when he could pull himself up to standing, but he is held in the upright position long before this. At about 6 months infants held upright enjoy feeling their feet and for several moments will tense their leg muscles and make their legs into strong supporting pillars before relaxing and flexing them. This leads to stabilization of pelvis and trunk upon the legs which is an essential precursor of normal gait. Further opportunities to improve pelvic stability occur towards the end of the year as the child is side-stepping whilst holding on, the so called *cruising* action.

As the infant becomes increasingly aware of sensory stimuli he learns to locate their source and acquires greater understanding of what they convey. This knowledge is further enhanced by his increasing manipulative skills. All these abilities are utilized to help him to come to terms with his surroundings.

6 Weeks Old

At 6 weeks of age a baby is still a 'babe in arms,' and when carried requires adequate support for the head. The general flexed posture still predominates, and limb movements are still gross and purposeless. The fists may be open from time to time. From his usual comfortable, well-wrapped position the 6-week-old explores the world around him with his eyes. His most characteristic response is a steady fixation of gaze upon his mother's face and a spontaneous smile in response to her overtures. He responds to sounds by either quieting or stilling or by a startle response, according to their intensity.

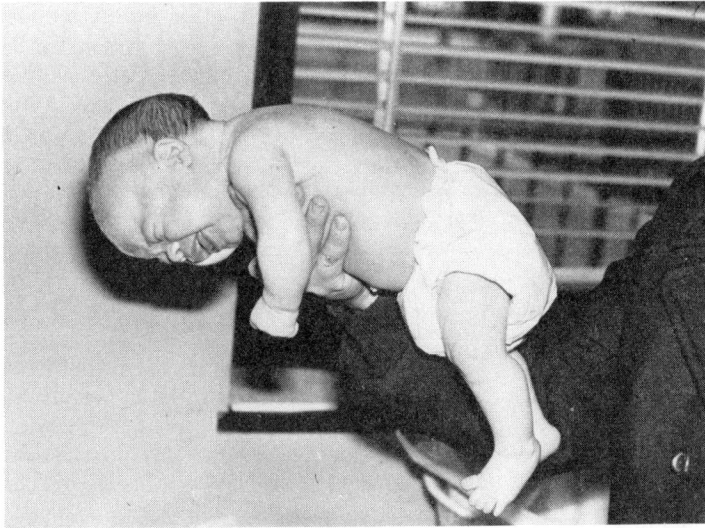

(a)

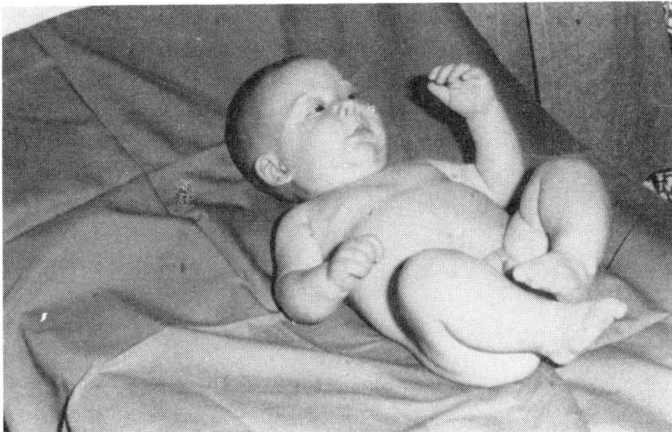

(b)

Figure 32. 6 weeks old: (a) ventral suspension (compare Figure 29 (b)); (b) posture in supine

When he is laid prone the pelvis may still be high, but the legs are now extended backwards. The head may be raised momentarily. When supine the limbs, especially the arms, may assume an asymmetrical tonic neck reflex posture with the arm on the face side being extended and the other arm flexed. Headlag is present when he is raised to sitting from supine, but is much less marked than in the earlier neonatal period. In a supported sitting position the back is smoothly rounded and the head raised momentarily. When held in ventral suspension the arms and legs are flexed and do not hang down limply, as they did a few weeks earlier, and the head is raised to the same plane as the trunk. When held upright no appreciable degree of weight-bearing occurs. It is now less easy to elicit a stepping reflex.

Some vocalization may be heard during observation and examination. This may consist of some rather gutteral grunts of contentment or lusty cries of distress or hunger.

3 Months Old

Although still very much a baby, considerable control over posture and muscle activity has been acquired in the intervening weeks. Head control is usually good and the mother gives support at the shoulders when lifting the baby rather than behind the head. Visual and auditory interest have increased and the eyes move around to look at nearby objects even if the head is not turned.

When supine the flexed posture is less marked and the limb movements are smoother and more controlled than previously. The hands are loosely open most of the time. Most babies at this age will anticipate being lifted to sitting either by a pleasurable social response, or by tensing the neck muscles and raising the head, or in both these ways. As the baby is raised to sitting the head should be firm on the shoulders most of the time with little head lag, if any at all. When held sitting the back is straight and the head is bobbingly erect. When prone the pelvis is quite flat and the head and chest are raised for short periods as weight is taken usually on the forearms. In ventral suspension limb flexion is now only slight. The head is raised to look forwards.

Visual alertness is considerable. The baby may stare fixedly at nearby objects as if he were 'taking hold of them with his eyes'. He turns his eyes and head to follow moving objects. He also shows awareness of and interest in sounds, and his own vocalizations are becoming interesting coos and gurgles. He begins to recognize familiar people and situations and to react pleasurably at the sight of his mother, bottle or bath.

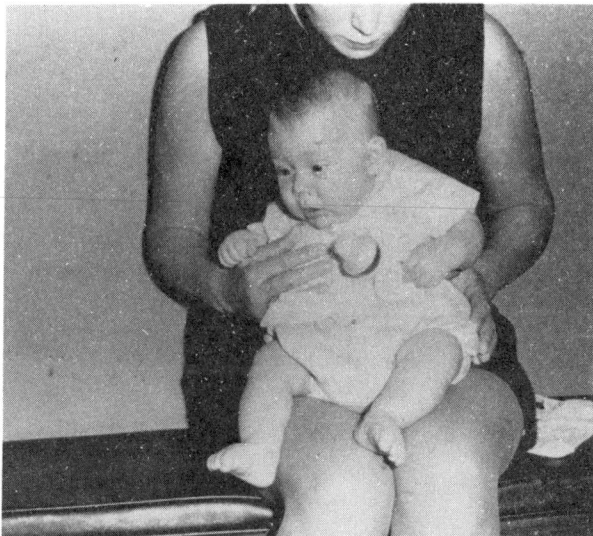

(a)

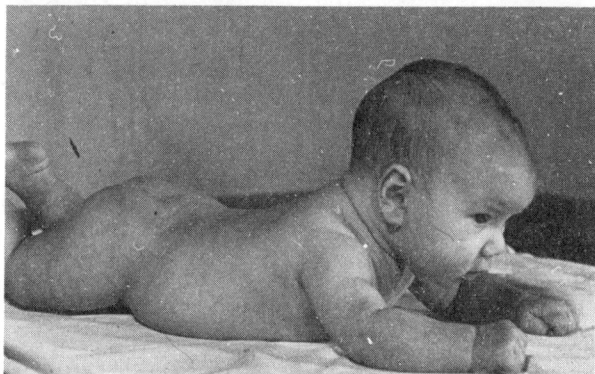

(b)

Figure 33. 3 months old: (a) supported sitting on mother's knee. Visual interest. Holds rattle placed in hand momentarily; (b) posture prone

6 Months Old

By 6 months of age considerable muscle control has been acquired and an infant of this age is able to take up several different postures. He has acquired some awareness of and familiarity with his immediate environment and is preparing for the development of mobility.

He is seen no longer as a baby in arms, but as a definite individual sitting up in his cot or high chair, or on his mother's lap. He enjoys the supported sitting and standing postures where he can use his hands, and strives to get out of the supine and prone positions.

When supine he raises his head from the pillow, and with relatively little assistance raises himself to sitting with a straight back and steady

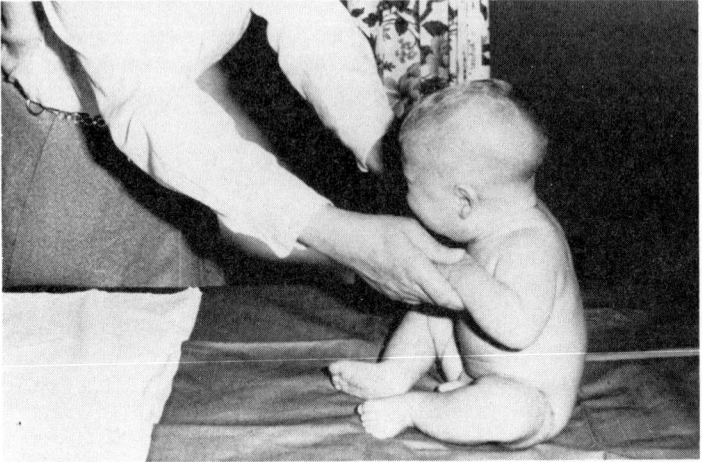

(a)

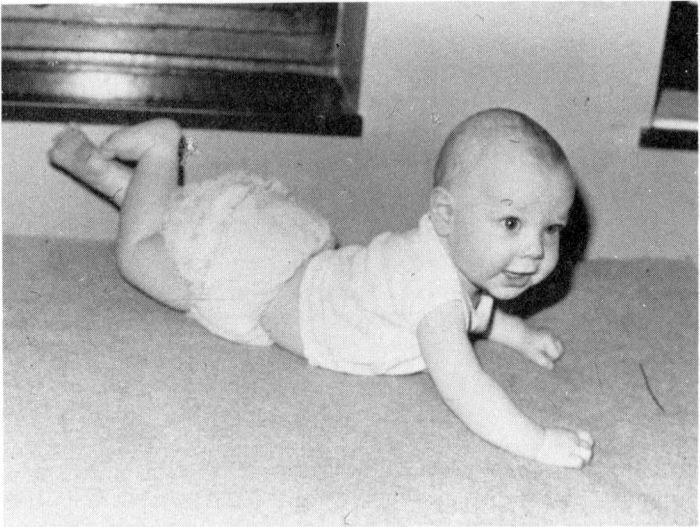

(b)

Figure 34. 6 months old: (a) posture sitting; (b) prone development

head. He may sit alone for a brief moment, and can certainly be sat in a high chair. When prone he raises himself on his extended arms and may show various manoeuvres to move from this position such as 'swimming' (with back arched and arms and legs raised), 'pivoting' (rotating around on abdomen) and 'scooting' (dragging himself forward with his hands). When he is held upright his legs extend and adduct slightly (parachute reaction); then as the feet contact a firm surface he contracts his leg muscles, turning his legs into strong supporting pillars as he supports most of his body weight. He enjoys this, and bouncing up and down in this position is often a great delight especially at bath time. He holds his arms out to be lifted up. He reaches out spontaneously and accurately with either hand, taking objects with a palmar grasp and bringing them to the midline and transferring them from hand to hand.

Conjugate movement of the eyes and binocular fixation are now established so squint is not normally seen after this age. Visually he is busy identifying objects and learning to distinguish them from the immediate environment. He is interested in sounds, appears able to distinguish familiar from strange noises, and turns towards sounds. His own vocalizations show a wide range of sounds and a tuneful sequence effect called babbling. He is just beginning to show a little coyness with strangers.

9 Months Old

One of the most distinctive changes which occur about this age is social responsiveness. Before 9 months infants are happy little 'buddhas' who sit contentedly on the floor for periods of ten minutes or more and give a spontaneous benign response to all who approach. After 9 months infants show growing awareness of strangers and their responses are controlled and reserved for those who are familiar to them. The appearance of a stranger with an unusual voice or pair of spectacles can easily precipitate a bout of crying. This is just one aspect of a rapidly blossoming social awareness and responsiveness. He enjoys personal attention which he will seek by attracting attention using vocalization or pulling clothes, and will reinforce it by participating in games of imitation, such as hand clapping, peekaboo, and vocal play. He tries to help when being fed. He is aware of the emotional content of speech, especially pleasurable approving sounds and regulatory 'No's'.

The 9-month-old infant is more aware of the world around him because he has a concept of the permanence of objects and will look for toys which drop from his hands or the tray of his high chair, and will resist attempts to take a toy away from him. Manipulation is now much more skilful. His fingers are active. The index is used to prod and poke, he picks up small objects (e.g. string, Smarties) in a pincer grip between thumb and index. He uses his increased manipulative skill to satisfy his exploratory interest in searching for objects inside other containers. This exploratory activity is helped by his increased motor ability. He is very stable in independent sitting and may even attempt to shuffle around in this position. He readily changes from sitting to prone from where he moves about by rolling and squirming and may even creep and crawl.* He will usually stand holding on when placed in that position and may well attempt to pull up to standing. Control in lowering is not well developed and it is always amusing to watch infants of this age drop back on to their well padded rears. Coincidental with this increased motor activity is the appearance of protective responses which increase the infant's safety. When he falls (or is made to fall) forwards or sideways the arms or arm reflexively extends in a protective response.

Awareness of the surrounding world now extends beyond his mother's lap for several feet. He is aware of sounds in this extended environment and localizes them immediately and accurately. He visually searches the

* The terms 'creep' and 'crawl' are sometimes used differently in American and British literature. In Britain 'creep' refers to quadrupedal progression in prone with the abdomen flat, whereas in 'crawl' the abdomen is raised.

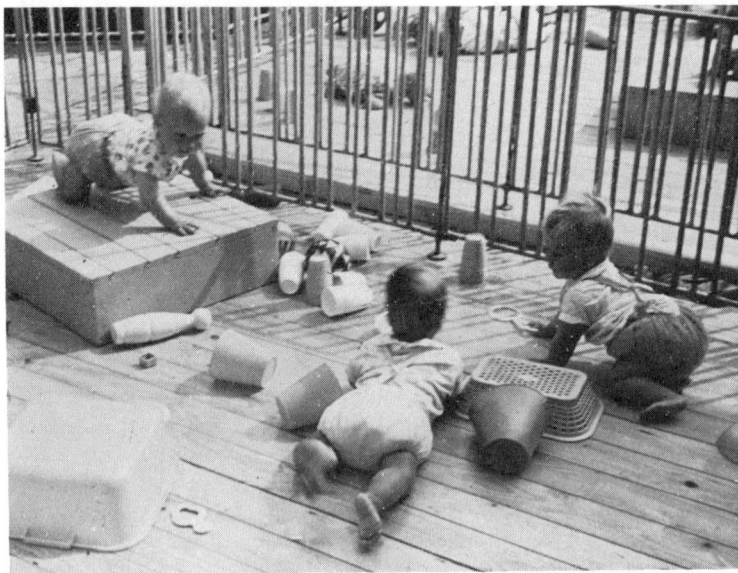

(a)

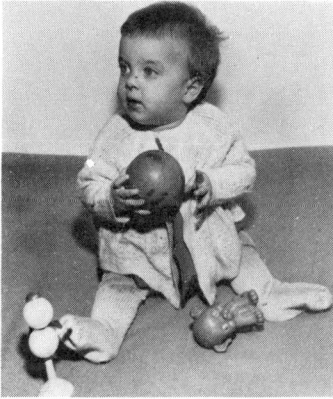

(b1)

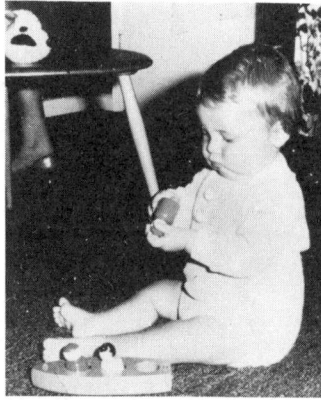

(b2)

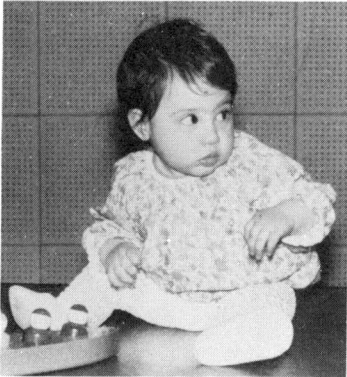

(b3)

Figure 35. 9 months old: (a) prone posture at 3, 6 and 9 months; (b) sitting posture showing (1) visual interest, (2) manipulative play and (3) awareness of strangers; (c) looking for dropped object

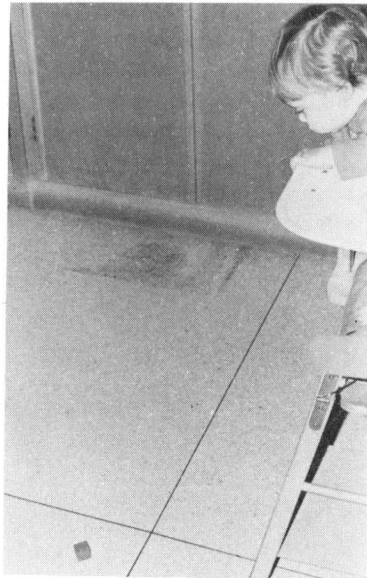

(c)

area and visually directs and controls his motor actions with considerable maturity.

12 Months Old

The first birthday marks the end of a year of intensive progress which has brought the child to the stage of readiness for big advances in

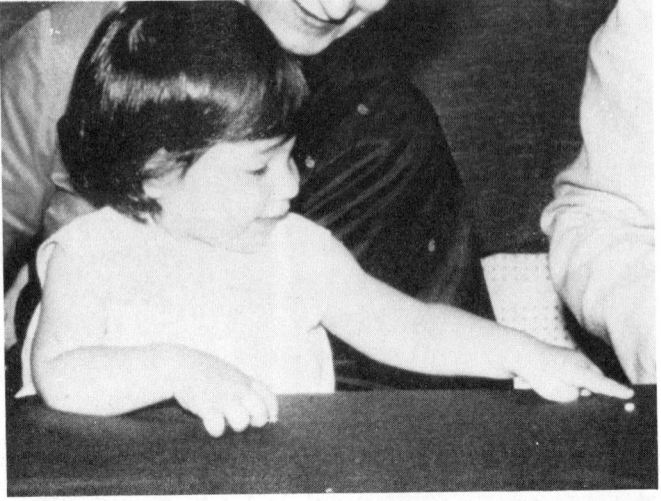

(a)

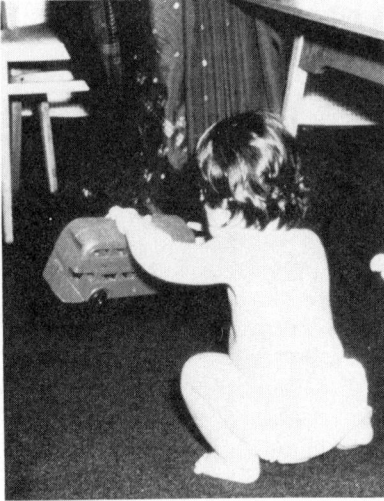

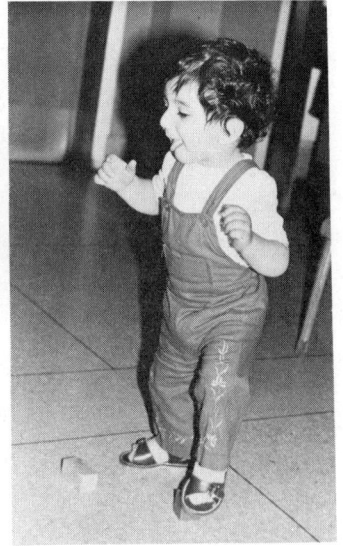

(b)   *(c)*

Figure 36. 12 months old: (a) index approach well established; (b) squatting in play; (c) early steps. Note posture of hands; (d) use of hands at 6, 9, 12 and 15 months, exploring, comparing, giving, building

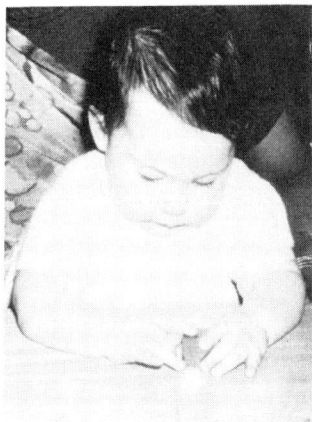

(d)

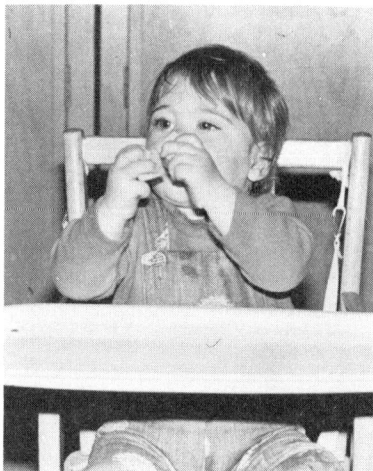

(d)

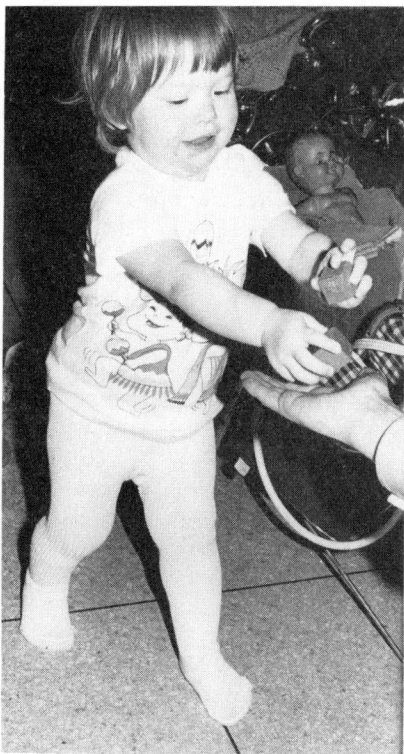

(d)

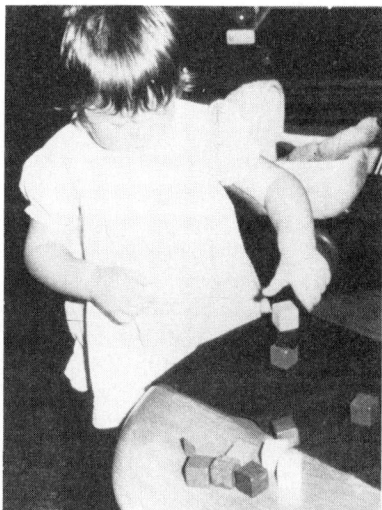

(d)

mobility and motor skills, language development, and exploration and domination of the world around.

One-year-olds like to be on their feet. Some will take a few steps with support, often with just one hand held, and a few are already walking independently. Pulling to stand and lowering down again, and cruising, are usually evident skills. Supine lying is now usually reserved for sleep because an active infant in a supine position soon rises to sitting, or rolls to prone and hence to crawling.

Manipulative skills are now performed much more easily than at 9 months. The index finger is used for poking and pointing, objects are picked up between the thumb and fingers, and the thumb index pincer grip is neat and precise. Manipulative exploration and play occupy much of the daily activity. Simple objects such as blocks may be taken into each hand simultaneously and inspected, compared and knocked together. He shows great interest in playing give and take, searching for hidden objects, and pat-a-cake. He may recognize objects and will even attempt to use them for their correct purpose, for example trying to feed himself with a spoon, to brush his hair, and to co-operate in dressing.

Visual exploration is well developed and manifest both with nearby objects and more distant surroundings. Auditory discrimination is developing, so enhancing interest in speech. His verbal understanding is exhibited by his behaviour in response to a few familiar words (e.g. daddy, dinner, walk). Learning is a very important part of his activities and clues to his ability in this respect come from seeing what use he makes of his newly acquired skills.

Significance of Changes in the First Year

The developmental changes occurring in the first year are highly significant because they are so very considerable; because they establish a firm basis for many skills and activities; and they also prepare the individual for a wholly independent existence.

The great magnitude of the changes is obvious. With respect to motor function the infant has gone from being a totally dependent neonate to literally standing on his own feet at one year of age. Visual and auditory stimuli, which initially produced only reflex responses, have been found by the infant to convey much information from which he has learnt to recognize and to identify the features of his environment. Objects and people become meaningful and tangible. The striking observation of an 8-month-old infant looking for a dropped cube illustrates the beginning of his sense of permanence of objects and of continuity in his environment.

Whereas the neonate is at the mercy of his environment and has to depend upon his reflexes for preservation, an infant who has begun to recognize his environment begins to react to it and to control it. Thus, with inanimate objects he attempts to use them appropriately, and with people he begins to interact, communicate and modify his responses according to the situation.

The acquisition of each new perceptual skill and the performance of each new motor action during this very busy 12-month period appears to follow a characteristic pattern. Each new task at first calls forth intense concentration while other activities are inhibited or ignored. For example, early visual awareness is characterized by prolonged visual fixation with suppression of motor activity and response to sounds; and early tactile exploration is such an intense activity that the infant shows little interest in other activities. After this initial stage the infant learns to deal with each particular task with less and less effort. During this period infants show increasing ability to switch from the task in hand to other tasks and then return to the original one. Ultimately, a stage is reached when the task requires little effort and can be performed quickly. For example, the visual preoccupation of the initial period is ultimately superseded by a quick visual glance; and turning towards a sound each time it is repeated does not occur in this later stage because the infant has analysed and identified the first sound stimulus and further interest is lost. At this stage other new tasks can now be given intense attention, and attempts can be made to link tasks together. Thus an infant becomes able to listen whilst playing with toys. This linking of skills which appears towards the end of the first year develops considerably in the following years.

The physical separation of a baby from his mother occurs at birth—a brief and dramatic event. The neonate is still dependent, however, and the purpose of development during the first year is to prepare the infant for independence. This is achieved by the development of mobility and the emergence of his individual personality. At one year of age the infant is ready for the second major step forward—his emancipation from his mother towards his own independence. The succeeding years are spent in building up this independence.

Variation and Signs of Abnormality in First Year

All too often it is suggested that paediatricians need to be familiar with the characteristics of normal development only in order to be able to detect serious abnormalities. This is important, but it is only one of his tasks. He is often required to examine infants in order to

confirm that all is well and to give advice about their future development; he is required to be familiar with and to evaluate the significance
of variations in the usual pattern of development which may be normal
but which nevertheless cause considerable worry to parents, and he
must advise about the management of these cases so as to relieve worry
and avoid more serious distortions later on; finally he is required to be
alert to those variations of development which indicate definite and
serious disorder.

Knowledge of the features and pattern of development enable the
paediatrician to perform these tasks. Development follows a similar
pattern in most infants. Variations do occur, however, in both the
pattern and its rate of evolution.

Not all individuals do things at precisely the same time and in
exactly the same way. There are therefore natural biological variations.
Variations also occur according to the experiences and opportunities of
the child. The descriptions in the preceeding pages referred to the
normal healthy mature infant, but allowances must be made for both
unhealthy and immature infants. In the case of premature babies a
useful working rule is to deduct a period equal to the length of time
short of full gestation when making developmental calculations. Thus,
a 6-month-old baby born 8 weeks prematurely will be expected to show
the developmental features of a 4-month-old baby.

DEVELOPMENTAL DIAGNOSIS

Developmental diagnosis is based upon six features:-

  (a)   delay in developmental pattern;
  (b)   distortion of developmental pattern;
  (c)   quantitative changes;
  (d)   qualitative changes;
  (e)   application of abilities;
  (f)   other signs.

Delay in Developmental Pattern

So much happens so quickly during the first year that the characteristic
developmental picture changes every few weeks. Consequently delayed
development should be detected fairly easily. Consider the situation of
a baby whose development is 25 per cent behind normal expectations.
This is equivalent to a week behind at 1 month, six weeks at 6 months,

and three months at a year. It is not easy to be certain about a week's delay at 1 month of age although suspicions may be raised if the baby seems to be unusually limp and to make insufficient attempts to raise his head. By 6 months there should be little difficulty because the infant will behave more like a 'typical' 4½-month-old. Thus, full head control will have been acquired only recently and the head may still be insecure when the trunk is shaken; voluntary reaching will be just developing and transfer will not be seen; when held upright there will be little support from the legs; and chewing actions will not be seen.

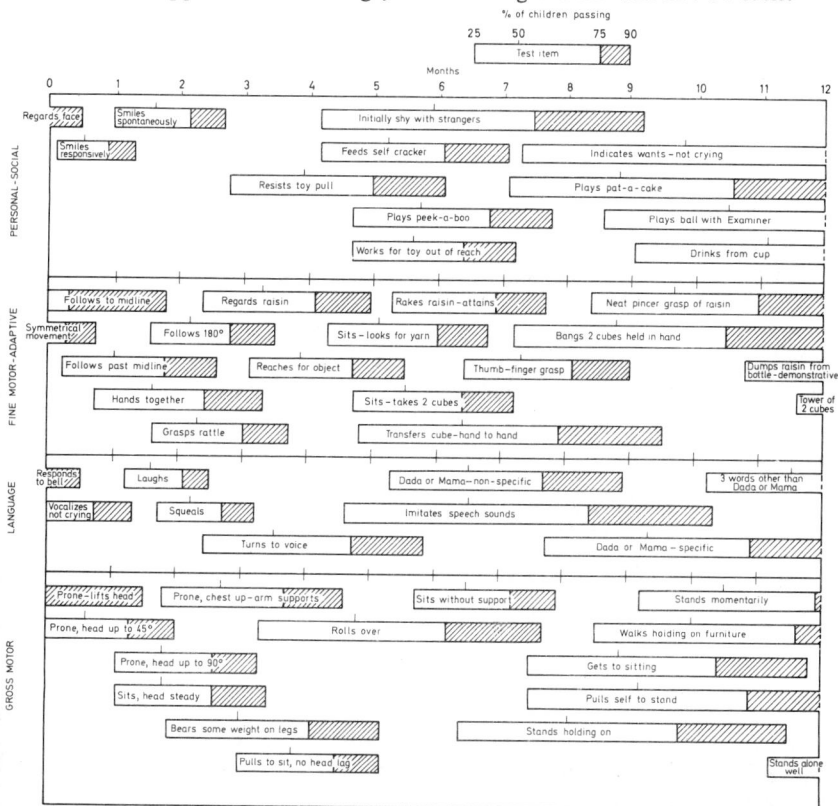

% of children passing

| 25 | 50 | 75 | 90 |

Test item

Months

PERSONAL-SOCIAL
- Regards face
- Smiles spontaneously
- Smiles responsively
- Initially shy with strangers
- Feeds self cracker
- Indicates wants – not crying
- Resists toy pull
- Plays pat-a-cake
- Plays peek-a-boo
- Plays ball with Examiner
- Works for toy out of reach
- Drinks from cup

FINE MOTOR-ADAPTIVE
- Follows to midline
- Regards raisin
- Rakes raisin – attains
- Neat pincer grasp of raisin
- Symmetrical movements
- Follows 180°
- Sits – looks for yarn
- Bangs 2 cubes held in hand
- Follows past midline
- Reaches for object
- Thumb–finger grasp
- Dumps raisin from bottle – demonstrative
- Hands together
- Sits – takes 2 cubes
- Tower of 2 cubes
- Grasps rattle
- Transfers cube – hand to hand

LANGUAGE
- Responds to bell
- Laughs
- Dada or Mama – non-specific
- 3 words other than Dada or Mama
- Vocalizes not crying
- Squeals
- Imitates speech sounds
- Turns to voice
- Dada or Mama – specific

GROSS MOTOR
- Prone – lifts head
- Prone, chest up – arm supports
- Sits without support
- Stands momentarily
- Prone, head up to 45°
- Rolls over
- Walks holding on furniture
- Prone, head up to 90°
- Gets to sitting
- Sits, head steady
- Pulls self to stand
- Bears some weight on legs
- Stands holding on
- Pulls to sit, no head lag
- Stands alone well

Figure 37. Denver Developmental Scale (Cardiff modification)

An infant of one year showing a 25 per cent delay of development will show actions considered to be typical of a 9-month-old.

The greater the delay in development, the more serious it is. Lesser degrees of delay may not even be abnormal, but represent normal variations. It must always be remembered that the various developmental features do not appear at precisely the same age in all children; in some they occur earlier and in other cases later than the average age. This is shown well in the Denver Developmental Scale which was designed for use by paediatricians and ancillary child health personnel. It shows the age range of many developmental features in the first year (Frankenberg and Dodds, 1968). *Figure 37* shows a slightly modified D.D.S. based upon its use with children in and around Cardiff (Bryant, Davies and Newcombe, 1974). On this basis any developmental feature which appears outside the normal range should be considered to be abnormal until proved otherwise. The decision is less easy with infants whose developmental performance appears to be slow but is still within the normal range. In these cases the correct answer is usually found after examination of some of the other components of developmental diagnosis, as discussed below, or by continued observation.

Distortion of Developmental Pattern

Everyone who studies child development soon becomes aware of the smooth integration which normally exists between the various features, and when this pattern is distorted they suspect the presence of some abnormality. The greater the distortion from the usual developmental pattern shown by the majority of infants the more likely is it that a serious abnormality is present. Nevertheless variations are frequently seen which are not due to any abnormality and they should not be labelled and treated as if they were. Developmental paediatricians need to be aware of these normal variations in order to protect infants from wrongful diagnoses and to be able to give sound developmental guidance to parents.

Quite considerable variations occur in behaviour. Mothers soon recognize that their baby has a characteristic personality. If their baby is very different from others, for example, if he is exceptionally irritable, they will need to be reassured that he is perfectly well and normal, assuming that examinations show this to be so, and they will need guidance about his rearing.

Interesting variations occur with respect to infants' responses to visual and auditory stimuli; whereas most infants learn to respond to both types of stimuli some infants develop an intense fascination for one or the other. This is usually a temporary phase; but it may last several months, and during this time the infants' behaviour is influenced by his particular sensory preference.

The greatest normal variations in the first year are seen in motor activity. Rearing patterns influence the infants' motor performance in the early months. It is possible to distinguish babies who spend most of their time in the prone position from those who spend most of their time supine by their behaviour during developmental examinations (Holt, 1960). Babies who are placed prone for most of the time from birth onwards behave more confidently in the prone position and appear to be advanced for their age. They soon begin to 'scoot',—an activity in which they push or pull themselves with their hands and so begin to move about in the prone position, and later they often favour crawling for mobility and use this for quite a long time. In contrast their performance in the supine position and when pulled to sitting appears to be immature, inept, and delayed when compared with the performance of babies who spend most of their time in a supine position. These early posturally induced variations of motor performance do not appear to have a lasting effect upon other aspects of development.

Robson (1970, 1975) has made some particularly interesting studies of early motor development. He describes normal variations in which prolonged crawling and bottom shuffling are the principal means of mobility. He considers that familial influences are important in these cases because a history of similar variant patterns is obtained from other members of the family. These variations do affect later development. Independent walking, for example, occurs later than usual. He suggests that late onset of walking should not be considered to be abnormal for particular patterns of early motor development (Table 19).

Quantitative Changes

Observing the quantitative aspects of behaviour is useful. Does the infant spend too little time on tasks? This might be abnormal. Does the infant spend a lot of time on any particular task? This might be acceptable and normal if the particular activity was acquired recently and is appropriate for his age. Too much interest upon one activity at the expense of other activities is as worrying as too little interest in anything. For example, hand regard is commonly seen at about 5 months of age. Much of this activity might be considered useful if it lasted only a week or two because during that time it could indicate reinforcement of eye-hand co-ordination. Its persistence for a long period and its presence at a later age would however alert one to the possibility of abnormality for why otherwise should this action be long continued and not replaced by something more constructive?

Qualitative Changes

Doctors should be familiar with the quality of the normal performance of infants and should always observe this aspect. For example, excessive separation and extension of the fingers as the infant grasps may be a clue to neurological disorder. Useful clues may come also from observing the quality of visual function—a prolonged regard usually indicates the recent acquisition of a new visual awareness, a quick glance which appears to provide useful information to the infant usually represents a fairly advanced level of development, and gaze avoidance is an early sign of emotional disorder.

Application of Abilities

Doctors should observe what use the infant makes of every stimulus he perceives and every action he performs. Suspicion is immediately raised in the case of any infant who fails to make use of his opportunities. If an infant can reach out to take hold of objects, does he do so? and what does he do when he has got the objects? If an infant can roll does he indulge in this activity randomly or does he use this motor skill to get from place to place, or to reach his toys? Constructive use of activities is an encouraging feature.

Other Signs

A developmental paediatrician's great asset is his ability to use information from his general examination in the interpretation of his developmental observations. For example, in the case of an infant showing minor developmental variations he will view these more seriously if he also finds in his general examination abnormal variations of muscle strength and tone, and of the tendon reflexes.

Developmental diagnosis in the first year of life can be very rewarding, but in many cases observations need to be continued in later years. The developmental characteristics of the toddler and pre-school periods are described in the next chapter.

REFERENCES

Apgar, V. (1953). A proposal for a new method of evaluation of the newborn infant, *Curr. Res. Anesth. Analg.* **32,** 260

Amiel-Tison. C. (1968). Neurological examination of the maturity of newborn infants. *Archs Dis. Childh.* **43,** 89

Barlow, T. G. (1962). Early diagnosis and treatment of congenital dislocation of the hip, *J. Bone Jt Surg.* **44B,** 292

Beintema, D. J., and Prechtl, H. (1968). A neurological study of newborn infants, *Clinics Dev. Med. 28.* London: Heinemann

Braselton, T. B. (1973). Neonatal behaviour assessment scale, *Clinics Dev. Med. 50.* London: Heinemann

Brett, E. M. (1965). The estimation of foetal maturity by the neurological examination of the neonate. *Clinics Dev. Med. 19,* 105, London: Heinemann

Bryant, G. M., Davies, K. J., and Newcombe, R. G. (1974). The Denver Developmental Screening Test: Achievement of test items in the first year of life by Denver and Cardiff infants, *Devl Med. Child Neurol.* **16,** 475

Dargassies, S. Saint-Anne. (1954). Methode d'examen neurologique du nouveau-ńe, *Etud neo-natal.* **3,** 101

– (1971). Value of assessing clinical neuropathology at birth, *Proc. R. Soc. Med.* **64,** 468

Drage, J. S., and Berendes, H. (1966). Apgar scores and outcome of the newborn, *Pediat Clins N. Am.* **13,** 625

Dubowitz, V., and Goldberg, C. (1970). Clinical assessment of gestational age in the newborn infant. *J. Pediat.* **77,** 1

Farr, V., Mitchell, R. G., Neligan, G. A., and Parkin, J. M. (1966). The definition of some external characteristics used in the assessment of gestational age in the newborn infant, *Devl. Med. Child Neurol.* **8,** 507

– Kerridge, D. F., and Mitchell R. G. (1966). The value of some external characteristics in the assessment of gestational age at birth. *Devl. Med. Child Neurol.* **8,** 657

Frankenberg, W. K., and Dodds, J. B. (1968). *The Denver Developmental Screening Test Manual.* University of Colorado Press

Holt, K. S. (1960). Early motor development: posturally induced variations, *J. Pediat.* **57,** 571

– (1963). In *The Development of the Infant and Young Child Normal and Abnormal,* Illingworth, R. S. 2nd edn. p. 251. Edinburgh: Livingstone

– (1965). Age, growth and maturity of the neonate, *Clinics Dev. Med.* **19,** 100. London: Heinemann

Paine, R. S. (1961). Neurological examination of infants and children, *Pediat. Clinics N. Amer.* **7,** 471

Prechtl, H. F. R. (1965). Prognostic value of neurological signs in the newborn infant, *Proc. R. Soc. Med.* **58,** 3

–and Beintema, D. (1968). The neurological examination of the full term newborn infant, *Clinics Dev. Med. 12.* London: Heinemann

Robinson, R. J. (1966). Assessment of gestational age by neurological examination, *Archs Dis. Childh.,* **41,** 437

Robson, P. (1970). Shuffling, hitching, scooting or sliding: some observations in 30 otherwise normal children. *Devl. Med. Child Neurol.* **12,** 608

– (1975). Personal communication

Smith, D. W. (1970) *Recognisable Patterns of Human Malformation.* Philadelphia: Saunders

Thomas, A., Chesni, Y., and Dargassies, S. Saint-Anne. (1960). The neurological examination of the infant, *Little Club Clinics 1.* London: Heinemann

CHAPTER 4

Observable Development: Pattern, Range and Variations—1 to 5 Years

During the four years from the first to their fifth birthday children rapidly develop many motor and language skills and use them to explore and to control their environment. There are so many new things to discover, and so much to do that there is never a dull moment—life is activity or sleep. These activities enable them to wean themselves from their close maternal attachment. Although all is 'child's play', adults have an important role during these years. The early development of self-awareness and self-importance finds expression in control of the limited everyday world they comprehend. Wider exploration of their surroundings, and growing awareness of others helps them through this stage towards a willingness and desire for co-operative play with others. These transitions require many adjustments which are often accompanied by varied reactions. Much of this period may be spent in rebellion which is expressed against a background of dependence, but these problems are usually resolved as they approach 5 years of age.

The years from 1 to 5 are eventful in other respects. The children's environment expands and moves from the confines of the home to include the playgroup and nursery school. More siblings may appear in the family. Other children, both older and younger, and both from within the family and without bring many interests to the developing children.

Table 9 summarizes the main features of development during this period.

18 Months Old

The 18-month-olds should be walking. Many have been doing so for a few months and are now effective toddlers, seldom falling, able to bend

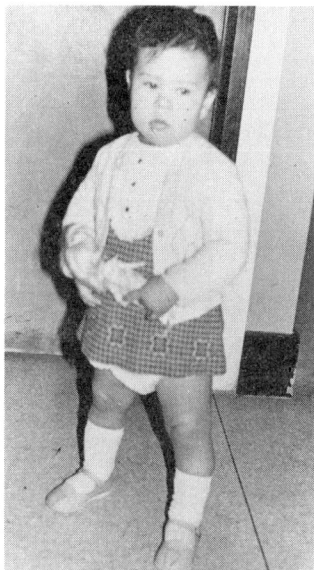

(a)

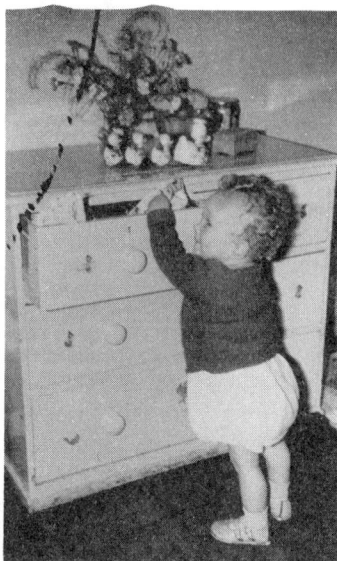

(b)

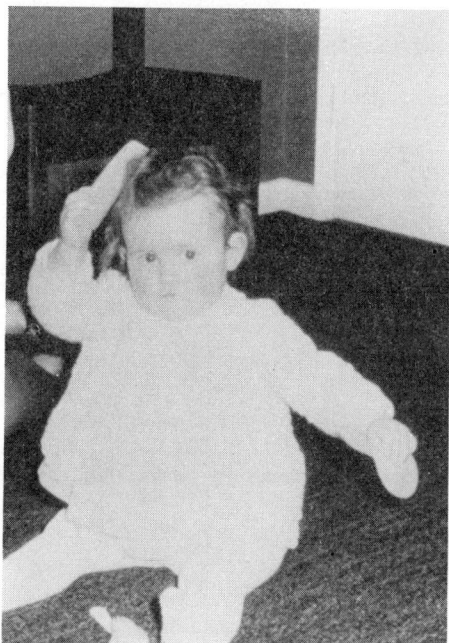

(c)

Figure 38. 18 months old:
(a) toddling with toy
which is still just an object;
(b) exploration of shelves
and drawers made pos-
sible by acquisition of
mobility; (c) demonstra-
tion of appreciation of
purpose of object by use
should be well established
by 18 months

TABLE 9

Summary of Developmental Progress, 1 to 5 years

Age	Motor	Vision and Manipulatic
12–18 months	Independent walking develops. Likes to push and pull wheeled toys. Often squats when playing. Climbs on to chairs. Goes up stairs usually with hand held and may attempt coming down, sometimes by bumping down on bottom.	Enjoys picture book points with finger. Mu practice of eye-hand c ordination. Sees sm objects and picks them with thumb and ind finger. Does not yet turn bo pages individually.
18–24 months	Earlier motor skills more proficient. Beginning to attempt kicking and throwing ball. Shows better judgement of size and position of objects, e.g. chairs.	Likes to scribble w pencil, imitates vertical stroke. Turns book pag singly.
2–3 years	Very mobile, using this ability for exploration. Likes nursery climbing frame and large boxes to climb into and out of. Rides tricycle. Much more nimble. Walks sideways and backwards.	Responds to Stycar sin letter vision tests and go visual acuity is demons able. More mature hold crayon. Copies circ Beginning to thread be and use scissors.
3–4 years	Now skilful in motor activities. Modifies speed and negotiates skilfully. Likes to try new skills, e.g. standing tiptoe, hopping.	Beginning to make recognizable two- dim sional line drawings, e house, man.
4–5 years	Walks on straight line. Stands on one leg. Hops and skips with alternating feet. Responds to rhythm and music and movement group activities enjoyed.	Hand skills developing rapidly. Colours pictu Much neater and quicl

TABLE 9 (contd)

~aring and Language	*Social*
pid development of vocabulary)ecially of concrete nouns and ~bs of action. Likes jingles. derstands single simple mmands.	Becoming independent in feeding. Aware of and disapproves of wetness. Plays alone, but needs adult nearby. Vulnerable in unsuitable environment.
ginning to join words. holalia often normally sent, rries out verbal requests.	Responds to adult guidance and control. Not yet co-operative with peers although may play alongside them. Domestic mimicry.
nguage well developed. May be pressed so quickly that elligibility is reduced es language for questioning d to direct actions. Repeats d sings nursery rhymes.	Clings to mother. Often has favourite toy or rag. May rebel over feeding. Beginning to help with undressing and dressing. Will help with tidying away.
vious verbal skills and ivities increased. es to hear and to relate long ries.	Imaginitive play in which everyday activities are imitated and children take adult roles. Tolerance of short separation and waiting developing. Beginning to share. Understanding good and bad.
ent speech free of infantile terns.	More confident and independent. May like to be 'king of the castle'. Likes small groups but group identity not strong. Play influenced by sex of child and culture.

in order to pick up an object from the floor, to modify the speed of walking, and often carrying some plaything as they move about. They play with the large push and pull toys which they are often given at this age. They will explore and play with almost anything, but seem particularly to enjoy everyday household objects with which they demonstrate their understanding of purpose by imitating domestic activities.

Awareness of different parts of the body is just developing and they show this by pointing to their shoes and taking off their hats and socks.

At 18 months manipulative skills are developing rapidly as shown by their successful use of a spoon in feeding, which they do without tipping it over and spilling. They are also able to build cubes into a small tower of 2 or 3, and given a crayon they will scribble on paper.

Their language is developing and most will have a few words which they use correctly, and which are usually the names of everyday objects. They enjoy pointing out familiar items in pictures. Their vocalizations, however, are seldom limited to just a few words. Long babbled conversations—jargon—are heard frequently, and singing may be attempted. Simple games of 'peekaboo' and 'give and take' are enjoyed and may lead to peals of laughter. They carry out simple single instructions, e.g. 'Bring Mummy's handbag'.

2 Years Old

Two-year-olds are extremely energetic. They are able to walk and run, to stop and start with ease, to avoid colliding with objects, and to squat to play with an object and to rise again. They climb on to furniture, crawl upstairs, seat themselves at table, and go wherever they can contrive to get to. Doors and drawers may not be barriers. They are just beginning to attempt to throw and to kick. They still tend to misjudge sizes and distances, for example, they may try to sit in a doll's chair, or walk into a ball when trying to kick it. But these mistakes are being corrected. Considerable variations are seen between children depending to some extent on their experiences.

Language has developed a lot in the preceding 6 months. They now understand many words and will use 50 or more different words, many of which are articulated clearly. They will put 2 or 3 words together. They ask for things by name. Jargon is disappearing, and *echolalia** is appearing. They like to listen to stories and to join in songs and nursery

*Echolalia: the automatic repetition of words or phrases, usually those recently heard. Normally echolalia occurs occasionally and never so frequently as to dominate expressive language.

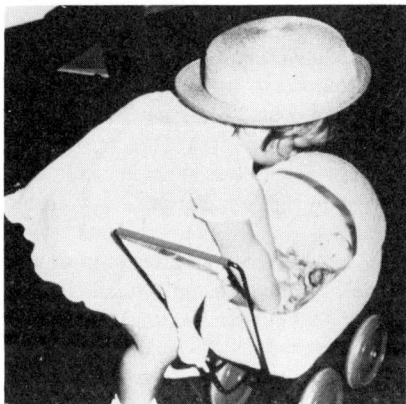

(a)

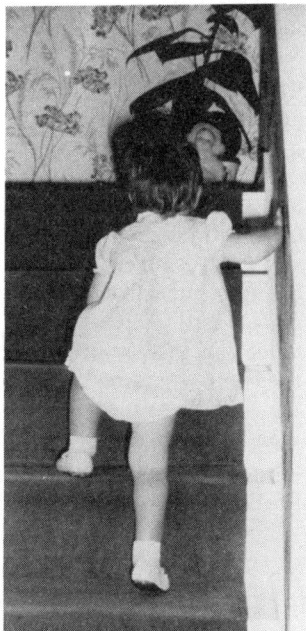

(b)

Figure 39. 2 years old: (a) early imaginative play; (b) beginning to use stairs; (c) pencil and paper: immature grasp, scribble

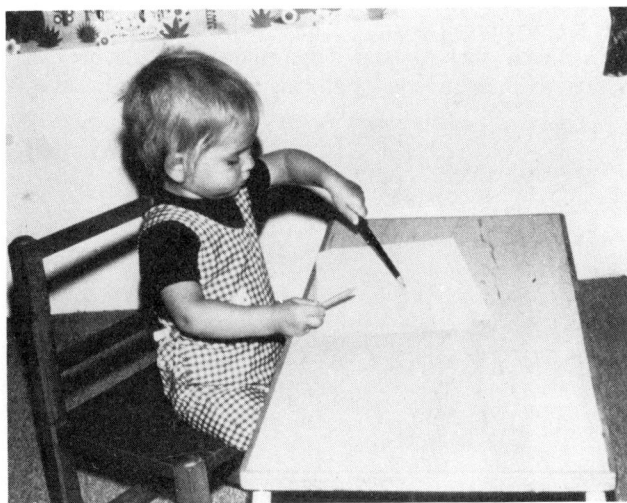

(c)

rhymes. They will hold a book and turn the pages one by one. They understand requests and enjoy doing little errands.

They have a strong sense of their own identity and possessions. They resist anything being done to them, e.g. medical examinations, and they safeguard their possessions and will often have a tantrum if a favourite one is taken away.

Many children of this age are feeding themselves and some are clean and dry, but others may still be having intense battles over one or other of these items.

In play, domestic mimicry is very evident; so is an interest in simple building and screwing tasks. They are beginning to understand that an object can be represented by its name (verbal labelling) and by a model, picture or drawing (symbolization). This new appreciation of the identity and representation of objects may result in their distress if they see them incomplete or broken and they will attempt to make them whole again. Preferred hand use is usually evident. They will hold a pencil like a rod and scribble on paper. They build up cubes and usually succeed in making a tower of six or seven before it falls.

3 Years Old

Children are not miniature adults, but anyone meeting a three-year-old child for the first time might be forgiven for thinking he was. The three-year-old is no longer a toddler. Boys play with tools, cars and engines, but girls are often seen talking to their dolls. It is interesting to speculate how much their greater opportunity for playing with dolls contributes to their superiority in language development as compared

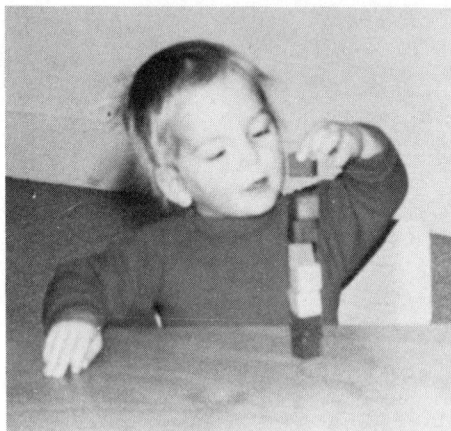

(a)

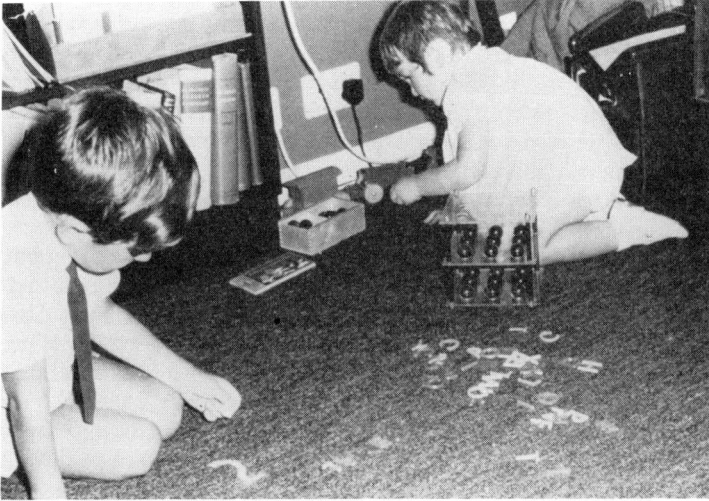

(b)

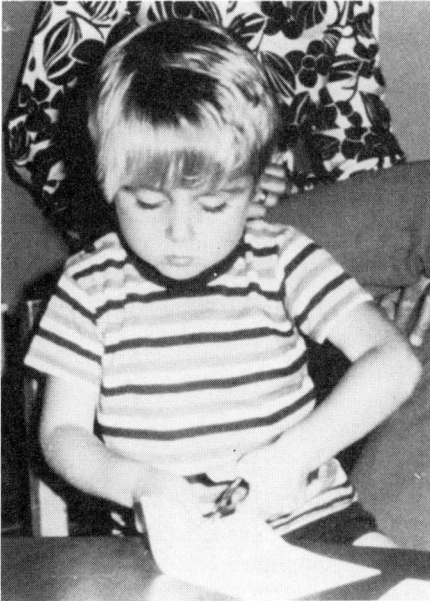

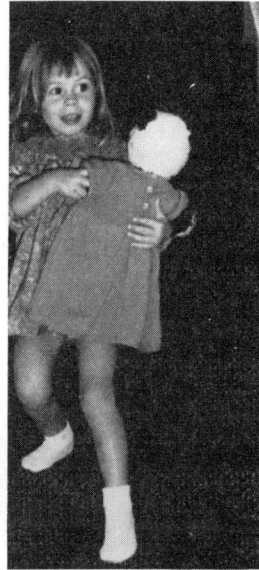

(c)   (d)

Figure 40. 3 years old: (a) greater proficiency with blocks; (b) parallel play—
alongside older brother; (c) play—cutting with scissors; (d) increasing skill on
stairs

with boys at this age. They hold conversations with both adults and their playthings. They identify themselves with adults, especially their mothers, with whom they are affectionate and confiding. Their engagement in domestic tasks is no longer simple imitation, but acting out their mothers' rôles. This rôle adoption is extended further and is shown in the vivid make-believe play which appears at this age and which they may share with playmates and siblings.

Very often observation of play reveals a child's expressive language development. Speech is well developed, is supported by an extensive vocabulary, and is fairly clear apart from some persisting infantile phonetic patterns. He tells his name and sex, asks questions, recites nursery rhymes, and converses about many things including absent objects and past experiences. Language is used to direct and to control play. So rich is language development at this stage and so valuable for play and intellectual development that it seems amazing that some children who do not develop speech and language until quite late do not suffer more general effects and frustration than they appear to do.

Counting, and a sense of quantity, are just beginning to appear, as is also an understanding of sharing and taking turns.

The three-year-old is independent with regard to some aspects of undressing, dressing and washing, but still needs some assistance and supervision.

He is nimble on his feet, and is fairly accurate in judging positions and sizes of openings. Motor skills are now well established and proficient. He negotiates steps, going up with alternating feet. but going down he may still put two feet on each step. He likes to jump, and can stand on one leg momentarily. He is now beginning to ride a tricycle and to throw and catch a ball, albeit very immaturely.

Manipulative skills include building a tower of 8 or 9 cubes; holding a pencil in a conventional way and copying a circle; cutting with scissors; threading beads.

4 Years Old

Four-year-old children walk and run skilfully, turning and negotiating objects at speed. Stairs no longer present problems; they go up them easily with alternating feet without needing support, and in most cases are as nimble going down. They climb whenever they get a chance. Many are now able to balance on one leg for a few seonds, and this leads to hopping. Those who have had the opportunity to practise may now be expert tricycle riders.

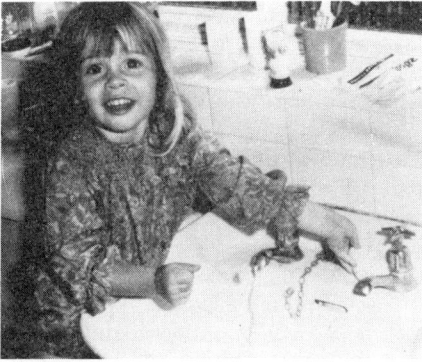

(a)

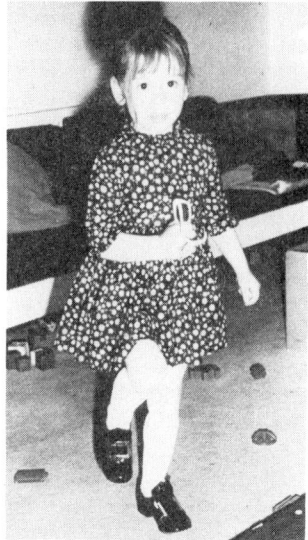

(b)

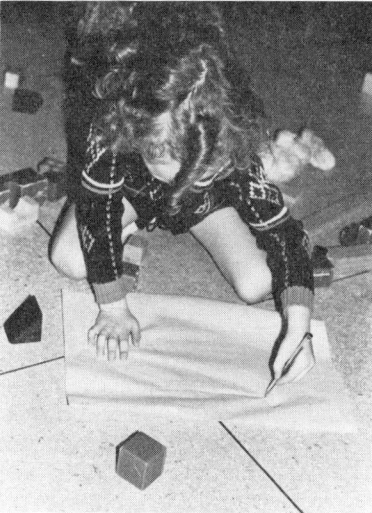

(c)

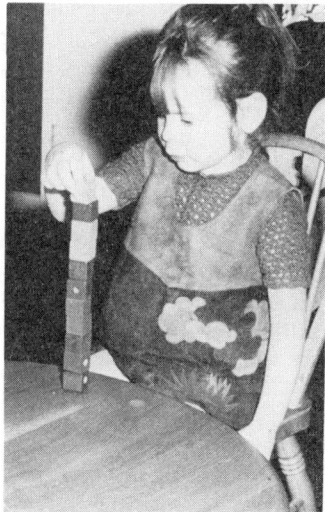

(d)

Figure 41. 4 years old: (a) increasing independence—washing; (b) standing on one leg; (c) drawing. Note mature grip of pencil; (d) steady hand to complete tower of 11 cubes

A four-year-old should be able to eat well with a spoon and to use a knife when required. Knowing the front and back of clothes, he should be able to undress and dress completely except for buttons, back fastenings and laces. He should wash and dry his face and hands and brush his teeth.

Four-year-olds are aware of their own toilet needs and most will attend to these themselves. Boys will stand to urinate in imitation of their fathers. Both boys and girls should be able to sit on a normal size toilet seat, but they may still need to be checked and helped with wiping themselves.

His grip upon a pencil is now almost at the mature dynamic tripod stage with the thumb and first two fingers flexibly controlling the pencil point as he copies a circle and a cross and attempts to draw a house and a man.

They can exhibit skill and understanding in numerous ways: with cubes, by building a bridge from a model, and a 3-cube pyramid; with pencil and paper, by copying a circle and a cross, and by folding a piece of paper twice or three times; with formboards, by completing them within a specified time; and with various objects by selecting them according to differences in size, weight, length and colour.

His speech is now free of most of the earlier infantile phonetic substitutions. He is constantly questioning, and also recounting his own experiences. He is apt to exaggerate and enjoys fantasy stories, incongruities and jokes.

In social activities he likes companionship both with other children and with adults. He has bouts of quarrelsomeness as well as close co-operation. He appears to have some feeling for others. Now that he has an understanding of time he looks forward to treats and trips.

5 Years Old

Almost all five-year-old children enjoy exhibiting their motor skills— hopping, skipping with alternate feet, dancing rhythmically to music, sliding, swinging, showing his big muscles, and playing ball games with sufficient ability to begin to join in group games. These characteristics are utilized at childrens' parties and ballet lessions.

Manipulative skills have advanced and are put to many uses. A 5-year-old will hold a pencil maturely and enjoy drawing and painting. He draws a recognizable person and house. The figures he draws have limbs and facial features, and his houses have doors and windows. He now copies a triangle and a square. Some five-year-olds are even able to write a few letters.

He should be almost, if not completely, independent in everyday skills such as dressing, washing and eating. He goes simple errands and will help his mother in the house.

In play he enjoys dressing up and make-believe. He shows understanding of the needs of others and plays companionably with other children. He picks his friends. He both understands something about rules and also finds them acceptable.

His language shows evidence of his understanding. His speech is fluent and grammatically correct. He asks the meaning of abstract

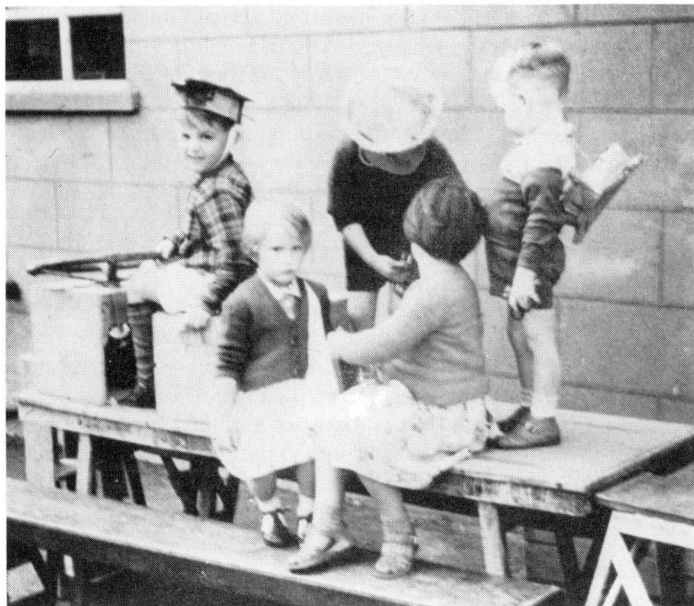

Figure 42. 5 years old. Pre-school group activities and make-believe play

words, distinguishes parts of the day, counts to 20, carries out complex commands which require 3 or 4 actions, names coins and colours, and appreciates similarities and differences.

Significance of Development 1 to 5 Years

These years witness a great increase in mobility and motor skills, the development of complex language, an acquisition of a fuller understanding of a much wider environment, and the establishment of independence of actions and personality. At the end of this period the child is one of a herd about to be schooled. He is able to join this herd as a result of his new found understanding, skills and independence.

The first independent steps of the one-year-old are the beginning of a rapid spurt of motor activity. Many new motor skills are acquired, including running, hopping, skipping, climbing, throwing, catching. With practice these are performed with greater and greater ease and precision. These skills enable the child to explore his environment which he does with great satisfaction. His environment widens and he feels himself to be the king of his domain. These activities open up possibilities for learning and opportunities for social play.

This is also the period in which children develop much understanding which is so distinctly human and so important for later intellectual development. They learn to understand the basic attributes of objects—their size, shape, weight, nature and colour. Add to this an ability to recognize similarities and differences between objects and they have the foundation for systems of classification and coding which contribute to later learning. Most important is the acquisition of the ability to understand that objects can be represented by models, drawings, and words. This whole process of symbolic representation and identification enhances the child's learning potential and means of communication.

The development of language during this period enables children to understand and to follow verbal messages and commands and also to formulate their ideas and wishes with verbal components, and also to express themselves in speech. They use expressive language to tell their experiences and wishes, and to control the activities of themselves and others. Language bears many resemblances to mobility in that its acquisition also widens their world, enhances social interaction, and provides them with a tool with which they can control their world.

Independence develops in many ways. The development of loco-motor and manipulative skills makes each child independent so far as choosing their own position and seeing to their own needs of washing, dressing and feeding, are concerned. Personal independence also requires emancipation from parents, an ability to make a voluntary choice of friends in the group with which he identifies himself, and these abilities are acquired in this period. The extensive development of these four years produces children who are ready to enter the wider world of school life. They are ready to take their first steps to be men and women of the world, but many years of training and development pass before this adult stage is reached.

Signs of Abnormality, 1 to 5 Years

These are years of very rapid development. Many new skills appear, and each day presents numerous opportunities (or should do) to practise these skills and to elaborate upon them. Lateness of develop-ment, clumsy, inept and bizarre performance of actions, and failure to utilize opportunities may all indicate abnormality. Parents seek help when their child is noticeably slower than his contemporaries, and especially if he is not walking or talking when other children are doing so. They may also seek help if their child's actions and behaviour seem to be different from other children, or from what they expect, and also if they find difficulty in understanding and relating to their child. All these worries must be taken seriously and appraised according to the history and circumstances and the results of examinations.

However, not all delayed and deviant development is due to serious abnormality. With such rapid advances occurring in many aspects of development considerable individual variations can be expected and do in fact occur. During this period, perhaps more than in any other, is seen the influence of environmental factors and opportunities upon the richness of development. Before deciding that any particular aspect of development is abnormal the possibility that it may be due to normal variations or to reduced or unused opportunities must be considered.

Developmental delay should be suspected in the following circum-stances.

(1)   The existence of measurable delay

A quantitative measure of developmental delay in this age range can be obtained from a variety of tests such as the Bayley, Gesell, Griffiths and Merrill—Palmer tests (Chapter 9). The Reynell Language Scales are particularly useful because they explore several aspects of language development, which is such a prominent and important feature of this period (Chapter 7).

(2)   The detection of changes in the quality of performance

Observation must be made of how a child performs a task as it often reveals abnormality. Uncertainty, clumsiness, tremor, posturing of the hands and poor eye-hand co-ordination may be noticed.

(3)   The persistence of earlier patterns of behaviour

Abnormality should be suspected when some earlier aspect of behaviour persists longer than should be the case. Some activities not only persist too long, but are exaggerated and dominate the child's behaviour.

Casting, for example, is normally seen at the beginning of the second year and does not normally persist more than a month or two. Casting is the name given to the activity in which the child delights in dropping his toys off the tray of his high chair or out of his pram. It is as if he were practising his newly acquired awareness of the continuity of objects in space and time as he throws them from one place to another. Normally, during the few months casting is present it can be used by an understanding mother as a game. Each time she picks up the toys she talks, laughs and tickles her baby. In this way the opportunities for reinforced interpersonal relationships which it provides are fully utilized. However, persistence of casting beyond 18 months, its exaggeration, and the failure of the child to develop more fruitful activities indicate probable abnormality. Similarly, a certain amount of echolalia is normally heard around 2 to 2½ years, but its persistence should make the doctor very suspicious of abnormality.

(4)   *The exhibition of extreme patterns of behaviour*

Very wide variations of behaviour with adults are seen during this period. A shy timid child may be just as normal as an uninhibited extrovert. Nevertheless, persistent marked extremes of behaviour, sudden change in the usual pattern of behaviour, and behaviour inappropriate to the circumstances may all indicate abnormality. The very withdrawn child should be easy to spot, but may be overlooked because he is no problem. The uninhibited socializer who goes to anyone yet fails to make any deep and lasting relationships may be seriously abnormal, despite the fact that his parents may think he is very bright. Gaze avoidance is particularly significant of probable abnormality.

Further Reading

It is possible only to summarize the main features of development during this very active period and further reading is essential for all who would learn about young children. There are many suitable publications. The following are mentioned as suitable starting points.

Brackbill, Y., and Thompson, G. G. (1967). *Behaviour in Infancy and Early Childhood* (a book of readings). New York: The Free Press
Isaacs, S. (1964). *Social Development in Young Children*. London: Routledge and Kegan Paul
— (1966). *Intellectual Growth in Young Children*. London: Routledge and Kegan Paul
Matterson, E. M. (1965). *Play with a Purpose for the Under 7's*. London: Pelican Books

Mussen, P. H., Conger, J. J., and Kagem, J. (1974). *Child Development and Personality*. 4th Edn. New York: Harper and Row
Newson, J. & E. (1970). *4 Years Old in an Urban Community*. London: Pelican Books

Observable Development: Pattern, Range and Variations–The Younger and Older School Child

THE YOUNGER SCHOOL CHILD: 6 TO 10 YEARS

These are years of steady progress. They are 'the benign years' because they come between the fervour of rapid development in the first five years and the turbulence of adolescence.

At the beginning of this period the child possesses many motor and language skills, and a considerable degree of independence both in self-care activities and sense of personal identity. He is ready for systematic training to perfect his skills and to use them to increase his knowledge and understanding. It is customary to arrange his training in similar age groups. Entry into this new world of peer groups within school and adjustment to the situation is a characteristic feature of the beginning of this period.

Physical growth proceeds at a steady rate during these years with almost identical increments of height and weight each year. Strength increases. Sex differences are present. The boys are bigger and stronger than the girls and on the whole succeed better in motor skills requiring strength. Girls tend to be lighter and more nimble.

Motor skills are developed for useful activities, for example, running, jumping, climbing, swimming, riding. Both unorganized frolics such as tree climbing, as well as organized games promote the steady evolution of motor abilities. So many activities can be developed that it is not always possible to have the time to become skilful in all of them. Even so some junior school children do remarkably well in this respect. A good foundation of motor skills in the early years is a help to them, and they are also urged on by the natural competitiveness of this period and a desire to gain approval from their peers. Personal interests and opportunities determine which skills are favoured and there is a strong culturally determined sex difference; for example, girls skip and knit and boys climb and do woodwork.

A great ability to absorb information both auditorially and visually develops in this period. No opportunity is lost by school teachers and sometimes parents to pour knowledge into the receptive youngsters. Evidence of these pressures may be seen sometimes in the children's performance and reactions. For example, it seems possible that the switching of the focus of attention in recent years from what the child says and how he speaks to his ability to read has led to a decline in problems of stuttering and to an increase in reading disabilities.

One of the most important developments in this period is an increase of conceptual ability. There is an increase in concept formation, the complexity of the conceptualization, and the ability to formulate hypotheses. These all arise from the language development of earlier years. To form concepts the child has to have the ability to categorize and to group his impressions. Then he is able to begin to understand their meaning, purpose and interrelationships. He develops concepts of quantity (mass), number, distance and spatial relationships; of values in money; and of more abstract ideas of good and bad and beautiful and ugly. He comes to have ideas about life and death, and of past, present and future. As with all emerging abilities he likes to practise his mastery of concepts whenever he can. He enjoys fantasies in which real and unreal situations merge; is fascinated by extremes such as the grotesquely huge and minutely small; and is intrigued by riddles which introduce possible misconceptions. His concepts of good and bad often create a fear of being bad and of being disapproved of by his parents, or by a more remote parent figure of God.

Conceptualization helps him to learn about and to understand his world and himself. To match this broader comprehension his world expands as he enters school and does much more outside the home. He achieves greater emancipation from adult support and direction, and develops identification with and reliance upon peer groups. This great change widens his experiences considerably.

Children who fail to gain acceptance by a peer group lose more than the widening of experiences which comes from such association. They carry their own thoughts and feelings, feel sad and lonely, and may brood.

At the end of this period the child has gained physical, intellectual, emotional and social strengths. His understanding of the world and his abilities make him a pleasant companion for adults, and even encourage moments of cheekiness. Carried to extremes these features

THE YOUNGER AND OLDER SCHOOL CHILD

TABLE 10

Overview of Development, 5 to 10 Years

Age (years)	Area of activity	Motor abilities	Manipulation
5	Home Infant school	Stands on one leg Hops Jumps off step	Draws with dynami tripod
6			
7	Junior school	Runs, climbs	Prints large irregula letters
8			
9	Increasing activity outdoors, parks, etc.	All skills per- formed more smoothly and efficiently; competitive games	Joined up, neat writing; bat and ba games

create the aggressive single-sex groups of this age. Puberty is not far off, however, when many changes will take place.

The overwhelming characteristic of this period appears to be a striving towards certain goals—physical, intellectual and emotional. Many things enhance, inhibit or distort these changes and in consequence great variations are seen between children of similar ages. Clear cut developmental levels are not as evident as in the earlier years. Any individual child should be judged by the relative strength of these developmental features. For example, peer-group identification develops during this age period. In any particular child this characteristic may, or may not be well marked, and may occur early or late during this period, but usually peer-group identification is shown only weakly by most 7-year-old children, and is much more evident with 9-year-olds. The following descriptions of 7-year-olds and 9-year-olds are compiled to illustrate the dynamic evolving nature of development during this period, with some abilities fading and others appearing for

TABLE 10 (contd.)

aily activities	Personal–Social	Language
oes simple rands	Parents and adults held in awe; active imagination, fears and fantasies, exaggerations, tells tales	Increasing ability to express thoughts and use language directively
anages own ily care, e.g. essing, going bed	Increasing link to peer group, but still needs adult support and direction	New concepts developing rapidly; greater understanding of size, shape, weight, distance, etc.
ay get self to nool	Ideals of right; God as punitive super-father	
	Needs acceptance by peers; resents social isolation	Ability to hypothesize and solve problems beyond the here and now
ginning to lp in house- ld tasks, e.g. shing up, aking tea; creasing iability when ing tasks	Tendency to brood; single-sex gangs	

the first time, and still others being present throughout in various strengths.

A summary of these features is shown in Table 10.

7 Years Old (*Figure 43*)

Seven-year-old children are typically active, happy and biddable. They find a lot to interest them and a lot to do. They still respond to each idea by doing it rather than by thinking about it, so they seem to be hustling about all the time. Play and chatter absorb them until they sag from fatigue, but a sound sleep restores them and they are off again. They eagerly respond to doing things for parents and teachers who are still regarded as all-perfect and all-powerful.

The years since 5 have provided the practice for them to become really independent in daily care activities. This is accompanied by greatly increased confidence and associated willingness to defend their rights by fighting. But some of their fights seem really to be no more than a sheer mutual enjoyment of the activity by the participants. They boost their own self esteem by derogatory comments about friends and may still run to tell tales to adults.

Most 7-year-olds should be able to read and to write to some extent; the pattern of reading will depend very much upon the type of training they have received. Those trained by the 'look and say' method will read whole words, but may be completely stumped by an unfamiliar word. Those taught by the older phonetic method usually read more slowly as they sound out the syllables, but have more success in sounding out unfamiliar words. Writing usually consists of printing in rather large and irregular letters.

Boys especially enjoy physical activity and racing, climbing and tumbling can develop spontaneously when there are a few together. Football and hand-ball games are played with more efficiency, but some organization by adults may still be necessary.

This is an age when imagination is active; sometimes they will exaggerate their impressions and ideas and quite frighten themselves. Fears of the dark and of frightening films and television can be troublesome.

Their confidence in adults which make them easy and biddable, may also lead to them copying and attaching themselves to older children. Unless one is careful this can lead them astray.

The 7-year-old is at a point of change, with the strength of parental attachments declining and those to the peer groups increasing. Having been with peers for two or so years he is confident in the situation and from now onwards he will increasingly identify with them and hate being different from them in dress, actions and thoughts.

9 Years Old

The nine-year-old child is growing up and is aware of it. Girls especially are aware that puberty is only a year or two ahead and with it the approach to womanhood. They are beginning to abandon some of their earlier activities as childish. They are less interested in fairy tales. They have a wider interest in everyday affairs and enjoy adventures beyond their everyday world, for example, trips to museums. An increasing cheekiness is noted sometimes backed up by reference to friends or 'the gang'.

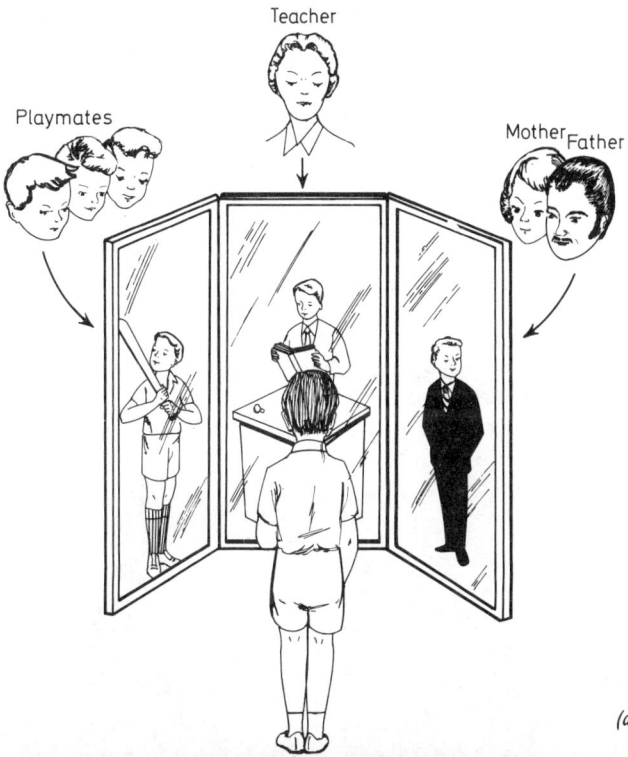

(a)

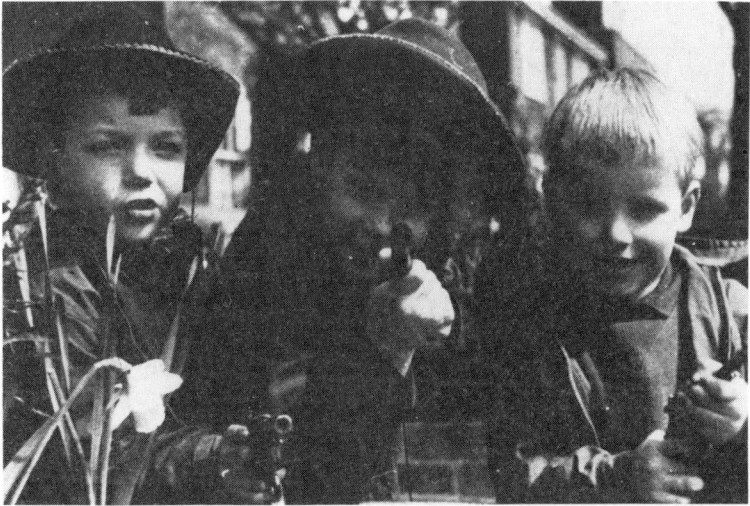

(b)

Figure 43. 7 years old: (a) development of self concept (Hurlock, 1956); (b) play

All motor skills are more assured and quicker than at 7 years. Interest in team games is increasing and is often fostered by interest in a local professional team. Manipulation is good, as shown by neat joined-up handwriting, and by such activities as the making of wood-work articles and the mending of others such as bicycles.

Group identification is very strong. Not only do boys gang to-gether; they positively discourage, deride and reject girls at this stage, and *vice versa*. Many children of this age are Cubs or Brownies and such activities fulfil their gang interests.

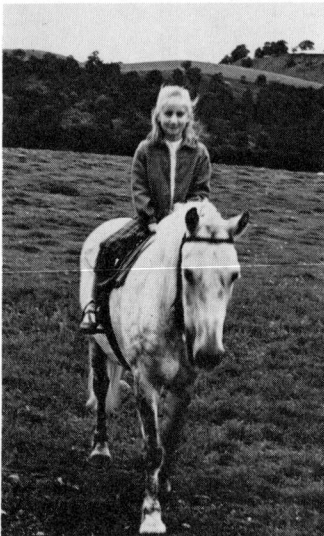 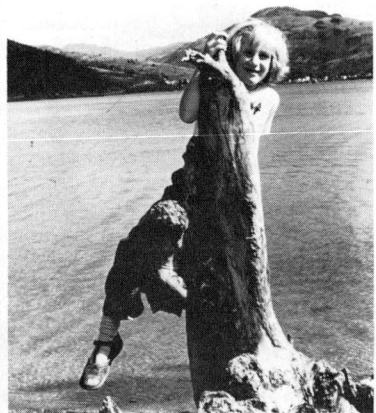

(a)   *(b)*

Figure 44. 9 years old: (a), (b) typical activities of the 9-year old

Intellectually the 9-year-old is able to deal with many subjects in school, but his powers of understanding abstract relationships are still fairly limited.

Socially, 9-year-old children are still too young to be wholly inde-pendent and so they are expected to join in family activities, but they may rebel on occasions. They are capable now of doing more to help and should be encouraged to lay the table, help wash up, clean the car and other suitable activities.

Significance of Development: 6 to 10 Years

This is a period of solid learning and steady progress. All skills are practised and are utilized both for learning and reaching independence.

Once the child has settled in school he shows increasing desire and ease in working in peer groups. This is ideal for training the developing minds and greatly facilitates the task of the school teacher.

Everyone recognizes that education does not consist just of pouring in facts, but includes stimulation of the child's interest and exploration and understanding. This is no easy task, and a good appreciation of conceptualization during this period is essential for all who desire to help children of this age. Quite often educational failure is found to be due to an omission or error in some basic concept formation at an earlier stage.

It is all too easy to see the educational aspects of development during these years and to ignore all else. The teacher is teaching and the child is learning. But the child is also learning in the playground and in his home as well as in school, and he is learning about more than is covered by the school curriculum. This helps to explain the ample evidence which exists to show that the more socially advantageous children make better progress than others.

During these years the child is learning to understand himself and his own emotions, and to manage his relationships with others, and this must be taken into account when evaluating any aspect of development and behaviour in this period.

Many abilities develop during this age period. Reading and writing are especially important because they are the basis of school work, and provide evidence of ability which is much sought for by parents. Reading and writing also open up channels of communication and expression for each child. In addition to these two basic abilities many motor skills emerge during this period which greatly increase the range of children's activities. It is pertinent, therefore, to consider all these abilities in more detail.

Writing

This skill requires that the child can steady the paper with one hand whilst holding the writing implement in an appropriate way with the other one. He must recognize the nature of the task and then reproduce the letter symbols on the paper. He has to learn the correct shape and orientation of the letters, how to make them of appropriate size and place them in a suitable position on the paper. At first the letters are poorly formed, of varying inappropriate sizes and arranged irregularly. All these gradually improve until an ability to produce mature, neat, legible joined-up writing emerges.

Writing is a means of expression, so that what is written is more important than how it is written. Nowadays encouragement of expression takes precedence over drilling in penmanship. Nevertheless, it is not possible completely to separate these two aspects. Some children experience considerable frustration because they cannot write as quickly as they think and in these cases helping them to achieve an easier, simpler and quicker technique of writing is of value.

With so many factors involved in the development of writing it is to be expected that wide variations will be encountered. The pattern of evolution of writing skills shown in Table 11 should, therefore, be used only as a general guide and in no way at all as a test.

TABLE 11

Evolution of Writing Skills (Hurlock, 1956, Jarman, 1973)

Age	Characteristics of writing	Example
Up to 5 years	Enjoys using pencil to make patterns. Prints large irregular capitals anywhere on the page. Copies printed words.	*Figure* 45(a)
5–6 years	Prints first name. Letters large and irregular and frequently reversed. Makes erratic attempts at short messages.	45(b)
6–7 years	Prints alphabet and numbers 1–20. Copies words. Letters usually capitals. Still large and irregular and sometimes reversed.	45(c)
7–8 years	Most children can now write and many are struggling to make smaller letters and to set out the writing more neatly. Errors still occur.	45(d)
8–9 years	Some children are beginning to join letters together. There is often variation in neatness and legibility. Girsl tend to be more capable than boys.	45(e)
9–11 years	Writing should be well established and evidence of a joined-up style should be emerging.	45(f)
11–14 years	Gradual emergence of a fast, legible style of handwriting.	

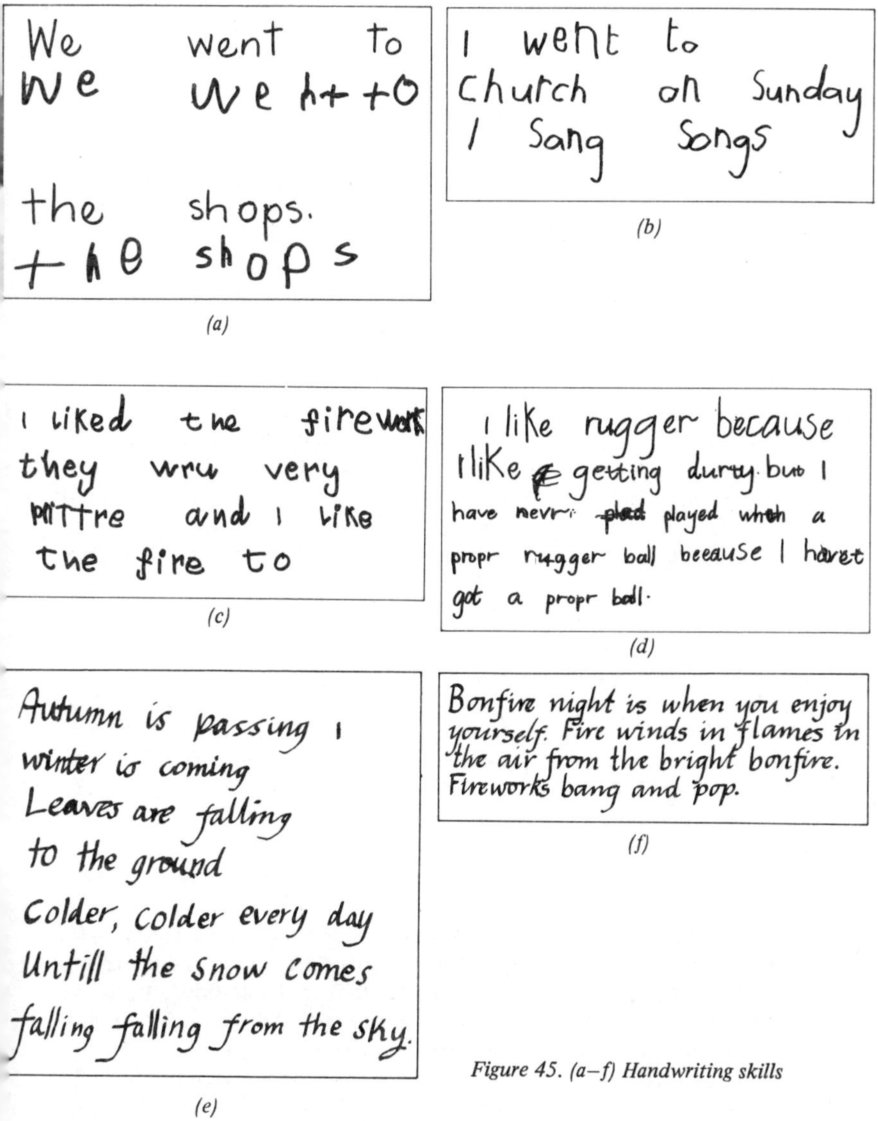

We went to
the shops.

(a)

I went to
church on Sunday
I sang songs

(b)

I liked the firework
they wru very
prttre and I like
the fire to

(c)

i like rugger because
I like getting durty but I
have nevr played played when a
propr rugger ball because I havet
got a propr ball.

(d)

Autumn is passing
winter is coming
Leaves are falling
to the ground
Colder, colder every day
Untill the snow comes
falling falling from the sky.

(e)

Bonfire night is when you enjoy
yourself. Fire winds in flames in
the air from the bright bonfire.
Fireworks bang and pop.

(f)

Figure 45. (a–f) Handwriting skills

Reading (Schonell and Goodacre, 1974)

Reading is another complex ability acquired during these school years. It requires the recognition of letters and words and the understanding of the meaning of groups of words in sentences. Evidence of ability to read and to understand written words and sentences is shown by the child responding to a written message. He might show such response by carrying out a request contained in the message, by laughing at the humour of the written sentences, or by answering the message. The ability to repeat the written sentence verbally as in reading aloud is an important attribute and is one of the tasks practised whilst learning to read. Nevertheless, it must be associated with comprehension, otherwise the so-called reading is nothing more than mechanical repetition. Unfortunately, emphasis upon learning to read in a narrow sense may produce this type of mechanical reading without comprehension, and this must be avoided.

Very many factors contribute to the development of reading ability so there are expectedly wide variations in children's abilities. The situation is affected also by the use of several different reading methods, and the opportunities and encouragement received by each child. It is difficult, therefore, to quote precise standards for reading.

There are three major phases which merge into each other. These are as follows:

    (a)   pre-reading phase—up to 6 years or thereabouts;

    (b)   reading practise—from about 6 to 9 years;

    (c)   use of reading—from about 9 years onwards.

In the pre-reading phase interest in stories and books is encouraged. Participation in word games both at home and in school promotes further interest in reading and encourages recognition of simple words. For example, the teacher talks about the day's weather and asks the child to identify the appropriate words as she mentions the sun and the rain.

Once the basic skills of reading are achieved considerable practice is required to enable reading to develop to the point at which it can be used by the child for his own purposes. A series of graded readers are used to provide this practice. The sentences are simple and short and there is much repetition of words and phrases. Large print, attractive illustrations, and other means are used to increase interest and simplify the task. As the child gets older these adjuvants are lessened.

The attainment of adequate proficiency in reading enables the child to use this ability for his own purposes—understanding written directions, communicating amongst his friends, learning all that is conveyed in the books, and also enjoying the stories. At this stage children are expected to use text books for classroom work, and some read for pleasure. A wide range of books are available for pleasure reading which can often be introduced to children through their interests and hobbies, for example, football, riding, and stamp collecting.

TABLE 12
Schonell Graded Word Reading Test

tree	little	milk	egg	book
school	sit	frog	playing	bun
flower	road	clock	train	light
picture	think	summer	people	something
dream	downstairs	biscuit	shepherd	thirsty
crowd	sandwich	beginning	postage	island
saucer	angel	ceiling	appeared	gnome
canary	attractive	imagine	nephew	gradually
smoulder	applaud	disposal	nourished	diseased
university	orchestra	knowledge	audience	situated
physics	campaign	choir	intercede	fascinate
forfeit	siege	recent	plausible	prophecy
colonel	soloist	systematic	slovenly	classification
genuine	institution	pivot	conscience	heroic
pneumonia	preliminary	antique	susceptible	enigma
oblivion	scintillate	satirical	sabre	beguile
terrestrial	belligerent	adamant	sepulchre	statistics
miscellaneous	procrastinate	tyrannical	evangelical	grotesque
ineradicable	judicature	preferential	homonym	fictitious
rescind	metamorphosis	somnambulist	bibliography	idiosyncrasy

118

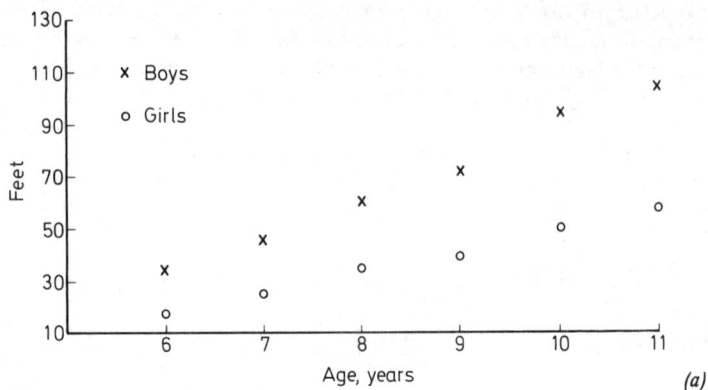

(a)

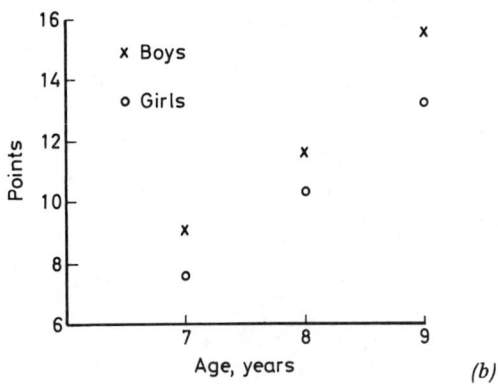

(b)

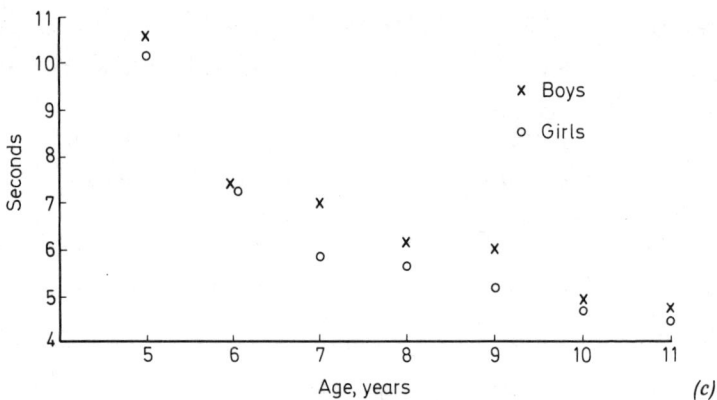

(c)

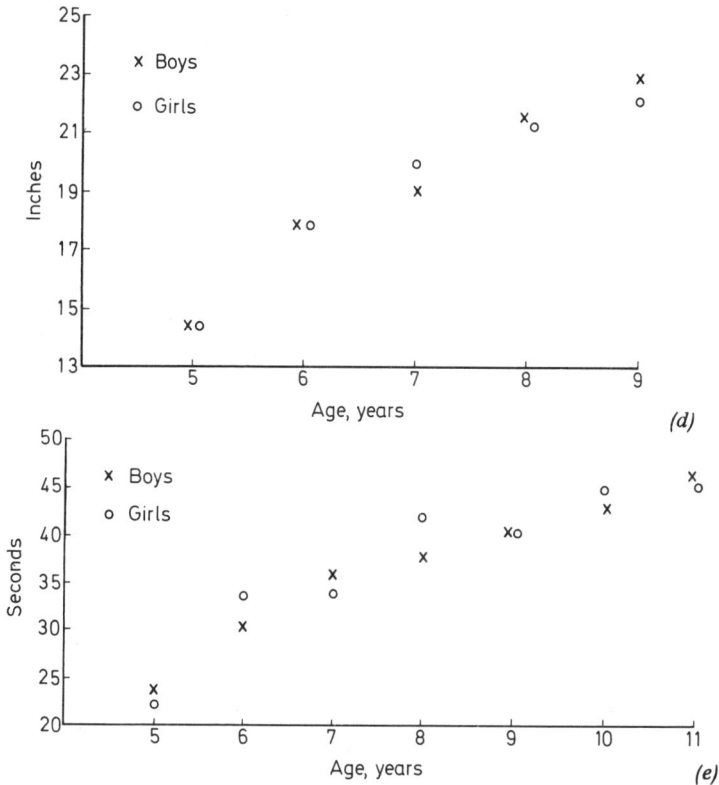

Figure 46. Some motor skills in school children (Keogh, 1965): (a) ball throw mean scores (age 6 to 11); (b) accuracy of throw mean scores (age 7 to 9); (c) 50-feet hop mean scores (age 5 to 11); (d) hurdle jump mean scores (age 5 to 9); (e) beam balance mean scores (age 5 to 11)

The evaluation of reading progress is a complex task which is best carried out by competent educationalists and psychologists. Children with reading problems are frequently referred to developmental paediatricians either to find out if there are any visual, neurological, developmental, emotional or other causes for the reading problem, or to decide the significance of associated phenomena such as clumsiness.

One of the most usual ways to test a child's reading ability consists of presenting a list of words of increasing complexity and finding how many he can read aloud (comprehension of the meaning of the word is not required in most such tests). Table 12 shows one of the most frequently used reading tests, the Schonell Graded Word reading test (McCulloch, 1965). This test has to be administered and scored in the prescribed way. As an approximation, however, each two lines of 10 words represent about one year's advance in reading ability between 6 and 15 years of age.

Motor skills

Between 6 and 10 years of age many motor skills develop and improve. Marked changes are seen as each year goes by. The strength, speed, accuracy and neatness of the various skills all improve and reflect the considerable amount of motor learning which takes place. *Figures 46 (a−e)* show the increasing proficiency of some motor skills during this age period (Keogh, 1965). The subject of motor skills is dealt with more fully in Chapter 6.

Signs of Abnormality: 6 to 10 Years

Signs of abnormality usually show themselves in one of three areas: in motor performance, as learning disabilities, or as behavioural disturbances.

Abnormalities of motor performance may be noticed by parents or teachers, and may consist of failure to acquire certain motor skills, or their performance in a clumsy or inept fashion. The range of variation in motor performance encountered normally is extremely wide; in consequence it is often difficult to determine the reason for a poor performance. Motor performance much inferior to that shown by most children of similar age may be still within the normal range, or it might be due to lack of opportunities to develop motor skills, or to general illness. These kinds of possibilities have to be considered before attributing poor performance to an organic lesion, especially a neurological lesion. The evaluation of the clumsy child is difficult and should always be done by an experienced clinician. Care must be taken, especially by psychologists and teachers, not to speak of brain damage and chronic brain dysfunction without having definite evidence to that effect from a specialist medical examination. The evaluation of poor motor performance rests upon a full medical examination, during which unsuspected abnormalities may come to light; upon finding definitely abnormal signs; and above all upon the *quality* of the motor performance and not just what is or is not achieved.

Learning disabilities are more likely to be noticed first by a teacher. In the case of any child who is failing to make educational progress three areas have to be explored, namely, the child, the content of the teaching, and the teacher and his or her teaching technique. Learning disabilities are far too large a subject to deal with here, but it is sufficient to state that all too often these difficulties are not fully investigated, but are dealt with in an *ad hoc* manner.

Behavioural disorders are extremely difficult to evaluate. Attempts have been made to quantify them, but these have not been very satisfactory. The essential point is that any particular behaviour must be seen in the light of the individual child, his past experiences and present circumstances. Two children may behave similarly; the behaviour may be in one case abnormal, yet in the other case the identical behavioural pattern may be normal. The following behavioural features may indicate abnormality and so call for further attention: extremes of behaviour; changes of behaviour; behaviour which is disturbing the child's activities and learning; and behaviour which is out of keeping with the child's background and circumstances.

THE OLDER SCHOOL CHILD: 11 TO 15 YEARS

This period of development is concerned with the transition from childhood to adulthood. Hormonal changes produce a considerable spurt in growth during which the rate of growth is often as great as that seen in the second and third years, and they also bring about the appearance of the secondary sexual characteristics. These physical changes of puberty, and a growing awareness of their significance, are associated with emotional changes and reactions which characterize adolescence and of which the most noticeable are an increased self-awareness and sexuality.

Motor activities become more organized during this period. There is a peak of interest in team games and competitive events. Personal participation becomes more selective and the choice strongly reflects the child's sex and personality.

Intellectually there is increasing development in complexity, especially of abstract thought and reasoning. Bright children revel in any intellectual challenge and will join in quiz games and intellectual puzzles. This is just as well because this is a period of intense educational activity in which those with academic prowess are distinguishable (and distinguished) from the others. All too often preoccupation with educational needs leads to neglect of all the other aspects of development at these ages. It is not surprising that the educational demands of this period are often associated with problems. At present insufficient attention is given to the medical aspects of these problems, but perhaps this will be remedied in the future.

Although the gang may still have strong appeal at the beginning of this age period, it sooner or later gives way to friendships in smaller groups of two or three. These groups are usually of the same sex, but a desire for heterosexual friendships either singly or in groups begins to appear.

The period of gang friendships coincides with rebellion against authority, both parental and also other forms. As the gang period fades each individual teenager appears to rebel against parental authority in particular. This often leads to parents considering their children to be thoughtless and difficult, but in fact the children are usually much concerned with ethics and values and are thinking things out. In this process of thinking out they may develop extreme views and intense passions for causes. Religious fervour may occur.

Increasing independence will be seen during this period. Teenagers begin to take responsibility for choosing their own clothes, making their own personal arrangements, and performing more and more responsible tasks. They respond well to responsibility, for example, when made school prefects. Their increased self-awareness has many repercussions. For example, on the one hand it gives greater insight into the actions and motives of others and, on the other hand, leads to periods of introspection.

12 Years Old

In Britain this is the first year of the senior school. Puberty comes at different ages and some 12-year-old children will be more physically advanced than others. Quite wide differences in height are encountered. Differences in physique and interests between boys and girls are becoming more apparent. Girls are beginning to appear more mature than the boys. There is relatively little mixing between the sexes. Both prefer groups of their own sex and usually shun and scorn the other sex: boys appear to be coarse and clumsy to girls, while girls seem to be silly and giggly to boys. Organized activities, as in Scouts and Guides, are popular and provide the combination of opportunities for adventure which the 12-year-old craves, with the structure and support which he still requires.

12-year-old children tend to be critical of their parents and may even be openly rebellious. This seems to be largely due to a desire to do things for themselves rather than an appreciation of themselves as adults which becomes more evident later.

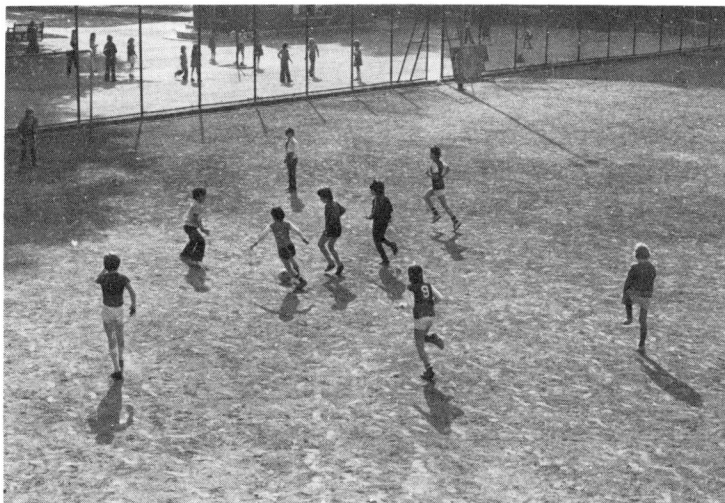

Figure 47. 12 years old: skills and play

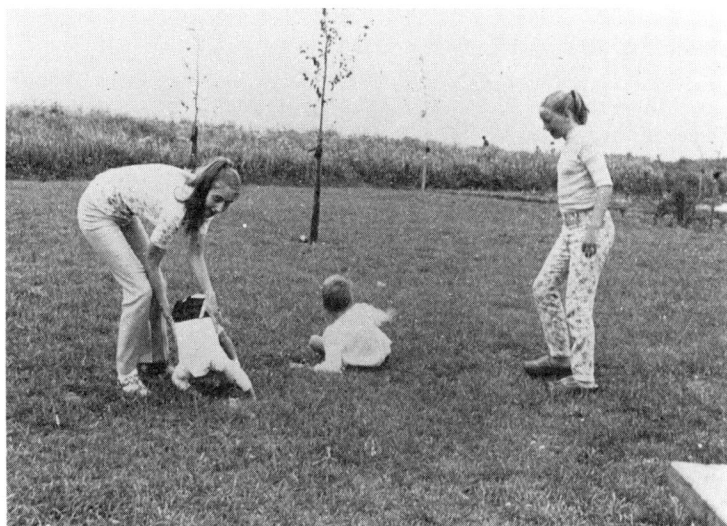

Figure 48. 14 years old: activities

14 Years Old

Most 14-year-old children are well advanced into puberty and, in some, the physical changes will be complete. Both sexes are much nearer to their adult characteristics and in consequence appear to be considerably more mature than 12-year-olds. Personal interests and social activities are also more definite and allied to their future adult roles. At this age they like to be treated as emerging young adults and to have opportunities for increasingly independent action and responsibility. These periods last for varying lengths of time and in some 14-year-olds may be relatively short and interspersed with periods of return to childishness. This fluctuation between the independence of their adult-like rôle and the dependence of childhood confuses parents, teachers and, most of all, themselves, in whom it leads to distress and irritation.

The two sexes are quite distinct at this age. Boys are strong and enjoy physical activities. Team games are important, and also opportunities to go adventuring in groups, for example on camping expeditions. Many boys see girls as individuals who cannot attain comparable abilities, and who, when present, disrupt the cohesiveness of the gang. Some regard girls with awe and trepidation as they sense their future relationships.

Girls at this age are more self-possessed than boys and are more aware of their sexual attractiveness. They often find boys of their own age unattractive because of their lesser maturity. Girls explore the possibilities of self-adornment and will often spend long periods upon this activity. This, together with spells of brooding and day-dreaming, makes them seem to be remote from everyday events. In a way they are preparing themselves for a stage when they inevitably will have to deal with everyday events.

Significance of Development and Signs of Abnormality: 11 to 15 Years

Although the speed of growth and the other physical changes are obvious features of this period the really significant events are related to the establishment of personalities. Children of this age think about themselves, who they are, why they are, and so forth. They learn much by comparing and contrasting themselves with their parents, their friends, and with idolized figures from the world of entertainment and sport. The processes are not easy and many side effects may be observed. Fluctuations of behaviour, unpredictable reactions and contrariness may all occur frequently during this period. Not surprisingly educational effort and results may show similar fluctuations.

It is strange that apparently so little attention is given to the developmental needs and stresses during this period which is so often regarded only as an opportunity for more and more teaching. Both physical and emotional adjustments are necessary, and whether the accompanying manifestations are mostly internal or external, severe or mild, they may still be completely normal.

It is particularly difficult to differentiate between normality and abnormality during this period. Gross extremes, both of failure to make the necessary adjustments and of behaviour, should be considered abnormal, if for no other reason than that they require investigation and treatment. Otherwise it is probably far better not to attempt to grade every aspect of behaviour as either normal or abnormal, but to regard it as an expression of the ongoing development.

REFERENCES

Hurlock, E. (1956). *Child Development*, 4th Edn. New York: McGraw-Hill
Jarman, C. (1973). Is children's handwriting neglected? *Where*, January, 5
Keogh, J. (1965). *Motor Performance of Elementary School Children*. Berkeley: Department of Physical Education, University of California
McCulloch, R. W. (1965). Review of Schonell tests in O. K. Buros (ed.) *The Sixth Mental Measurements Year Book*. New Jersey: Gryphon Press
Schonell, F. J. and Goodacre, E. (1974). *The Psychology and Teaching of Reading*, 5th Edn. Edinburgh: Oliver & Boyd

CHAPTER 6

Some Theories of Child Development

Many approach the subject of child development with a belief that it is simple and uncomplicated, but this is far from the truth. The 'obviousness' of child development and belief in its simplicity probably go a long way towards accounting for the relative sparsity of original research in the subject. There are notable exceptions, but on the whole child development has not received the attention of research workers which it requires and deserves. Several hypotheses about development have been put forward, but until recent years little sound experimental work had been carried out to substantiate them.

Although it is not yet possible to put forward a complete theory of development and a clear explanation of all the mechanisms involved, it is profitable nevertheless to examine some of the views which have been propounded. Doing so should provide a deeper understanding of child development, and may also cause each of us to review his own current views about development. Such an exercise is especially valuable because, whatever views one has, and however incomplete and controversial they are, they will profoundly influence our attitudes towards children. Therefore, at this stage of incompleteness of understanding of development, it is particularly important to study the strengths and weaknesses of the various schools of thought.

No attempt is made in this chapter to provide a comprehensive review of all the theories of child development. Mention will be made of four important and very influential views, and an attempt will be made to summarize the present situation. It is hoped that this attempt may provide clinicians with a perspective and a sound basis for understanding child development, and stimulate them to explore further and deeper into the subject.

All theories of child development lie between two extremes. On the one hand there is the idea that the infant is completely naive and the brain is like an empty sheet. Every character and thought has to be introduced by indoctrination and training, and this learning and experience are engraved upon the blank sheet of the brain. In the past, such views led to some very harsh training routines for young children, but at the present time such extreme opinions are not widely held.

On the other hand there is the view that all abilities and understanding are contained within the brain, and that as the brain grows there is a gradual unfolding of a predetermined pattern of development. This view emphasizes the inherent capacity of the nervous system and denies the influence of environmental experience. Maturation is all! This view was supported by the work of Gesell; it received much support in the earlier part of this century and still has some adherents. Adoption of this outlook leads to a passive attitude towards children with developmental difficulties. It is assumed that they will be capable of performing the missing abilities when the brain is sufficiently mature, and that in the meantime nothing need be done.

Neither of these two extreme views is acceptable today. Arguments about the relative importance of nature and nurture which these considerations provoke are not very fruitful. What is required is an appreciation of all the mechanisms concerned in human development. As our understanding of these increases we begin to realize that the maturation of the nervous system and the results of external experience are intertwined and interrelated. It is hoped, by considering some of the major theories of child development, to provide a deeper understanding of the processes involved and to lead the way to an acceptable synthesis of the various views.

GESELL'S APPROACH TO CHILD DEVELOPMENT
(e.g. Gesell, 1948, 1966; Gesell and Amatruda, 1947; Gesell, Amatruda, Castner and Thompson, 1930).

Arnold Gesell was the founder of the Child Development Center at Yale University and was its inspiration for many years. He and his colleagues observed and recorded the responses and behaviour of babies and children when they were placed in standard pre-arranged situations. Their subsequent detailed analysis of the ciné film and written records form the basis of their descriptions, statements of principles, and hypotheses about the mechanisms of child development.

Their descriptions of child development are as vivid and comprehensive as any which exist. They recognized that various responses and behaviour patterns emerged gradually following a preparatory build-up. Some responses are of a *permanent* nature, that is, once they have appeared they persist as a constant feature of the child's behavioural repertoire. Failure of such items to appear at the expected ages indicates delayed development. Other responses are of a *temporary* nature, in that they appear for a period and then are superseded by another type of response. Failure to observe a temporary type of response at the appropriate age may indicate a delay in development; but alternatively it may be due to an acceleration of development in which case the temporary item was present earlier (and has been superseded already), or to relative weakness of the temporary item so that it is overlooked.

Gesell described the features of development as it occurred in several channels or pathways, thus, gross and fine motor, adaptive, language and personal-social pathways. This separation assists in the analysis of observed development and has been followed, with various modifications, by many subsequent workers. He emphasized that, despite the usefulness of such a separation into pathways, in order to obtain an understanding of child development it was necessary to appreciate its integrated wholeness and its flowing continuity.

On the basis of his observations Gesell considered the pattern of development to be so uniform that he felt that it must follow several principles. These include the following.

(a)   Development follows a definite sequence.
(b)   Development shows a cephalocaudal progression.
(c)   Development proceeds from gross undifferentiated skills to precise and refined ones.

These aspects were considered to be relatively immutable. Many subsequent workers interpreted these principles as laws which every child must obey, and this led to recommendations that children who show deviant development must be made to repeat earlier developmental sequences in correct order so as to include all the features previously omitted.

The one aspect of development which Gesell accepted might vary was its rate, which was slowed in certain conditions and circumstances.

Gesell was a paediatrician who wrote for paediatricians in order to help them in their clinical work. Consequently, having described the observed stages of development and defined the principles of development, it was a relatively short step to the concept of developmental diagnosis. The major abnormality which may be diagnosed is, of course, developmental delay, but other types of developmental abnormality to be found are:

(a)   an abnormal quality of performance;
(b)   the undue persistence of temporary responses;
(c)   a disordered sequence of development.

Another type of abnormality, developmental dissociation, has been described by Illingworth, an ardent follower of Gesell (Illingworth, 1958).

Gesell considered that the observed developmental phenomena reflected maturation of the central nervous system. This hypothesis received much support from observations and experiments which were being reported about this time. These experiments fall into two categories. The first group is concerned with evidence that restraint does not prevent the development of responses. The responses studied were motor skills, and observations were made on children who were swaddled (Greenacre, 1944), anaesthetized tadpoles (Carmichael, 1926) and restrained birds (Dennis, 1943). In all these cases the organisms walked, swam or flew when released. The interpretation made from these observations was that maturation of the nervous system had continued during the period of restraint so that the appropriate skill was there and ready for use at the appropriate time and was demonstrated when the restraint was released. Development thus depended upon maturation. These studies did not examine in any depth the quality of performance of the skills in these circumstances, the effect of the restraint upon other aspects of development, or the developmental value of the experiences which the individual would have undergone had he not been restrained. These studies show that maturation of the nervous system is important in the development of motor skills, but it is unjustified, on the basis of this evidence, to conclude that maturation is the only influence of importance in the development of motor skills in particular, or of all aspects of development in general.

The second group of observations is concerned with evidence that practice prior to the usual time of appearance of a particular skill does not hasten its appearance. Several studies were reported in which one member of a set of identical twins was given early training and practice, and when both twins were examined at a later age the untrained one possessed the same motor skills as the trained one (Gesell and Thompson, 1929; McGraw, 1935). The interpretation of these observations was that abilities develop irrespective of training and when the nervous system is ready for them to do so, and, therefore, that development is dependent upon maturation of the nervous system. These are undoubtedly important observations and it is reasonable to accept that a certain level of neurological function is necessary for a particular ability to be possible, but the conclusions have been applied more widely and rigidly than is justified. They have been responsible for a very widespread negative attitude amongst clinicians towards therapy for young handicapped children. It is maintained that nothing need be done to help a child showing delayed or aberrant development because the missing abilities will appear as the brain matures. This attitude assumes that: (a) the results of relatively crude observations upon a few healthy twins apply to all children and in all circumstances; (b) when the nervous system has reached a level of maturity appropriate for the appearance of a particular ability this ability will manifest itself whatever the circumstances; and (c) no attention is necessary to ensure the persistence and elaboration of any ability once it appears. It is very doubtful, therefore, if these extreme views are acceptable and justifiable.

The weaknesses of the Gesell approach to development are that it does not include sufficient experimental work to back up the conclusions drawn from the excellent descriptions, that it emphasizes the motor aspects of development more than the others, and that it is too rigidly adherent to the concept of maturation.

The strengths of the Gesell approach to development lie in its wealth of accurate clinical descriptions, the concept of the dynamic continuity of development, and its clinical applicability to developmental diagnosis.

The Gesell approach to child development appeals particularly to clinicians; the Piaget approach appeals particularly to educationalists.

PIAGET'S CONTRIBUTION TO CHILD DEVELOPMENT
(Brearley and Hitchfield, 1967; Maier, 1969; Flavell, 1963)*

Piaget is a Swiss who trained initially as a zoologist, but later turned to psychology. He has revolutionized thinking about cognitive development in childhood. His work is based upon extremely detailed and precise observations of children, especially his own children, the results of which he then subjected to intense logical reasoning and, following this, he tested his conclusions in simple experimental ways.

He was interested in the cause and effect of every action and every response. He wanted to find out what the responses meant to the child and how they helped him to adapt to his environment, because he considered such adaptation to be a fundamental feature of development. His methods and reasoning will be understood better by considering the steps taken in the acquisition of a mature concept of an object.

* These references provide a good introduction to the many writings of Piaget and colleagues, and all contain bibliographies to Piaget's works.

An individual with a mature object concept 'sees' objects as entities in their own right, existing and moving in space and persisting in time. They are independent of any activity on the part of the observer or others such as looking at the objects or manipulating, smelling or listening to them. As the individual conceptualizes objects as separate entities in this mature way, he also conceives object-like properties in relation to himself. How is this mature concept reached? Piaget described the following stages.

Stages 1 and 2

The object presents sensory impressions which may be 'seen' by the child. Continued looking (or touching, smelling or listening to) is encouraged by the pleasure evoked by the sensory impressions, which may persist after the object is moved.

Stage 3

The child begins to extrapolate in time and space by a series of manoeuvres.

(a)   He shows visual anticipation of movements of the object.

(b)   He searches for the object. Visually this is a roving search over the whole immediate area.

(c)   He plays with a 'there—not there' situation. He looks at the object, then turns away, then looks back at the object again, and does this repeatedly.

(d)   He anticipates the whole object when seeing a part.

(e)   He will remove an obstruction to see the object.

Stage 4

He searches for hidden objects with increasing degrees of sophistication.

Stage 5

He focuses his search upon the place where the object was last seen.

Stage 6

He searches for objects by imagining a series of possible positions which they might be occupying. In this way he demonstrates his awareness that objects have an existence apart from himself.

These conclusions are drawn from numerous careful observations like this one:

'At 0.7 (months) Jacqueline tries to grasp a celluloid duck on top of her quilt. She almost catches it, shakes herself, and the duck slides down beside her. It falls very close to her hand but behind a fold in the sheet. Jacqueline's eyes have followed the movement, she has even followed it with her outstretched hand. But as soon as the duck has disappeared—nothing more. It does not occur to her to search behind the fold of the sheet, which would be very easy to do (she twists it mechanically without searching at all)'

The simple but very neat experimental studies devised by Piaget and his colleagues can be illustrated by describing the investigation of understanding of quantity. The examiner makes a ball of clay and the subject makes another one just like it. One ball is kept as a standard of reference and the other is distorted in various ways. The child is then asked if it is the same substance, same weight and same volume. Experiments of this type revealed that at first there is no sense of conservation of matter, volume or weight; then occurs a transitional period during which some transformations are recognized; and then finally comes a stage when all transformations are recognized. Appreciation of conservation of matter becomes common at 8 to 10 years, of weight at 10 to 12 years and of volume only after 12 years.

Piaget and his colleagues accumulated a vast amount of data upon which they based descriptions of the processes and patterns of development of cognitive reasoning in infancy and childhood. Development is considered to occur as a result of the interaction of four processes:

Maturation   Differentiation and elaboration of the central nervous system.

Experience   Interaction with the physical world.

Social transmission   The effect of care and education upon the nature of experience.

Equilibration   Self-regulation.

The essence of development is seen in a biological sense as the individual's adaptation to his environment. In development, differentiation is made bewteen two aspects of adaptation, namely, *assimilation* which consists of the individual's experiences at his level of ability to accept and integrate those experiences; and *accommodation* which consists of the modifications provoked by the experiences. For example, a cube placed in front of a baby provides visual and tactile stimuli which are assimilated, and they provoke visual regard, manipulation and mouthing as accomodative responses.

Development is a continuous process built up stage by stage in a developmental hierarchy. Time is required for each process to be practised, to be perfected, and to be used as the basis for the next succeeding stage.

This method of thinking about development led to the differentiation of *horizontal* and *vertical* features. When a new task appears which requires the same level of organization as an earlier one a horizontal expansion of development is said to have taken place; but when a new task appears which requires a higher level of organization than previously, this is said to be vertical development.

Development is dynamic in that a child is never anything, but is always becoming something. Actions are important in Piagetian development since they are the expression of cerebral processes and since thoughts are essentially internalized actions.

Piaget and his co-workers showed that each reasoning process leads on to the next more complex one. They described the following stages, each of which contains several substages, and arranged them in chronological sequence.

1. Sensorimotor Stage (Up To Approximately 2 Years)

In a sense this period of development involves the whole infant. He is coming to grips with his physical world—learning to deal with the sensory experiences, fulfilling his physical needs, and using his whole self for expression and communication. During this period the infant learns to perceive his environment and to control his actions.

The sub-stages are as follows:
(a)   Use of reflex actions (0–1 month).
(b)   Development of habituation of actions (1–14 months).
A response is repeated until it becomes an established schema. This is the beginning of repetition in sequence. The repetition of a response is

called a *circular action*. The actions which develop during this period are called *primary circular reactions*. These lead to the appearance of the first voluntary action.

    (c)   Co-ordination of actions (4–8 months) e.g. vision and pre-hension.

The primary circular reactions are now extended beyond the immediate basic needs to have a secondary function, now called *secondary circular reactions*. This opens up the possibility of developing imitation, play and emotion.

    (d)   Co-ordination of secondary schemata in which previous experiences are used to influence actions (8–12 months).

This is an important transitional substage. The child's greater mobility is an important influence. This stage opens up new dimensions such as ability to recognize signs, to anticipate response, and to observe.

    (e)   Differentiation of action schemata in which new ways are found by experimentation (12–18 months).

The circular reactions are further developed to a *tertiary stage* in which repetitions are modified when new objects are met and are further modified to explore the object purposefully.

    (f)   Internalization of schemata in which all the earliest reactions become incorporated into automatic spontaneous responses (18 months onwards).

The last substage (f) is the third and most complex of the goal-directed behaviour responses seen in the period of sensorimotor development. The first was seen in substage (d) and consisted of the co-ordination of existing and familiar schemata. The second was seen in substage (e) and consisted of experimentation to discover new ways to use existing schemata. In substage (e) possible solutions to new situations are worked out internally before being put to the test. Existing schemata are now internalized and the most appropriate one is selected to deal with new challenges. At this time the child also becomes aware of the independent existence of objects and to some extent of his own identity. These are vital changes for the development of his personality and social relationships.

2. Stage of Concrete Operations (From Approximately 2 to 12 Years)

The study of concrete operations in cognitive development from 6 to 12 years is one of the most complete aspects of Piaget's work. The preceding years of preparation and transition also possess much richness of their own with the development of symbolization, language, play and personality being important parts.

(a)   Symbolic function: pre-conceptual (2 to 4 years).

At this sub-stage the child knows the world as he sees it and experiences it. He lives in the here and now and knows no alternatives. The sensori-motor stage equipped him to explore further as he does in constant play. He is further helped in this by recognizing that objects may be represented by models or can be identified in various ways, but most particularly by verbal symbols.

(b)   Intuitive thought (4–7 years).

      (i) representational organization;

      (ii) articulated representational regulation.

The child's world expands considerably at this age. He starts school; he has many playmates. He relies upon imitation of the behaviour of others (especially adults) to deal with the many new experiences. It is as if he intuitively knew what to do, but all the time he is learning. He replaces acting-out of his thoughts and reasoning with talking-out; much of his play is verbally controlled. Much of this period is occupied with learning how to deal with an increasing number of concepts and to order them in place and time. Language is an essential help in this process. It is used as a tool of intuitive thought, to help to order the various concepts and to deal with social relationships.

(c)   Concrete operations (6–12 years).

      (i) simple operations, e.g. classification;

      (ii) whole systems operations, e.g. co-ordinates.

This is the period during which the child achieves mastery over his physical world. He has learnt about many properties possessed by objects in his environment and now he begins to compare and contrast different objects and to classify them. He recognizes the relationships of parts to the whole, and he groups similar items together in time and space. To deal with all this information the child develops a series of logical strategies of increasing complexity which enable him to deal with an increasing number of concepts.

3. Stage of Formal Operations (Approximately 12 Years Onwards)

(a)   Hypothesis-deductive operations.

(b)   Lattice operations.

The characteristics of this stage of Piaget development are the replace-ment of random cognitive behaviour by a systematic approach to problems, and the acquisition of abilities to hypothesize, to reason deductively and to understand and work out complex interrelationships. Understanding of the physical properties of objects has proceeded in the sequence, (a) space, time, reality and causation; (b) number, order, measure, shape and size; (c) motion, speed, force and energy. The experiences of past opportunities to compare and contrast have led to concepts of equality and balance between concepts and actions. This understanding is applied to social relationships as well as to physical entities and underlies much of the awakening of personal awareness which characterizes adolescence.

It is quite impossible to do justice to all of Piaget's thinking in this brief summary, but I hope sufficient has been written to show that this is more than just a description of observed development. It is an exploration in depth of the processes involved in the child's cognitive reasoning. Its great value is that it provides an insight into the child's strategies of problem-solving and provides a sound basis for developmental intervention and teaching programmes. It does not cover all aspects of development, and it has been criticized for not taking more account of the Freudian views of childhood. That Piaget did consider this aspect a great deal is reflected in his writings. It is possible that the detailed analysis of cognitive reasoning does not readily lend itself to psychoanalytical appreciation, which requires an understanding of the global effects of experience. For this we need to turn to the appropriate literature.

THE PSYCHOANALYTICAL APPROACH TO CHILD DEVELOPMENT WITH PARTICULAR REFERENCE TO ERIKSON'S CONCEPTS
(Maier, 1969; Winnicott, 1957; Erikson, 1967)

Freud and his followers revealed those strong influences, of which we are not normally aware, which control an individual's emotional development and stability, his attitudes and reactions, and his interpersonal relationships. They showed the continuity of these influences and demonstrated that early childhood experiences might have profound consequences much later on. Their studies showed that the direction of the child's psychic orientation changes at different ages. Thus, in the first year there is a predominance of the oral orientation, of elimination (or anal-urethral) orientation in the second and third years, and of sexual (or genital) orientation in later years.

The vast literature on these subjects cannot possibly be covered in this brief review. Nevertheless, there is much in the psychoanalytical literature which is pertinent to child development and of which developmental paediatricians should be aware. Some familiarity with the writings of Anna Freud and of Donald Winnicott would serve as a sound beginning. The latter's popular lectures of the early 1940's on child-rearing are excellent reading for practising paediatricians. The work of Erikson has been selected for further comment because he of all psychoanalysts has ordered his views towards an understanding of child development.

Following a sound training in Freudian concepts Erikson moved from Europe to America where he added to his psychoanalytical views additional information derived from observations of children, anthropological data, and studies of child-rearing practices. He then elaborated his ideas into a theory of child development.

Erikson believes that it is important for children to have an awareness and stability which is appropriate for their level of development; that this is achieved by balancing opposing influences; that children's behaviour at any age is a reflection of their success in achieving this balance; that the direction of the orientation of their equilibrium varies at different ages; and that periods of transition from one orientation to another are times of crisis and stress.

Erikson describes the following 5 phases during childhood:

1. Infancy—Sense of Trust

The infant is vulnerable and needs to acquire a sense of security or trust. His attractiveness and dependency help by provoking strong feelings of tenderness. The unfamiliarity of everything around him creates uncertainty and mistrust. He is very dependent upon all the strengths derived from the mothering situation to balance the contrary doubts and so achieve equilibrium.

2. Early Childhood—Sense of Autonomy

Awareness of his own will stimulates a child to exercise it to create a sense of autonomy. This positive drive forwards is associated with apprehension about the strength of his will and exploration of the unknown, and shame over abandoning the ties of phase 1. This sets the scene for the conflicts of phase 2. The end result is determined by the balance achieved by the child and the environment created by his parents.

3. Pre-school—Sense of Initiative

Having achieved a sense of autonomy, and coming to believe that he is what he thinks he is, he now explores new worlds in which he tests himself. He goes into the sphere of other children's activities and behaviour: this is well seen by observing young children at play. His drive to initiate activities, to explore and to exert himself meets rebuffs, frustrations. This conflicting situation often extends into his rich fantasy world where many problems are worked out. The efforts of the struggle to achieve a balance may provoke resentment and rebellion against trusted parents who let him get into this situation.

4. School Age—Sense of Industry

The child has now reached a stage of considerable physical and intellectual energies which he applies in order to master all he can. The school child is receptive to all he is taught and responds accordingly. Contrary influences consist of a fear of failure and a sense of inferiority with respect to his peers. He struggles to achieve a balance between industry and inferiority in his intellectual and physical pursuits and his social relationships.

5. Adolescence—Sense of Identity

The individual now moves forward to reach a readiness to face the entire world. On the one hand there is his awareness of his many abilities and skills and confidence in them, and on the other hand there is his awareness of the many uncertainties in the world and a reluctance to plunge ahead on his own. Some of the conflicts of this period as identified by Erikson are as follows.

(a)   Time perspective and acceptance in contrast to time diffusion. Doing the good things on time, hoping the bad things will never come.

(b)   Self-certainty in contrast to self-uncertainty and self-consciousness.

(c)   Acceptance and evasions of rôles and identities.

(d)   Persistence and anticipation of achievement in contrast to sporadic activity with periods of work paralysis.

(e)   Sexual identification and acceptance in contrast to bisexual diffusion and conflicts.

(f)   Leadership versus diffusion of authority.

(g)   Uncompromising idealogical polarization in contrast to tolerance for diffusion of ideals.

Erikson's approach to child development creates an impression of a dynamic situation, and it provides clinicans, especially child psychiatrists, with a structure which can be the basis of therapeutic intervention. For example, his views of basic trust in phase 1, a trust which needs to be achieved by all babies, help one to understand the difficulties of a malformed baby who cannot find that security from his distraught mother. This then provides a basis for therapeutic help for both mother and baby. In some respects Erikson can be said to have done for the clinician what Piaget has done for teachers.

Studies of the global behaviour of children are not limited to the psychoanalytical approach as is soon evident when we study the ethological approach.

THE ETHOLOGICAL CONTRIBUTION TO CHILD DEVELOPMENT
(Barnett, 1962, 1967, 1973; Blurton Jones, 1972)

Ethology is the scientific study of animal behaviour and is said to be especially pertinent to an understanding of the manners of man and animals. The methods used by ethologists include observational techniques, experimental procedures, and deductive reasoning. Most of the studies have been centred upon birds, fish and animals. This has several advantages. Certain responses are more readily seen in some species than others so that, by selecting an appropriate species to study, lessons can be learnt more easily. The faster rates of growth and maturation of some species mean that the full effects of experimental procedures are seen more quickly. Furthermore, there is in any case greater scope for experimental work in animals then in humans.

Ethologists have been criticized for assuming too readily that what they observe in artifical experimental procedures gives a true picture of what occurs naturally, and that the conclusions from animal studies can be trasferred directly to humans. Despite these reservations, there is no doubt that ethology contributes much of value to our understanding of child development.

Ethological studies revealed the complexity of human development by providing evidence to support both the maturational and the environmental hypotheses of development. On the one hand, the very complexity of many behavioural responses supports the maturational hypothesis in which there is an unfolding of abilities due to a predetermined plan, as it is difficult to conceive how such behaviours could otherwise develop. On the other hand, the variations of behaviour which ethologists have produced by environmental manipulation make it very clear that observed development results from the continual interaction of organism and environment.

Several ethological concepts are important in the study of child development. The term *instinct*, or instinctive behaviour, is applied to the usually complex stereotyped species-specific pattern of behaviour which is produced promptly and regularly upon appropriate stimulation or 'triggering'. These specific responses are elicited easily at certain periods, and less easily or not at all at other periods. The times of easy elicitation are called *sensitive periods*. Each specific pattern of behaviour has its own characteristic sensitive period (this term should not be confused with the term *critical period* which signifies an optimum period for all learning responses).

Studies of the factors which lead to an ending of the sensitive periods have contributed to our understanding of the evolution of behaviour. Age and maturation are important influences. With both ageing and maturation (not synonymous, but related processes) there often occurs a change in the specific response. Sometimes the particular response being studied is terminated by the appearance of other responses which interfere with the initial response. Learning effects also contribute to the extinction of the sensitive periods. The incorporation of a particular response into the learnt repertoire of an individual appears to inhibit the continued display of similar responses. If and when a response becomes incorporated into some other pattern of action, the instinctive aspect of the response ceases to be necessary, so it is both appropriate and desirable that it should fade away.

Closely linked with instinctive behaviour and the concept of sensitive periods is the phenomenon of *imprinting*. At an appropriate time an often rather bizarre, but nevertheless apparently biologically-determined stimulus will trigger off a complex pattern of behaviour which may thereafter become well established. For example, the newly hatched duckling responds to the first moving object it perceives by automatically following it, even if it is only a cardboard box pulled along the ground; and human babies a few weeks old show a smiling response to any disc-like object held before their eyes. The biological value of this phenomenon of imprinting will be clear.

Opportunities to experience many stimuli and to exhibit a variety of responses appear to be essential for the development of all organisms. Childhood play is a rich source of both stimulation and opportunities for exercising responses. Ethologists have demonstrated experimentally the value of play for learning in many species, and also the long-range effects of deprivation of these opportunities. Observations such as those of Harlow upon the rearing of monkeys (Harlow and Suomi, 1971) have important lessons for all concerned with human development. These areas are only now being explored and evaluated and much interesting material is expected in the near future.

Ethology is particularly attractive for its contribution to a biological view of human development, but, like the other views of development, it is most useful when interpreted with the other views to produce an integrated picture of development.

AN ATTEMPTED SYNTHESIS

Several aspects of child development have been reviewed. There is much, however, which has not been included, such as the vast field of learning theory and the influence of different child-rearing practices, to mention just two topics. Nevertheless sufficient has been said to show the complexity of child development and the need for developmental paediatricians to have some insight into the various theories. Some integration is necessary.

The contribution of these theories to our understanding of child development can be illustrated by considering a simple example—the response of a baby to a cube. Imagine a baby a few months old being placed in front of a table on which rests a small cube. Gesell's descriptions and our own observations tell us what happens. The baby looks around in front of himself. He may give fleeting attention to the cube, but then becomes more interested in it as it is moved, or tapped on the table, and especially if in doing this the examiner is seen and heard, and speaks encouragingly to the infant. The baby reaches forward and grasps the cube in the palm of the hand. He may move his hand to bring the cube more clearly into his visual field. He may then move his hand and take the cube to his mouth. After a short while he drops the cube onto the table and appears to ignore it. A little later he accidently touches the cube with his hand and responds as if this is his first encounter with the cube.

The baby's pattern of behaviour in such a situation is determined by the fact that he belongs to the human species, and also by his age, the stage of maturation of his nervous system, and by his previous experiences and what he has learnt from them. If he has had previous experience of manipulative exploration, he may recognize the cube as a distinct object, and he may then reach for it spontaneously without waiting for the additional stimuli of moving or tapping, or its demonstrated association with a familiar adult. Reaching became a volitional act and the baby's principal means of tactile exploration because early arm movements, controlled by neurological reflexes such as the asymmetrical tonic neck reflex, produced random contact with objects.

Repetition of the action producing these tactile contacts led to its reinforcement and later incorporation as a voluntary act. It is possible to see in this sequence Piaget's stages of sensorimotor development. Also, the fact that when the cube drops it leaves the child's awareness and that when next he encounters it he comes upon it as an original experience, shows that the infant has not yet attained Piaget's stage of the awareness of the permanence of objects.

The infant reaches for the object with his arms as these are the usual tactile exploratory limbs, but the essential drive here is for the infant to acquire knowledge of this external object; accordingly if his arms are paralysed or absent, he will attempt to reach by whatever means he has at his disposal—perhaps his leg, or his mouth, or even his eyes, and all these phenomena are shown by disabled children.

The mouthing of the cube is more than just another means of exploration. Erikson's views show how this oral exploration reassures the infant of the safety and security of the novel object in his environment.

The analysis of one simple situation, therefore, reveals much about the learning and development of the baby, and shows how the various views about development can be integrated.

Development occurs as the result of a biological drive which is characteristic of living organisms, and which follows a species-specific pattern. It is mediated by a succession of involuntary actions produced by the maturing nervous system. These are stimulated, or inhibited, or otherwise modified as a result of interaction with the environment and the individual's awareness and interpretation of the effects and results of this interaction.

Abnormalities of development arise in several ways. There may be slowing of the biological process so that the whole process of development follows its usual pattern, but at a much slower pace. This is *developmental lethargy*. It may be that as a result of physical or sensory disabilities the individual is unable to effect or appreciate the environmental interactions which provide the material for future learning, or the environmental opportunities may be lacking. These situations produce *developmental deprivation*. On other occasions it seems as if the biological drive persists unaltered in strength, but the individual is unable to make use of and to learn from the interactions with the environment. In these situations it seems as if the persisting drive is easily diverted into bizarre and purposeless channels, as, in the case of so-called hyperactive retarded children. This is really *developmental non-assimilation* and *developmental distortion*.

Although much more needs to be learnt about child development, an appreciation of some of the current theories does much to deepen one's understanding of this complex phenomenon of child development. It also permits the creation of a working synthesis of the various views, which provides a basis for better understanding of both normal and deviant development.

REFERENCES

Barnett, S. A. (1962). Lessons from animal behaviour for the clinician, *Clincs Dev. Med. 7*. London: Heinemann
– (1967). *Instinct and Intelligence*. London: MacGibbon and Kee
– (1973). Ethology and development, *Clinics Dev. Med. 47*. London: Heinemann
Blurton Jones, N. (1972). *Ethological Studies of Child Behaviour*. Cambridge: Cambridge University Press
Brearley, M. and Hitchfield, E. (1967). *A Teachers Guide to Reading Piaget*. London: Routledge & Kegan Paul
Carmichael, L. (1926). The development of behaviour in vertebrates experimentally removed from the influence of external stimulation. *Psychol Rev.* **33**, 57
Dennis, W. (1943). The possibility of advancing and retarding the motor development of infants, *Psychol. Rev.* **50**, 203
Erikson, E. H. (1967). *Childhood and Society*. London: Penguin Books
Flavell, J. H. (1963). *The Developmental Psychology of Jean Piaget*. Princeton, New Jersey: Van Nostrand
Gesell, A. (1948). *Studies in Child Development*. New York: Harper and Row
– (1966). *The First Five Years of Life*. London: Methuen
–and Amatruda, C. S. (1947). *Developmental Diagnosis*, 2nd edn. New York: Harper and Row
–Amatruda, C. S., Castner, B. M. and Thompson, H. (1930). *Biographies of Child Development*. London: Hamish Hamilton
–and Thompson, H. (1929). Learning and growth in identical twins; an experimental study by the method of co-twin control, *Genet. Psychol. Monogr.* **6**, 1
Greenacre, P. (1944). Infant reactions to restraint. *Am. J. Orthopsychiat.* **14**, 204
Harlow, H. F. and Suomi, S. J. (1971). Social recovery by isolation-reared monkeys, *Proc. nat. Acad. Sci. U.S.A.* **68**, 1534
Illingworth, R. S. (1958). Dissociation as a guide to developmental assessment, *Archs Dis. Childh.* **33**, 118
Maier, H. W. (1969). *Three Theories of Child Development*. New York: Harper & Row
McGraw, M. B. (1935). *Growth: a Study of Johnny and Jimmy*. New York: Appleton Century Crofts
Winnicott, D. W. (1957). *The Child and the Outside World*. New York: Basic Books

Awareness: Receiving and Seeking Sensory Stimuli; Examination of Receptive Functions

Living organisms survive by coming to terms with their environment. They are able to do so by possessing from an early stage some means of warning to avoid accidents and predators; methods of finding and obtaining food; and ways of learning about their environment. Human beings, like all other organisms, need to acquire these biological characteristics and this is reflected in the development of their sensory functions.

Infants possess the senses of vision, hearing, touch, smell and taste. Many of the responses of the very young child to sensory stimuli are survival mechanisms, but as the peripheral organs which receive stimuli and the perceptual processes of the brain which analyse and comprehend the sensory input develop more complex reactions appear and the child is able to build up an increasingly wide range of information about the surrounding world.

FUNDAMENTAL CHARACTERISTICS OF THE SENSES

The eyes respond to waves from the infrared to the ultraviolet parts of the light spectrum. They are able to receive stimuli from considerable distances and can distinguish between two separate points separated by a distance so small that it would subtend an angle of only 1' at the eye (at a distance of 6 metres this is equal to 1.74 mm). They can examine near objects and detect fine detail. Colours can be distinguished. Eye movements increase the range of vision. Accommodation and convergence permit frequent and almost instantaneous changes between close and distant viewing.

The ears respond to sound waves within the range of 20—20,000 Hz (cps). Their principal rôle is the detection of speech sounds within the range of 60—8,000 Hz, and especially sounds between 3,000—8,000 Hz because this range includes most of the consonants which give distinctive clarity to speech. The intensity of speech sounds varies by as much as 30 dB. Most powerful are the vowel sounds produced with the mouth wide open; least powerful are the voiceless sounds such as 'th'.

To understand speech a child has to be able to detect sounds of short duration and to recognize differences between sounds in frequency, duration, and rhythm. Martin and Martin (1973) studied auditory perception in a group of schoolboys. They found that differences of frequency of 10 Hz and of duration of 200 milliseconds were readily detected but smaller differences were detected less often. Sheridan (1958) summarized the situation aptly as follows:

> 'Every ordinary spoken phrase imposes upon the listening ear the necessity to appreciate a large number of complex sounds which swing rapidly over differences of 8 octaves in pitch and 30 decibels in intensity. For practical purposes one may assume that a quiet voice at 3 feet carries to the listening ear sound intensities varying between peaks at 60 dB and troughs at 30 dB.'

In addition, to utilize auditory sensation to the full children must also learn to listen and to localize the source of sounds.

The sensory organs for smell respond to stimuli from varying distances according to their nature and intensity, and the air currents. Although this sensation is not as well developed in humans as in some other species it sometimes evokes strong reactions as when children react to the smell of their food or to a perfume. The sense of smell becomes more important when other distance receptors—vision and hearing—are impaired. For example, the mother of a deaf-blind baby should use the same perfume all the time so that she can be more easily identified by her baby.

The senses of touch and taste are used for nearby exploration and do not respond to stimuli from a distance. Tactile sensations consist of touch, pressure, temperature and pain. Sensitivity to tactile stimuli varies in different parts of the body. Areas used for exploration such as the finger tips are biologically prepared by being provided with a greater concentration of nerve receptors than other parts of the body. Sensitive tactile areas can detect as little as 3 mm between two points.

The sense of taste is fairly crude. It is said to be possible to identify sweet, sour, salt and bitter, but most tastes produce composite pleasant or unpleasant reactions.

The Perceptual Part of Sensation

The peripheral sense organs are useless without the perceptual function of the brain. The baby is subjected to many stimuli; he has to learn to identify, distinguish and select those stimuli which are most useful to him for self-preservation and learning about the world around him, and having selected, has to learn to suppress the irrelevant stimuli. This perceptual development is a very demanding task. In the early stages of the development of sensory awareness babies tend to be wholly preoccupied with one single sensory channel at a time to the exclusion of other interests and activities. A good example of preoccupation with one sensory input occurred once when I tried to give a demonstration of auditory responses by infants before a rather heavily-jewelled audience. The infants were so visually attracted and occupied that the demonstration was unsuccessful! The stage of single sensory input concentration passes and then the infant can devote more time to other important learning processes associated with sensory function, such as the simultaneous use of more than one sense for one particular task; rapid switching from one sense to another; and the simultaneous use of two or more senses for different tasks.

Sensory functions equip a child to learn about the world around himself. Impairment of any of these functions impedes this process. Developmental paediatricians are concerned with learning about the complex mechanisms of sensory perceptual development and integration, and with the application of this knowledge to help children in whom these functions are impaired. It is not just a matter of deciding if a child has difficulty seeing or has a hearing loss or not, but of understanding how these losses affect him and what needs to be done to ensure full development despite the losses.

AUDITORY FUNCTION

The peripheral auditory sense organs develop early in fetal life, and are probably functional towards the end of pregnancy. There are many stories of fetuses *in utero* responding to external sounds (e.g. Walker, Grimwade and Wood, 1971).

Babies are born into a noisy world. The loudness of some everyday sounds is shown in Table 13. Sounds of different intensities arrive at babies' ears from varying distances. Sudden loud noises provoke blinking, grimacing and even crying. Quieter sounds, especially steady notes appear to be soothing. If everything is kept as quiet as possible, it is not difficult to show that a baby is aware of nearby sounds. Babies show

TABLE 13

The Intensity of Some Everyday Sounds (Decibels, approx.)

Whisper	15
Average comfortable house	30
Average comfortable office	40
Quiet car	50
Conversation	60
Busy street	70
Cocktail party	75
Loud shout or scream	80
Pneumatic drill	80
Train	90
Engine room	100
Jet engine	110
Thunder	120

the most consistent responses to sounds when they are made within a conical receptive area extending outwards from the infant's ears (*Figure 49*). The size of this area is influenced by the intensity of the background noise. It is much less easy for an infant to receive sounds which are not distinct from the background noises.

Various factors familiarize infants with certain sounds. Frequent repetition of sounds is one important factor. The mother's voice and certain frequently recurring household noises, such as the clink of crockery, are obvious examples of frequently recurring sounds. Sounds which are accompanied by other pleasant sensory experiences also become interesting to the baby. Examples are the mother's voice which is accompanied by gentle caressing and pleasant smells, and the rattling of a spoon in a cup which is associated with the pleasures of feeding. Some sounds appear to be more attractive to babies than others. The mother's voice of higher pitch and greater musicality than the father's usually receives more attention from baby. All these

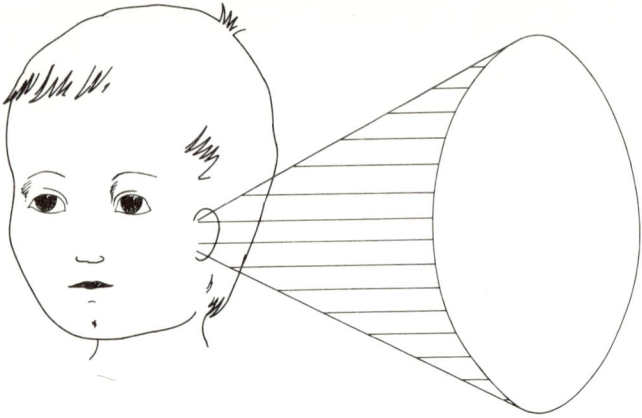

Figure 49. The sensitive auditory receptive area in infancy

examples show the importance of the mother's voice in the early
development of an infant's awareness of sounds.

The developing awareness of sounds is linked with turning of the
eyes and head towards the side of the sound. This directional response
is almost certainly reflex at first and is initiated by the reception of
auditory stimuli earlier and more intensely on one side than on the
other side. Occasionally turning of the eyes may be seen as early as
4 or 5 weeks. This is a reflex phenomenon which may even occur in
babies with poor vision. It must not be taken as an indication of visual
ability. Sheridan (1973a) stresses the importance of testing visual
fixation and following separately from response to sounds and the need
for the doctor to do the visual tests before the hearing tests. Consistent
signs of turning towards sounds appear at about 4 months of age.
Turning is soon associated with visual recognition of the sound-producing
object. This early audio-visual link may be centred upon a particular
rattle. Sometimes when babies are being tested they appear to be
reluctant to turn towards the sound. If they are first shown the rattle,
which they can then see and hear, they then appear more ready to turn
towards the sound of that rattle when the test is repeated.

In the six-month period from 4 to 10 months remarkable development occurs in this response of turning towards sounds. This is related
to the developing awareness of sounds as distinct entities with a source
of origin at a definite location. The maturation of auditory localization
is developing simultaneously with the acquisition of an awareness of the
permanence of objects, and the correspondence between these
phenomena will be obvious.

At first the infant turns towards the side of the sound. The developmental progression in acquiring more precise accuracy in sound localization was described by Murphy (1962). The infant develops a distinct two-phase action in which he first turns to the side of the sound and then makes a second movement of the head upwards or downwards towards the sound. Downward localization appears to develop before upward localization. These two movements gradually merge first into an arc-like movement towards the sound and then a single direct movement which by 10 months localizes the sound to within about 5 degrees (*Figure 50*).

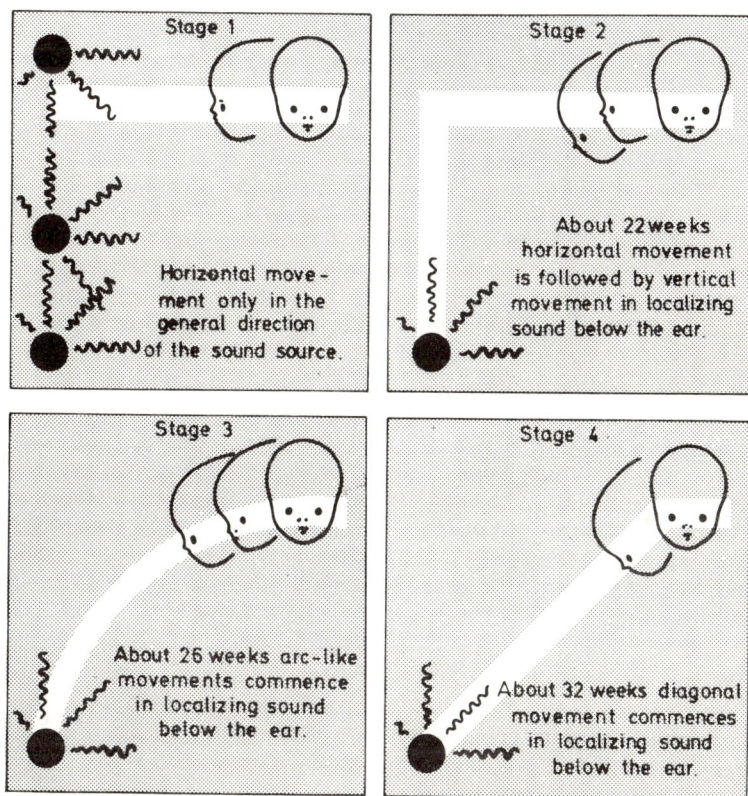

Figure 50. The maturation of localization of sounds

The ability to hear a sound and to turn directly towards it is no longer a simple reflex action. It is associated with the development of the concept of a sound, and with the ability to inhibit the response in certain circumstances. For example, a response may not occur if the infant is engrossed visually or tactilely, or if the sound is too familiar or uninteresting.

At this stage the infant is learning to identify and recognize sounds by their intensity, pitch, duration and association with other sounds and events, which, as described earlier, he must become able to do very quickly in order to be able to distinguish all the meaningful sounds of speech. Learning the characteristics of sounds greatly reinforces interest in sounds and promotes the development of auditory attention and listening. Each step in this process promotes others. The development of auditory alertness and the ability to listen is one of the most important attributes of the infant in the second half of his first year (Fisch, 1971). Failure to develop auditory interest and listening ability may be due to growing up in a noisy environment, or one in which there is little meaningful or interesting auditory stimulation. Such deprivation has a profound effect upon the development of language. In normal circumstances the most frequently heard sounds and also the most interesting ones should come from the human voice. Consequently close proximity to the speech source is important at the early stage when auditory discrimination is developing. Children usually learn all about sounds on their mother's laps. Once they are mobile and move away from their mother it is less easy for them to do so. A child playing at the far side of the room will be able to hear his mother's voice, but may not be able to distinguish the various speech sounds at that distance. He then loses interest in verbal communication. Many children are ready, from the point of view of auditory awareness and discrimination, for this distance separation when they achieve independent mobility, but some are not, and in consequence they may suffer a delay in their language development. Likewise, some mothers sense that their children still need close verbal stimulation and so move about with their actively mobile children and enjoy sessions of close contact, but other mothers do not appreciate these needs, and when their child seems to be uninterested in what they are saying they resort to shouting to them (and at them).

Screening, and Other Tests for Hearing Loss

Good auditory discrimination for speech requires good hearing ability over the whole range of speech sound frequencies, and particularly in the higher frequencies because these carry the distinctive consonant characteristics (as shown in *Figure 51*). Any evaluation of hearing ability must, therefore, include a demonstration of satisfactory hearing

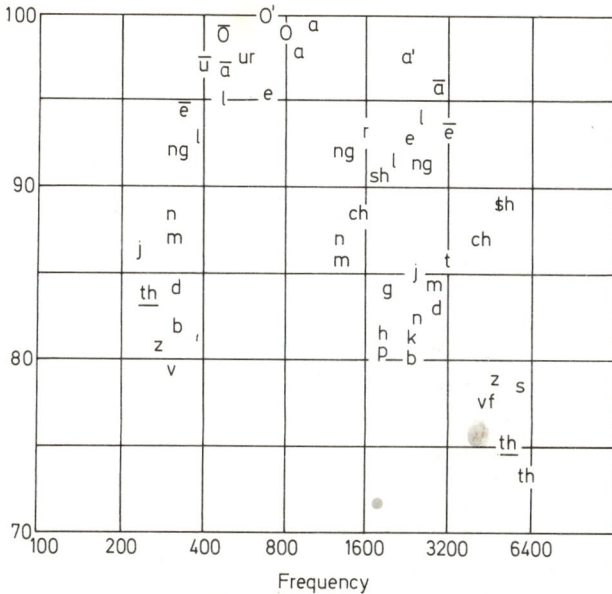

Figure 51. Sound frequencies of speech sounds (Fletcher and Harvey, 1953)

TABLE 14

Significance of Varying Degrees of Hearing Loss. (Fowler, 1939)

Hearing loss in better ear within speech range on audiogram (decibels)	Clinical effects
Less than 20	Usually not noticeable, may misunderstand whisper
20–40	Soft speech or poorly misarticulated speech misunderstood
40–60	Moderately loud speech often misunderstood
60–80	Even loud speech often not understood
Over 80	Shouted words often not understood
No hearing	Very loud shout not heard

at all these frequencies. The effects of various degrees of hearing loss are shown in Table 14.

Screening tests for hearing impairment provide an opportunity to explore a child's response to sound stimuli. In addition to noting any loss of hearing ability it is equally important to notice the degree of auditory alertness; the maturity and promptness of the responses; the ability to listen; the ability to detect sounds of short duration; the ability to discriminate between sounds; and the overall use the child makes of his ability to hear.

(1) Preliminary Examination in the First 6 Months

In a suitably quiet setting, sounds are made in the auditory sensitive cone area and the infant's responses noted. These responses consist at first of stilling, grimacing, blinking and even crying and later include turning of the eyes and head towards the side of the sound. The nature, especially the range of intonation, and the frequency of any vocalizations made by the infant during examination should be noted because abnormalities may provide a clue to diagnosis of developmental delay or deviation. The occurrence of early vocalizations does *not* exclude the possibility of deafness.

Cases of severe hearing loss may be detected as a result of screening tests in the early months, but many examiners prefer to rely upon tests carried out between 6 and 9 months when the infant's responses are more consistent and reliable and the tests are consequently easier to perform.

(2) Free Field Tests

Sounds are made in the air by the examiner at an appropriate position near the infant whose responses are being tested. The idea of these tests is simple and they are easy to carry out, but their value and reliability depend upon careful preparation, and failure to attend to several basic requirements can render the results useless. So much useful information can be learnt from these simple examinations if these are conducted properly that it is very sad to know that they are often done very casually and in quite inappropriate places.

The room used for the tests must be quiet and free from echo, but it need not be completely sound-free (in fact such a room is difficult to construct; is expensive; and is difficult to work in for long). Reflecting surfaces, shadows and draughts which might cause distraction and give false positive responses, should be avoided.

The examiner must be able to move about freely and quietly, hence there must be sufficient space, there must be a carpet on hard floors, and rustling clothes and rattling ornaments must be abandoned. It is necessary to be able to make sounds several feet lateral to either ear, so it is usually recommended that the room should be at least 10 to 12 feet long.

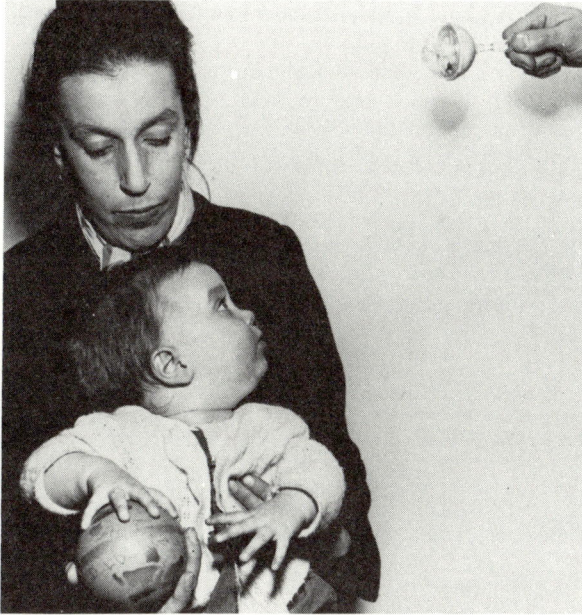

Figure 52. Free field hearing test

The infant must be comfortable, usually sitting on mother's lap and neither too sleepy nor too fretful (*Figure 52*). His attention is attracted by an assistant, who must learn to keep the stimulation at just the right level for the test and to avoid giving excessive visual stimulation or allowing tactile preoccupation with playthings both of which could lead to false negative responses in the test.

The tests are carried out using a variety of general sounds (e.g. scrape of spoon on cup, rattle, tap on wood, rustle of tissue paper, bell, voiced 's' or 'ff', or pure tones). In actually carrying out the test the sounds should not be too loud; for example, the spoon should be gently scraped along the inside of the cup (some examiners tap the cup sharply with the spoon but this is far too loud). It is possible to obtain a rattle which cannot produce sounds of more than 40 dB intensity. During the examination it is useful to have a sound-level meter near the child's ear in order to check the intensity of the sounds being received.

Adequate time must be allowed between test sounds to permit the infant to respond, and to avoid confusing him. Repetition of the same sound should be avoided because he may become bored and stop responding. It is also advisable to move frequently from one ear to the other.

The general sounds used in screening tests cover a wide range of frequencies so it is quite easy to miss a hearing loss affecting only certain frequencies. Consequently some of the high frequency voiced sounds should always be included, and a test with pure tones should be performed in every doubtful case.

A record is made of the promptness and type of the infant's responses; the maturity of localization; his vocalizations; and of any other features associated with this test.

The factors leading to fallacious results are listed in Table 15.

TABLE 15

Factors Leading to Fallacious Results in Hearing Tests

Hearing normal but deafness suspected because of lack of response

---

Tiredness or boredom of infant or examiner

Use of uninteresting or unfamiliar sounds

Use of same sound repeatedly

Making sounds in wrong position

Infant too preoccupied visually or tactilely

Examiner insensitive to minimal and delayed responses

Deafness present but missed because response observed

Infant visually alert and detects movements of examiner or his shadow

Examiner careless and makes movements in infant's visual field or touches infant's hair

Infant responds to draughts or vibrations

Examiner interprets chance movement as response

Examiner gives clues by facial expression

---

(3) Examination for Responses to Pure Tones

All the general sound-producing objects used in the free field tests produce sounds over a wide range of frequencies. To be quite certain that there is no impairment of hearing for certain frequencies, especially the high ones, it is necessary to obtain prompt responses to pure tones. In young children this may be achieved in several ways.

(a)   Pure tones from a hand-held audiometer may be used in free field tests.

(b)   Puppet audiometry (18 months onwards). The ear-pieces of an audiometer are placed inside glove puppets (*Figure 53*) and the child is encouraged to turn or point to the puppet producing the sound he hears. This technique provides a fairly accurate indication of a child's hearing ability and is useful for both young and handicapped children.

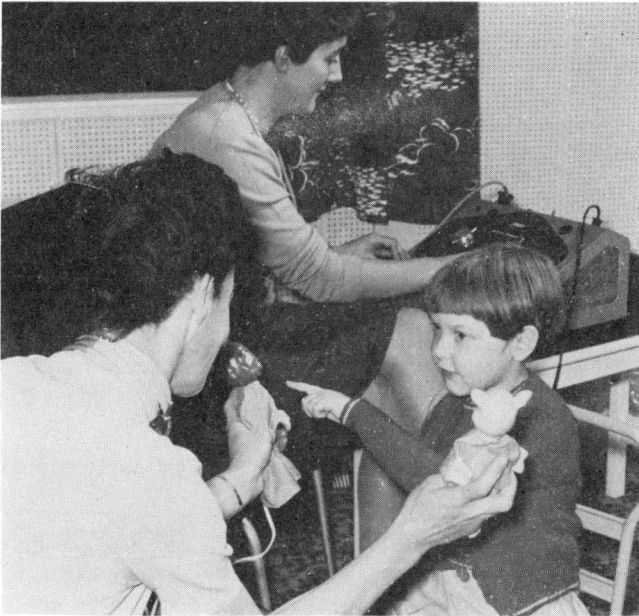

Figure 53. Puppet audiometry

(c)   Telephone audiometry (18 months onwards). The ear-piece of the audiometer is placed in the ear-piece of a telephone. A play situation is created. The child holds (or has held for him) the telephone to his ear and attempts to dial on hearing a sound.

(d) Formal audiometry. This requires acceptance of the head-pieces by the child, and his continuing co-operation throughout the test. It is usually feasible from 4 years onwards. The technique is described in standard otology references.

(4) Examination of Hearing for Speech and Auditory Discrimination

(a)   The examiner may use his own voice and note the response to particular words repeated progressively quietly. Usual words employed are 'go' and 'lift'. The latter is used to detect high frequency impairment. The child may be asked to make some action each time he hears the word: for example putting pegs into a board, or dropping cubes into a box.

(b)   The *Stycar Toys Test*. The child is asked to identify small toys placed on a table in front of him as their names are spoken quietly. There are three tests of increasing complexity. These tests must be administered according to the instructions and the name of the toy must not be altered. For example the ship is included because of the high frequency sounds associated with this word. To substitute boat invalidates the test. The three tests are as follows:
5-toy test: for normal children (18–24 months) —doll, ball, car, cup, brick;
6-toy test: for normal children (2–4 years) —spoon, doll, ball, car, cup, brick;
7–toy test: for normal children (3–7 years) —spoon, doll, fork, car, knife, plane, ship.

(c)   The *Michael Reed Picture Test* and the *Stycar Picture Test*. Pictures of familiar objects are placed before the child who must identify the correct one when the name is spoken quietly.

(d)   Word and sentence lists (e.g. *Stycar*). The child is asked to repeat words or sentences spoken quietly.

In all the above tests the pictures, words and sentences are chosen to be especially suitable for detecting auditory discriminative ability. Some contain high frequency sounds. Some sound very much like others, e.g. pin and pen, fish and dish. The tests should always be carried out in an appropriately quiet room, with the examiner saying the words at one side whilst the child's opposite ear is occluded, and holding a cover in front of his mouth to prevent the child seeing his mouth or feeling any draughts from it.

Techniques to Obtain Responses

Young children, retarded children and children with other disabilities may not be easy to examine. Two useful techniques in this connection are the following.

Conditioning   The child is assisted in carrying out some action every time an easily heard sound is made. This might be the dropping of a cube into a basket (a bowl is too noisy), or the placing of a peg into a board. The task should be kept as simple as possible, and sometimes the putting of pegs into a board is unsatisfactory because the child becomes too fascinated by the arrangement of the pegs. After a few trials he is encouraged to do this on his own. Once the procedure is understood testing can be carried out by presenting different sounds at lower intensities, a positive response being shown by the child performing the conditioned action.

Eye pointing and other actions   Severely disabled children may not be able to demonstrate any of the usual responses such as head turning,

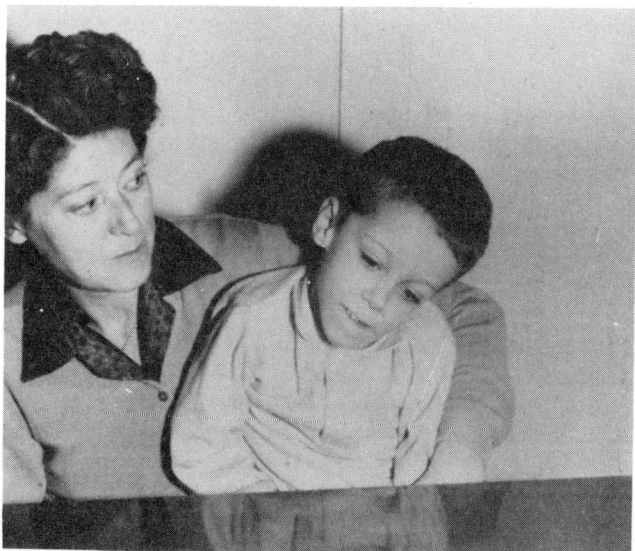

Figure 54. Eye pointing

speaking or lifting cubes. In these circumstances they may be able to show a response in some other way, e.g. grimacing, or moving toes. Eye pointing is a particularly useful technique which has enabled us to test many 'untestable' physically disabled children. This is shown in *Figure 54*.

EARLY VISUAL AWARENESS AND EXPLORATION

The essential visual element of the human eye, the retina, consists of two parts. The major, peripheral, part is spread out as a bowl-shaped light-sensitive receptor which is especially responsive to changes of light intensity and movement. The small, centrally situated part, the macula, is specialized for fine discriminative vision.

The peripheral retina is anatomically and functionally well developed at birth. A sudden increase in light intensity or a quick movement near the eyes cause the baby to blink protectively. This reflex mechanism soon becomes extremely sensitive and thereafter persists throughout life. The response may be so sensitive that the slightest movement or shadow in the peripheral visual field of a deaf infant during testing produces a response which is erroneously interpreted as due to the test sound.

The macula is not as well developed at birth as is the surrounding retina, but it soon becomes so. It is difficult to say just when a baby is first able to fix his gaze upon an object. This normally occurs in the first few weeks. Fixation appears to occur first upon objects of moderate size situated about one or two feet away from the eyes and which are clearly distinct from the background, such as when they are suspended on a string or placed on the end of a stick. Slight movement aids fixation, and the more interesting the object (e.g. the more pat-terned) the longer the duration of fixation, (Fantz, 1958). The infant's gaze is often first fixed upon his mother's face which possesses all the characteristics listed above and, in addition, the most valuable property of responsiveness. Consequently, what may begin as automatic or reflex visual fixation upon a nearby 'object' at about 5 or 6 weeks of age soon becomes the basis of a deeply significant and satisfying interpersonal relationship. The mother responds to the infant's gaze by animation of her face, movement of her eyes and vocalization. The baby responds to this global situation by smiling, and these actions and responses soon become mutually reinforcing.

The *doll's eye phenomenon* is observed in the first week or two of life. When the baby's head is turned to one side, the eyes lag behind. This soon disappears as head and eye positions and movements become associated.

In humans there is some overlapping of the two visual fields so it is essential that the eyes function as a single visual unit. The combined effective field of vision is available to explore the world to the front and sides of the child, but not posteriorly. Early fixation promotes conjugate action of the eyes which is further enhanced as visual following movements develop.

When an object upon which visual fixation has been obtained is moved slowly to one side, the eyes move to maintain visual fixation up to the limit of movement or interest. When fixation is lost the eyes return to their resting position. Such visual following occurs first in a horizontal plane over a limited range. The range of following increases rapidly with age, and simultaneously the ability appears to follow in vertical and oblique directions. Variations occur from infant to infant and so rigid criteria cannot be laid down, but any marked delay in fixation and following, and any failure to make progress, must be regarded with suspicion. Fixation and some horizontal following should be demonstrable at 6 to 8 weeks, and following in all directions should be well established by 6 months.

The early ability to visually fixate and follow is utilized in clinical tests of visual acuity in the early months of life. When an object consisting of contrasting fine black and white lines, or of black circles on a white background, is moved slowly in front of the eyes, nystagmus is induced providing that visual fixation upon the contrasting lines or shapes has occurred. The lines or circles are made smaller until fixation no longer occurs and nystagmus cannot be produced. This represents the limit of the infant's visual acuity. This subject was reviewed most recently by Catford and Oliver (1973). Using a specially designed portable nystagmus drum, they estimated that visual acuity in the young child was comparable to 6/18 at 5 months, 6/9 at 18 months, and 6/6 at 3 years.

The value of the abilities to fixate and to follow is greatly enhanced as stability of head posture is obtained. The visual field which the infant can explore is increased by controlled movement of the head and change of bodily position. Even so the range of the infant's visual interest seems to be limited to a few feet in the early months. If visual fixation is obtained upon an object or person which is then moved further away, the fixation will be lost after the first few feet. This appears to be a cognitive limitation rather than a visual one. The range of visual awareness expands more quickly than the range of auditory awareness.

One of the features of visual development at this early stage is the long steady periods of fixation which are observed. This is presumably a process by which the infant learns to visually identify familiar objects.

The development of visual recognition can be seen quite clearly when the infant gets excited upon seeing his bottle, or his mother. The process is stimulated by the linking of visual and tactile sensations. Many of the early tactile sensations occur by chance, as when a sweeping arm knocks the object under observation. If the infant is looking at the object as he knocks it the possibility of a visual-tactile link developing is present. Opportunities for this to occur at about 2 to 3 months of age are created by the asymmetrical tonic neck response which ensures that the arm on the side to which the child is looking is extended. From this simple beginning develops the following sequence:

      awareness of tactile contact—repetition of action, first accidentally then purposefully—visual control of movements—visual direction of active reaching—correlation of tactile impressions of objects with visual impressions of same object—development of ability to move object into visual field of interest.

Thus the infant rapidly acquires the ability to see—touch—take hold of—and bring towards himself objects within his immediate vicinity. Objects he can see are now in two groups. Those he can touch and those which he cannot touch. He is beginning to acquire an awareness of distance and of spatial relationships.

The visual and tactile exploration which has gone on in the early months helps the infant to achieve an awareness of the permanence of objects in the second half of the first year (Piaget). This further intensifies his visual searching. Many infants are extremely visually alert at this stage. Variations occur, but those who are most alert appear to be searching with their eyes all the time. They will look for every new object in their surroundings and will examine it visually with great preoccupation, often inhibiting responses to other stimuli (e.g. auditory) during this time. They enjoy playing games of looking for hidden objects.

The desire to visually explore stimulates mobility. The development of mobility, however this may be achieved (by rolling, shuffling, crawling etc.), enhances visual exploration and experiences. By this stage the infant's visuoperceptual world has expanded considerably. He is readily able to perform visual function tests at a distance of 3 metres (10 feet), as is especially well illustrated by the graded balls test of Sheridan (1969).

Graded Balls Test

Ten white polystyrene balls of different sizes from 0.3—6.25 cm (1/8 in—2½ in) are used. In one test they are rolled along a dark strip on the floor running horizontally to the line of the infant's gaze and 3 metres distant (*Figure 55*). They are rolled one at a time in random order and not always in the same direction. It is easy to observe infants' ability to fixate and follow these rolling balls.

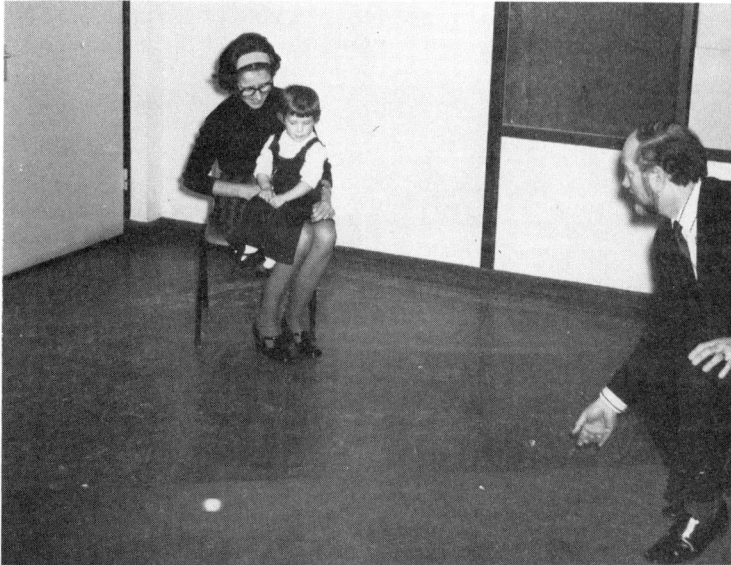

Figure 55. Rolling balls test

In another test the balls are mounted on thin rods and are presented from behind a screen placed 3 metres away from the infant (*Figure 56*). The background should be dark and non-patterned so that the balls show clearly as they are produced first at one point and then at another.

Infants from 6 months of age or so onwards respond well and enjoy these tests. Although the tests will reveal overall impairment of visual acuity they do not show the visual acuity of each eye separately. Sheridan (1973b) has related the results of the rolling ball tests at a distance of 10 feet to the visual acuity found by the nystagmus drum with the following results:

1/4 inch ball = 6/36
3/16 inch ball = 6/24
1/8 inch ball = 6/18 (after age of 18 months)

The development of visual exploration in infants may well be similar to the evolution of visual exploration of adults on encountering

new surroundings. At first new surroundings are searched visually in a
systematic manner, but as the scene becomes more familiar visual
searching is reduced to the identification of a few key items. Infants
similarly reduce their visual attention on objects, places and persons
with whom they are familiar. (Fantz, 1964). They now glance quickly—
identify the familiar object, and then pass on to other new and more
interesting items. The process has implications for the developmental

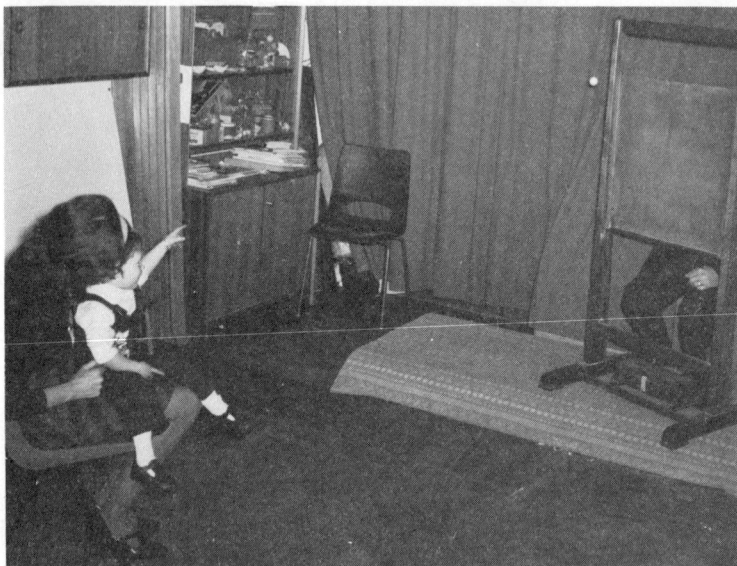

Figure 56. Mounted balls test

examination of children. If a child is very visually absorbed by a
particular object examiners must ask if this is because he is at that
stage of intensive visual exploration and learning, or, especially if it is
a very familiar object, if this stage is persisting longer than should be
the case. Similarly if an infant appears to pay scant attention to an
object examiners have to decide whether this is because visual acuity
is limited, or visual attention is poorly developed (as might be if he
were retarded), or if he is so familiar with the object that a quick
glance is all that is needed to identify it (and hence that he might be
a particularly bright child).

The developmental paediatrician is concerned with ensuring that a
child's eyes are healthy; that he is enjoying opportunities for visual
exploration of his world; and that these functions are developing
normally. He has a number of techniques at his disposal:

Screening, and Other Tests of Eyes and Vision

(1) *Examination of the neonate*

Ensure that the eyes are of normal size and appearance, lens and media are clear, that pupils are round, central, are responsive to light, and that the blink response is present. The examination can usually be done quite easily. If there is difficulty then observation during feeding or after the infant has been slowly rotated two or three times may help. Forceful opening of the eyelids should not be necessary. Nor is ophthalmoscopy part of the routine examination.

(2) *Examination in first 6 months*

Ensure that the eyes are of normal appearance, lens and media are clear, pupils are round, central, and responsive to light, and that the blink response is present. Observe fixation and following in both horizontal and vertical planes, noting range. Avoid using a sound-producing object for visual following at this age in case the eyes move reflexly to the sound and so give an erroneous response. Observe conjugate movement of eyes, convergence, and any visually directed reaching. Check visual acuity by nystagmus drum.

(3) *Examination: 6 months to 2½ years*

Repeat examination of the eyes as previously. Observe visual exploration, attention and preoccupation. Note fixation and following at up to 3 metres in the fixed and rolling graded balls tests. Observe conjugate movements of eyes, and convergence. Examine for strabismus (squint) by the reflected light test and cover tests (Stanworth, 1969).

In the *reflected light test* a small light of suitable intensity—i.e. bright enough for the reflexion of the light on the pupils to be seen easily, but not so bright as to be intolerable and cause screwing up of the eyes—is held about 12 inches in front of the child's face. As the child looks at the light the corneal reflections of the light should be symmetrical and situated in the centre of the pupils.

In the *cover test* each eye in turn is covered and then uncovered whilst the child visually fixates upon an appropriate object. As the eye is covered note is made of the following.

(a) Objection to the covering which if not due to apprehensiveness may indicate very poor vision in the uncovered eye. This is especially likely to be so if the response occurs when only one of the eyes is covered.

(b)   Readjustment of fixation by the uncovered eye indicating probable latent squint.

(c)   Unsteady fixation by the uncovered eye possibly due to poor visual acuity.

(d)   Latent nystagmus.

As the eye is uncovered note is made of re-adjustment of fixation by that eye which indicates probable latent strabismus.

Strabismus is abnormal from 6 months onwards and must receive attention. Note excessive intolerance to unilateral occlusion which may indicate contralateral amblyopia.

(4) Examination: 2 to 3 years

Repeat examination of previous period. Carry out the Stycar Miniature Toys Test. In the *Stycar Miniature Toys Test* the child is given a small tray or box lid containing seven small toys (chair, doll, car, plane, spoon, knife, fork). The examiner lifts similar toys one at a time from another box and the child is encouraged to copy this action. As soon as

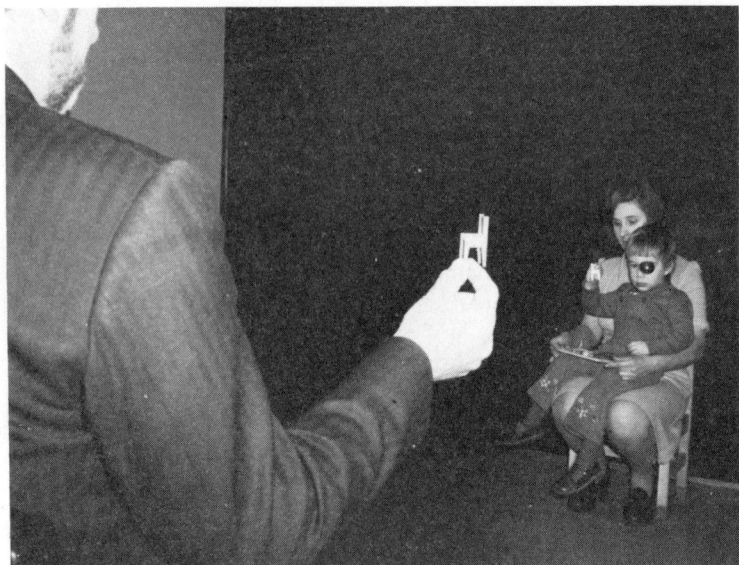

Figure 57. Miniature toys test of visual acuity

the child understands the procedure and is able to co-operate the examiner retreats to 3 metres, still retaining rapport, and holds each small toy in turn against a dark background. As the child picks out an identical toy he shows he has seen and identified the test object (*Figure 57*). *Ability to distinguish between the small fork and the small spoon and knife are crucial parts of this test* because it is thought that ability to recognize the small prongs of the fork corresponds fairly closely to the Snellen standards and represents a visual acuity of about 6/6.

Each eye can be examined separately with this test. Occlusion should be done as carefully as possible. The mother's hand, a wooden spoon, or a very light occluding disc on a spring fitting over the head are usually accepted by the child.

(5) *Examination: 2½ to 5 years*

The earlier examination can be repeated. The Stycar letter cards are used to test acuity of each eye separately at a distance of 3 metres and the Stycar or Sheridan–Gardiner near-vision cards are used to test the near vision of each eye separately.

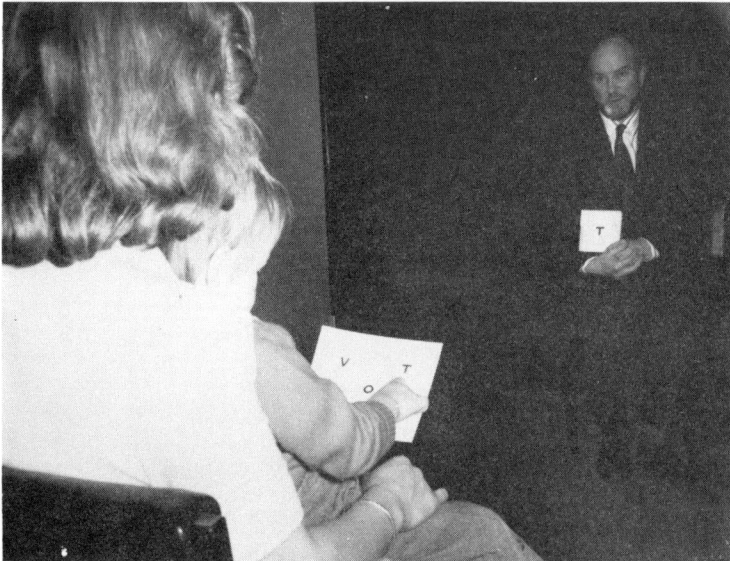

Figure 58. Stycar test of visual acuity

The letter card tests are particularly useful because each letter is on a separate card, the letters are chosen because they are those most easily recognized by young children, and the tests are arranged in a 5-, 7-and 9-letter series allowing selection to be made according to the child's age. The child is shown how to indicate his responses—either by pointing to the letter on the key card; by drawing the letter in the air; or by saying the letter if he knows it. After obtaining rapport by doing the test close to the child, the examiner retreats to 3 metres and carries out the full test at this distance (*Figure 58*). In order to be certain that distance visual acuity comparable to 6/6 is present, the test must be continued down to the smallest letters (3/3).

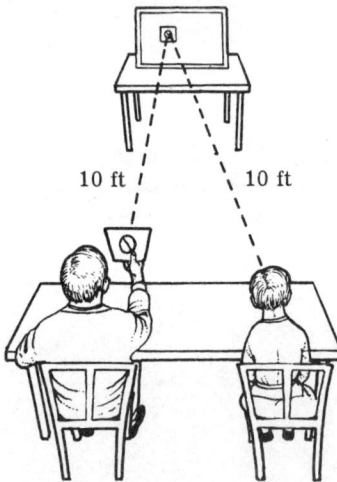

10 ft   10 ft

Figure 59. Special technique for the examination of distance vision in a young and apprehensive child

Very apprehensive children, or those with whom it is not possible to maintain rapport can be tested through a mirror with the examiner sitting next to the child (*see Figure 59*).

Near vision must always be tested.

(6) *Examination over 5 years*

This consists of visual acuity tests on each eye separately, for both near vision and distance vision at 6 metres (20 ft).

Colour vision can be tested in young (5 years of age approximately) and handicapped children by using Gardiner's test (Gardiner, 1973), and older children can be tested on the fuller Ishihara tests. Abnormalities occur more frequently in boys, and it is more pertinent therefore, to test colour vision in the examination of disabled boys. Tests of colour vision are even more essential nowadays when much greater use is being made of colour in educational equipment. Any child whose visual function appears to be abnormal or doubtful should receive a full ophthalmological examination, including refraction.

Gaze Fixation and Avoidance

A most important aspect of visual development is not really concerned with visual function as such but with emotional development. Gaze fixation and alignment are important aspects of interpersonal communication. Every mother attempts this gaze contact with her newborn baby (Klaus and Kennell, 1970; *Figure 60*) and the intense visual fixation and smiling in response which occurs in the early weeks is an

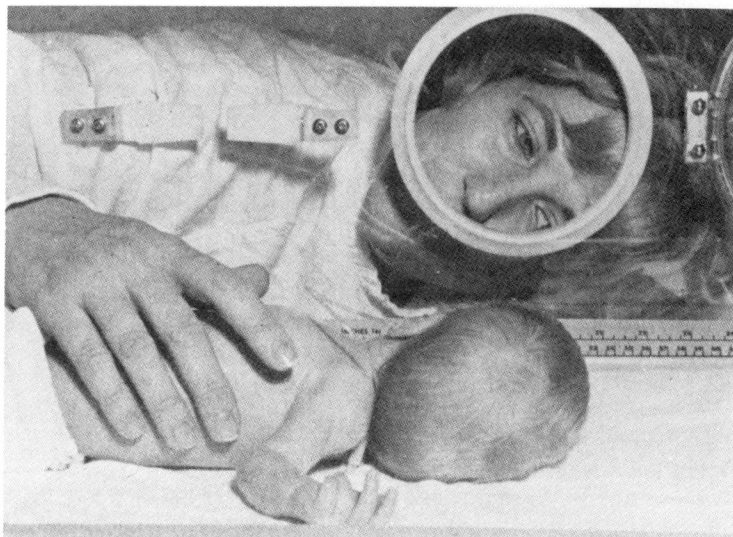

Figure 60. Gaze alignment by a mother with her newborn baby

extremely rich bond between baby and mother. One of the early stages of severe emotional disturbance in infancy can be failure of the development of gaze contact, and even the appearance of gaze avoidance. This phenomenon is easily seen by someone who is aware of the possibility, but otherwise may easily be overlooked. The detection of gaze avoidance requires referral for psychiatric appraisal.

TACTILE SENSATION

Very few studies have been made of the developmental aspects of tactile sensation, and examination of such sensations is not part of a usual developmental examination. This subject would repay study.

Testing tactile sensation is usually done as part of a neurological examination, consequently details of such tests can be obtained readily from neurological texts. The intention is not to repeat these details here, but to emphasize certain aspects of sensory tests which are not always appreciated and so lead to difficult and erroneous interpretation. Furthermore, the feasibility of the tests and the significance of the results is affected by the child's developmental level. When testing young children, therefore, it is essential to be clear about the precise nature of the test and what the child is being asked to do and how the child's developmental level will affect the test and results.

Tactile sensations fall into four categories with respect to the testing situation. These are as follows.

   (a)   Awareness of sensation—touch, pressure, pain, temperature, vibration, and joint movement.

The child must understand clearly what he is being asked to experience and must be able to make a response to indicate that he is aware of the particular sensation. Provided care is taken it is usually fairly easy to test these sensations.

   (b)   Localization of sensory contact.

This requires more intellectual ability by the child, including a knowledge of body parts, than does awareness of sensation.

   (c)   Discrimination between two or more sensations of similar nature administered either concurrently or successively, e.g. two simultaneous pinpricks, or two temperatures felt one after the other.

   (d)   Recognition of objects by tactile means.

These are not so much tests of tactile sensations as of the recognition and interpretation centrally of the information derived from tactile exploration. The development of this 'gnosic' ability has received considerable attention from French workers. The tests require considerable intellectual ability on the child's part to be reliable, but do provide interesting information about central function.

REFERENCES

Catford, G. V. and Oliver, A. (1973). Development of visual acuity, *Archs Dis. Childh.* **48**, 47

Fantz, R. L. (1958). Pattern vision in young infants, *Psychol. Rec.* **8,** 43

– (1964). Visual experience of infants: decreased attention to familiar patterns relative to novel ones, *Science, N.Y.* **146,** 668

Fisch, L. (1971). The probability of response to test sounds in young children, *Sound* **5,** 7

Fletcher and Harvey (1953). *Speech and Hearing in Communication: Combined Characteristics of the Fundamental Sounds of Speech.* Wokingham: Van Nostrand Reinhold Co.

Fowler, E. P. (1939). *Medicine of the Ear.* New York: Thomas Nelson

Gardiner, P. (1973). A colour vision test for young children and the handicapped, *Devl. Med. Child Neurol.* **15,** 437

Herckman, B. and Bench, J. (1972). Tonal stimulation of the human infant, *Sound* **6,** 1

Hoverstein, G. H. and Moncur, J. P. (1969). Stimuli and intensity factors in testing infants, *J. Speech Hear. Res.* **12,** 687

Klaus, M. and Kennell, J. (1970). Human maternal behaviour at the first contact with her young, *Pediatrics* **46,** 187

Martin, J. A. M. and Martin, D. (1973). Auditory perception, *Br. med. J.* i, 459

Murphy, J. P. (1964). *Reactions of Infants to Sound in Research in Deafness in Children,* Ed. L. Fisch. Oxford: Blackwell

Murphy, K. P. (1962). Ascertainment of deafness in children. *Panorama, December 3.* Reading: Linco Acoustics Ltd.

Robson, J. (1970). Screening techniques in babies, *Sound* **4,** 9

Sheridan, M. D. (1958). *Manual for the Stycar Hearing Test.* Windsor:NFER

– (1969). Vision screening procedures for very young or handicapped children, *Clinics Dev. Med. 32,* 39. London: Heinemann

– (1973a). *Children's Developmental Progress.* Windsor: NFER

– (1973b). The Stycar graded balls vision test, *Devl. Med. Child Neurol.* **15,** 423

Stanworth, A. (1969). The diagnosis and management of squint, *Clinics Dev. Med. 32,* 62 London: Heinemann

Walker, D., Grimwade, J. and Wood, C. (1971). Foetal response to sound, *Am. J. Obstet. Gynec* **109,** 91

Action and Ability: Responsiveness and the Acquisition of Skills; Examinations of Motor Activity

THE BASIS OF MOTOR SKILLS

Movement is an essential characteristic of living organisms. The simplest of organisms make spontaneous and often rhythmical movements. Organisms possessing even a very simple nervous system show reflex movements. More complex organisms show more complicated patterns of motor activities. Human beings acquire abilities to modify and to control reflex movements; to incorporate them into voluntary actions; to select movements for particular tasks; to combine movements into a flowing sequence; and to reproduce new patterns of movement. The repertoire of movements available to the mature person is very great indeed. These various actions and responses develop rapidly from fetal life onwards.

The fetus *in utero* makes movements which are felt by the mother from the middle of pregnancy onwards. Newborn babies show some apparently purposeless gross movements, and other movements which are reflexly determined and often serve a protective function, such as reflex turning of the head to the side when the baby is laid prone. From this relatively undistinguished start individuals acquire very complex motor skills such as piano playing and acrobatics. Many attributes are required to make these achievements possible.

Many of the movements of a newborn baby occur automatically or reflexly. Their frequency and intensity are influenced by the internal state of the baby as well as by external stimuli. Reflex movements are usually widespread and involve many muscle groups. They occur consistently and follow a stereotyped pattern in response to an often relatively trival triggering influence. Some reflexes have a protective function and others have a rôle in setting the pattern for different motor actions. Useful as they are, however, the grossness, consistency and stereotyped pattern of the responses have to disappear to enable a wider variety of selective motor actions to develop. The abilities which have to be acquired for motor actions to develop include the following:

(a)   the development of chain responses so that one movement leads into the next;

(b)   the acquisition of control of the speed and strength of the actions, and of the sequence and timing of the muscle actions to ensure smooth effective movements;

(c)   awareness of the task involved;

(d)   selection of the movements to carry out the task;

(e)   selection of the muscle actions to perform the movements;

(f)   awareness of different actions which can be used to achieve one particular task, and the choice of one of these;

(g)   choice of whether and when to carry out the action.

Emphasis is placed in the above list on 'awareness, selection and control'. This is done deliberately to stress their importance. Although peripheral structures such as limbs, digits and muscles are needed for motor actions, these are only effective if there is control and direction from the central nervous system.

A very simple action such as picking up a 1-inch cube will serve as illustration. The cube is seen. The infant must be aware of the cube and have a concept of it as a separate entity although the concept will probably be relatively crude and rough. The infant must have some awareness that he can touch, grasp or move the cube. The young infant reaches out, takes the cube in a palmar grasp. An older infant will perform the same action more quickly and smoothly and will take hold of the cube with a more mature finger grip. An even older child has a wider choice. He may decide he does not wish to reach out for the cube and having once seen it then ignores it, or he may decide to get the cube by some other means than reaching for it directly, for example by tilting the table so that it slides towards him. Once he has got the cube he may then take it to his mouth for further exploration. An older infant shows many other actions with the cube.

Considerable time elapses, however, before the full level of motor skill is reached. The processes which occur during this time are as follows.

(a)   The same movement is made more quickly and precisely and with less effort as unnecessary actions are suppressed.

(b)   Additional movements are incorporated with the action to make it more complete and effective.

(c)   Less and less associative checking occurs as more components of the action become automatic and 'internalized'.

(d)   Whilst one movement is being carried out, the succeeding one is being anticipated and prepared for.

These aspects will become more apparent as aspects of manipulation and locomotion are considered.

MANIPULATION

Study of the evolution of manipulative skills provides a fuller insight into the many factors which are involved than is achieved by simply listing the chronological appearance of manipulative actions. The mechanism and significance of the actions have to be analysed. When this is done, the principal items will be seen to be as follows:

(i)   maturation of neuromuscular actions;
(ii)   increase of speed and precision;
(iii)   development of new perceptual awareness;
(iv)   development of new skills.

These items will be better appreciated by analysing a manipulative action, such as the handling of cubes.

Manipulation of Cubes (*Figures 35 (c), 36 (d), 61 (a–c)*)

(a)The infant's grasp of a cube demonstrates the level of neuro-muscular maturation, the disappearance of the grasp reflex, and the development of the control of thumb abduction and opposition. It is difficult to place a cube in a baby's hand in the first few weeks because the effort usually intensifies the grasp reflex and causes the fist to clench even more. A cube can be placed in the hand at about 2 months of age and more certainly by 3 months. It is retained by a palmar grasp in which the ulnar side of the hand usually takes the larger share. This grasp gradually becomes more certain and by 6 to 7 months the radial side of the hand plays the predominant role. As the thumb increases in size and can be brought into opposition with the fingers, the grasp upon the cube moves from the palm to between the thumb and fingers.

(b) The strategies involved in taking up one or two cubes reveals much about an infant's perceptual awareness. When it is said that an infant at the age of 5 months shows voluntary grasp, it means that he is visually aware of the cube on the table in front of him and that he can direct his arm and hand into the appropriate position and take hold of it. He does this consistently and without delay by 6 months of age. When there is a second cube on the table, the infant may appear to be unaware of it, or he may be aware of it but do nothing about it, or he

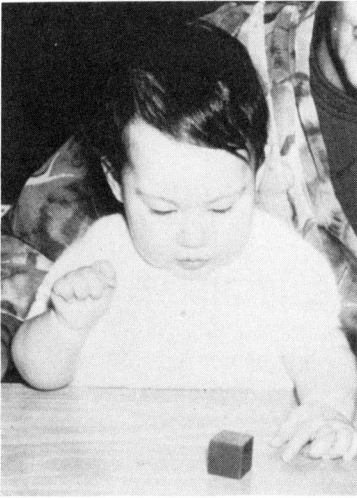

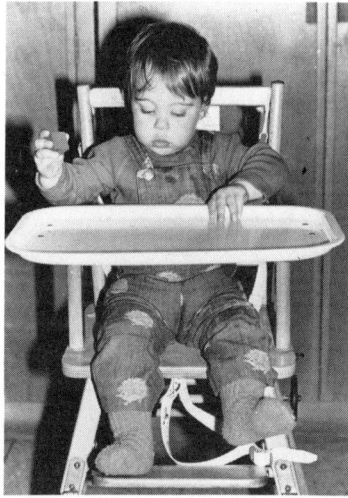

(a)

(b)

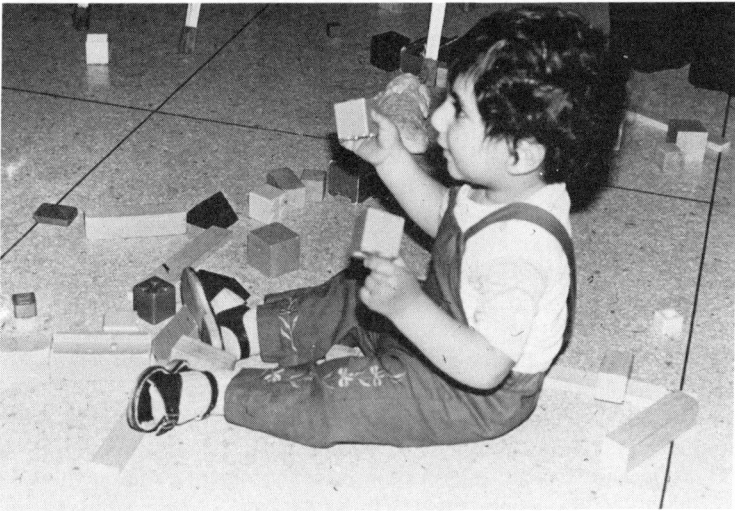

(c)

Figure 61. Handling cubes: (a) tentative approach to one cube; (b) secure thumb-finger grasp of cube in one hand; (c) grasps a cube in either hand, wonders how he can use them

may drop the first cube and take up the second with the same hand, or he may transfer the first cube to the opposite hand and then take up the second with the hand which had held the first one, or he may attempt to take up the second cube in the same hand as the first, or he may take up the second cube in his other hand. The possible actions are listed in the order in which they usually occur from 4 to 8 months, but individual babies sometimes show variations in the strategies which they employ.

(c) Study of an infant's reactions to cubes in either or both hands reveals more areas of developing perceptual awareness. Six months is usually accepted as the age at which most babies demonstrate their ability to transfer an object from one hand to the other. This is a different perceptuomotor skill to those described previously, and is one which promotes an awareness of cubes (or other objects) held by either hand. As this ability progresses infants will take cubes in each hand and then bring them together and compare them. This action may be seen at the age of 8 months, but many more months are required for infants to obtain all the information which is possible from such a comparison.

(d) Accidental release occurs early; voluntary release much later. It requires only relaxation of the flexor muscles of the fingers for gravity to cause a cube to fall from the hand. Voluntary release of a cube does not occur until the infant has an awareness of the object he is releasing and can voluntarily relax the flexor muscles. Consequently voluntary release of a cube is not seen until near the end of the first year.

Infants play at giving a cube before they are actually able to do so. An infant with a cube in his hand will push it into the examiner's hand as if giving the cube, but will then withdraw his hand still grasping the cube. As the ability to release develops the actions of giving, releasing and then withdrawing the hand are crude and exaggerated, but with practice more gentle release becomes possible. Once release is well established *casting* begins to appear. This consists of the deliberate dropping, pushing, and even throwing of objects from the cot, pram, or high-chair. It seems as if the infant wants to practise his new motor skill of release and to increase his awareness of space and the permanence of objects. Casting may seem to be an irritating habit, but its developmental value is considerable and this can be made even more important if the mother incorporates casting into play activity which reinforces the emotional links between herself and her baby.

(e) Introduction of a cup enables one to explore the child's ability to put cubes into and take them out of the cup, and his ability to detect a cube hidden by a cup. These actions explore developmental levels around 9 and 10 months of age. If an infant aged about 9 months is shown a cube which is then covered by an inverted cup, he will usually attempt to find the cube, revealing his awareness of its presence. Infants aged 10 months will usually take a cube out of a cup, and they may even put one in, but they keep hold of it and do not usually release it until they are a few months older.

(f) Building a tower of cubes requires considerable perceptual ability. The child has to be aware of the task, to be able to follow the demonstration, and to have the manipulative skill to carry it out. Some babies at one year of age understand what is required and make an attempt, but few succeed. Success comes a month or two later, and from then onwards they are able to build a higher tower at successive ages: 3 cubes at 1½ years, 6 at 2 years, and 9 at 3 years. With regard to this action, no new learning is involved during this time. The test is largely a measure of the child's manipulative ability combined with perceptual awareness of the task involved which was present from early in the second year. It is interesting to note the variations of the normal expectations in the test as quoted by different authors:

At the age of 2 years a tower of:

    2 or more cubes (Buchler & Hetzer, 1935; Stutsman, 1948) (Merrill–Palmer);

    4 cubes (Terman & Merrill, 1937; Valentine, 1958);

    5 cubes (Griffiths, 1954);

    6–7 cubes (Gesell & Amatruda, 1947; Illingworth, 1966; Sheridan, 1960; Bayley, 1965; Slosson, 1963).

These authors differ not only with respect to their expectations in these tests, but also in the way in which they are performed. For example, in the Merrill–Palmer test the child is expected to add 2 more cubes to a tower started by the examiner, or to build a 3-cube tower from the beginning. The Stanford-Binet requirement of a 4-or more cube tower is in imitation of the examiner's, whereas the Griffith's 5-cube tower is not so.

These simple examples show how much can be learnt from observing children building towers of cubes, and that reliance upon a precise score in a test may be misleading and dangerous unless the test and its method of administration are fully understood by the examiner.

(g) Other tasks with cubes. Once a child can build a tower of several cubes, his manipulative skill is quite good. More complex tasks with cubes explore both perceptual abilities as well as manipulative skills. Sometimes the child is asked to complete a particular task and is allowed unlimited time, but on other occasions his performance is timed or has to be completed within a time limit. These variations make interpretation difficult.

Examples are as follows: (*N.B.* This list is not compiled as a test and there are many more ways of utilizing cubes, but these examples should suffice to show how they can be used to explore various aspects of motor perception and skill)

Aligns 2 or more cubes as a 'train' (2 years, Gesell)
Aligns 3 or more cubes as a 'train' (2½ years, Bayley)
Adds 'chimney' to train   (2½ years, Gesell)
Builds a pyramid from 3 cubes in:
    17 seconds (3 years), 11 seconds (3½ years), 9 seconds (4 years), 7 seconds (4½ years) (Merrill—Palmer)
Builds a pyramid from 6 cubes in:
    35 seconds (4½ years), 20 seconds (5 years) (Merrill—Palmer)

Builds bridge by imitation (i.e. the child watches it being done and then does it himself) (3 years) and from model (i.e. child is shown completed item) (3½ years) (Gesell)

Builds gate by imitation (4 years) and from model (4½ years) (Gesell)

Manipulation of Pencil and Paper

Another aspect of manipulative skill which can be studied with advantage is a child's performance with pencil and paper. Several aspects will be considered;

Handling pencil and paper

Given an opportunity, children soon show an interest in using a pencil and paper in imitation of older children and adults. At first the grip upon the pencil is a cylindrical one with the pencil being treated rather like a rod (*Figure 62(a)*). The point projects from the lower, ulnar border of the hand and scribbling marks are made with a stirring-like action. If the pencil is taken into the hand the other way up, the child sometimes realizes that he can use it by pronating the forearm and so bringing the point into contact with the paper. Usually at this early stage when these grips are seen the child can do no more than scribble. This limitation is due mostly to immaturity and is not due just to the type of grip, because more perceptually advanced children are seen sometimes who for one reason or another retain this immature grip pattern, but are able, nevertheless, to make accurate reproductions on paper.

A big step forwards comes when the pencil is held between the thumb and fingers, especially the first two fingers (*Figure 62(b)*). These are usually held stiffly at first and only later do they relax so that the

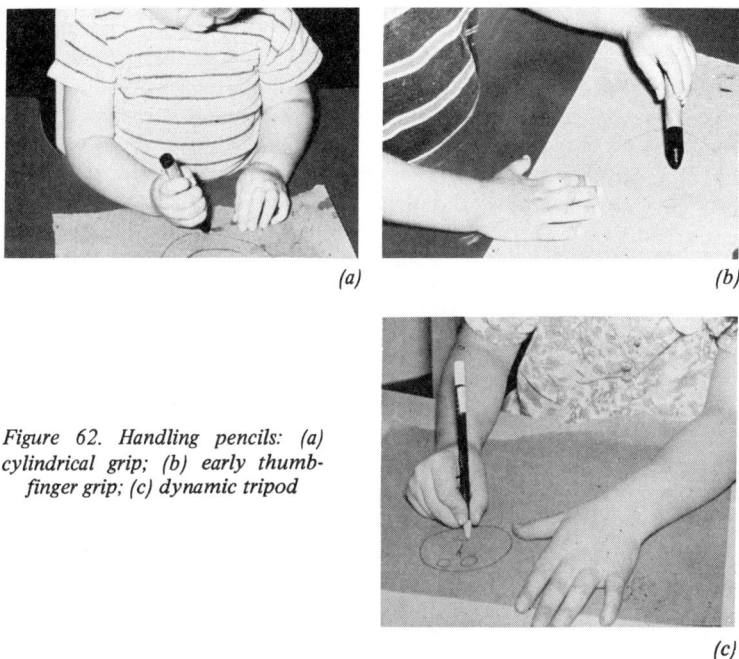

(a)

(b)

Figure 62. Handling pencils: (a) cylindrical grip; (b) early thumb-finger grip; (c) dynamic tripod

(c)

full benefit of the mature grip can be appreciated (*Figure 62(c)*). This grip is called the dynamic tripod in order to emphasize that three digits are involved together (thumb, index finger and middle finger) and that they are constantly moving to adjust the position of the pencil.

Handedness

Handedness is a very extensive and complex subject which can be discussed only briefly here. Children show a preference for one hand or the other during their second year, and they use this hand more readily and more frequently than the other one. As this preference becomes established, it is so well marked and consistent for some children that there is no doubt that they are right-or left-handed. In other cases the preference is not so marked, and in the early years, at least, there may be some variation from time to time.

Much has been written, often rather uncritically, about the implications of ill-defined hand preference and its relationship to cerebral dominance, neurological disturbance and learning difficulties. A more sceptical attitude to some of the sweeping assertions which have been made is now appearing, fostered considerably by studies which show little or no relationship between laterality anomalies and subsequent problems. A recent critical review of this topic by Touwen (1972) is especially useful. At the present time there are several generalizations which are widely accepted.

(a)   Any child showing extremely strong preference for one hand may have some neurological deficit of the other side.

(b)   Left-handed children have to make many more adjustments then right-handed children because many everyday articles are arranged for the right-handed majority of users, e.g. door handles. Also, writing from left to right across a page is easier for right-handed than for left-handed children. When writing with the left hand the writing already on the sheet is obscured by the hand unless, as often happens, some unusual posture is adopted. Barsley (1966) described the problems encountered by left-handed people very vividly.

(c)   Amongst children with uncertain and mixed preferences there is a greater than average number with neurological disturbances.

(d)   It is most dangerous, however, to attribute a child's difficulties to handedness problems without very careful evaluation.

Preferred handedness, footedness and eyeness can be determined by simple tests in which the child is asked to carry out simple actions, for example:

Handedness	Footedness	Eyeness
Pick up a pencil to write	Kick a ball	Look into a telescope held for him
Put a small object in a box	Tap a tune with a foot	Align a gun on target
Press a bell-push	Squash a small object with a foot	Examine a suitable object e.g. postage stamp, with a magnifying lens held for him

Although these are simple tests, care is required in order to avoid misleading results. For example, the objects for the child to pick up must be placed before him in the mid-line, and objects for the child to look into or through must be held for him; otherwise, if the child is allowed to take it up himself, he will do so with his preferred hand and will then be more likely to use the eye on that side because it is easier to do so whether or not it is the preferred eye. Also, whenever eyeness is being tested, it is important to ensure that visual function is equal on the two sides. Obviously, differences in visual function will affect eye preference, yet there have been scores of reports on laterality and crossed laterality which have ignored this point. More complicated tests exist for a full investigation of laterality such as those described by Benton (1959).

Imitating and copying symbols

Most children love to play with pencil and paper, and observing whether or not they can reproduce various symbols gives information about their perceptual awareness. Ability to draw straight lines running horizontally, vertically and obliquely, lines joining and crossing, areas enclosed by circles and by angulated figures and so forth are examined in many of the psychological tests for young children. In the performance and scoring of these tests, a clear distinction must be made between *imitation*, i.e. the child draws the symbol after seeing the examiner do so, and *copying*, i.e. the child draws the symbol from a picture of the completed symbol which is placed in front of him either throughout, or for a set period before he is asked to draw. A definite developmental sequence is seen in the reproduction of symbols and this is summarized in *Figure 63*. This figure is not meant to represent a test, but to show the developmental sequence observed and the approximate age levels.

Symbol		Approximate age level in years	
		Imitation	Copy
/	Stroke–random	$1\frac{1}{2}$	–
|	Stroke–horizontal or vertical	2	$2\frac{1}{2}$
○	Circle	2	3
+	Cross	3	$3\frac{1}{2}-4$
□	Square	$3\frac{1}{2}-4$	$4\frac{1}{2}$
△	Triangle	$4-4\frac{1}{2}$	5

Figure 63. The developmental sequence of symbol imitation and copying

When these abilities are examined in tests, definite criteria are laid down concerning the manner of presentation of the task, the number of attempts which are permissible and whether or not the symbol produced can be accepted. There is considerable individual variation in these skills and performance is affected by many factors, especially the environment of the test, the state of the child, and his previous experiences with pencil and paper.

Drawing

Children's drawings reflect their draughtsmanship, perceptual awareness, knowledge and understanding of the world around them, and their personal feelings. They are a rich source of exploration for any student of child development and behaviour. A child's awareness of body parts and their relationships is brought out in the Goodenough 'Draw a Man Test.' The child is asked to draw a man and is given all the time he requires to do so. He may be prompted to make sure that he has included everything. Then one point is awarded for each of the items of the drawing which is on the list below (no half points).

1.   Head present—any clear method of representing the head.
2.   Legs present—any method of presentation clearly intended to indicate legs. Number must be correct for the position.
3.   Arms present—any method of representation clearly intended to indicate arms. Fingers alone not sufficient—credit if any space left between base of fingers and body where attached. Number must be correct.
4.   (a) Trunk present—any clear indication of trunk, whether by straight line only, or by some sort of two-dimensional figure.
(b) Length of trunk greater than breadth—measurement should be taken at points of greatest length and breadth. If equal score minus.
(c) Shoulders definitely indicated—ordinary elliptical form never credited, score minus if trunk square or rectangular.
5.   (a) Attachment of arms and legs—both arms and legs attached at any point, or arms to neck, or at junction of head and trunk.
(b) Legs attached to the trunk. Arms attached to trunk at correct point. If (4(c) plus, point of attachment must be exactly at shoulders. If 4(c) minus, attachment must be exactly at point where shoulders should have been indicated.
6.   (a) Neck present—any clear indication.
(b) Outline of neck continuous with that of hand, or trunk, or of both.
7.   (a) Eyes present—either one or both.
(b) Nose present—any clear method of representation.

(c) Mouth present—any clear method.

(d) Both nose and mouth shown in two dimensions—2 lips shown.

(e) Nostrils shown—any clear method.

8.　(a) Hair shown—any clear method.

(b) Hair present or more than the circumference of the head. Better than a scribble. Non-transparent, i.e. outline of head not showing through the hair.

9.　(a) Clothing present—any clear method, e.g. buttons.

(b) At least two articles of clothing (as hat and trousers) non-transparent, i.e. concealing part of body supposed to cover.

(c) Entire drawing free from transparencies of any sort. Both sleeves and trousers must be shown.

(d) At least 4 articles of clothing definitely indicated—hat, coat, shirt, collar, tie, belt or suspenders, trousers.

(e) Costume complete without incongruities—a definite and recognizable kind of costume, e.g. suit. No confusion permitted. Hat must always be shown if part of costume, e.g. uniform. Sleeves and trousers must be shown, also shoes.

10.　(a) Fingers present—any clear indication.

(b) Correct number of fingers shown—5 or 10, according to hands shown.

(c) Details of fingers correct, 2 dimensions, length greater than breadth; and the angle subtended by them not greater than 180 degrees.

(d) Opposition of thumb shown—any clear differentiation from fingers.

(e) Hand shown as distinct from fingers and arms.

11.　(a) Arm joint shown—either elbow, shoulder or both—curve only at elbow score minus.

(b) Leg joint shown—either knee, hip or both—abrupt bend for knee. Hip, if inner lines of legs meet at point of junction with body, credited.

12.　(a) Proportion. Head—area not more than half or less than one-tenth of trunk. Score rather leniently.

(b) Proportion. Arms—equal to trunk in length or slightly longer, but not reaching knees. Width of legs less than trunk.

(c) Proportion. Legs—length not less than vertical measurement of trunk, nor greater than twice that. Width of legs less than trunk.

(d) Proportion. Feet—feet and legs must be shown in two dimensions. Length of foot must be greater than height from sole to instep. Length of foot not more than 1/3 or less than

1/10 total length of leg. Credited on full-face if · shown in perspective, provided foot separated in some way from rest of leg.

(e) Proportion. 2 dimensions. Both arms and legs shown in 2 dimensions.

13. Heel shown—any clear method. Credited in full-face drawings where foot is shown in perspective.

14. (a) Motor co-ordination. Lines A. All lines reasonably firm, meeting each other clearly. Degree of complexity of drawing to be taken into account—if few lines score more severely.

(b) Motor co-ordination. Lines B. All lines firmly drawn with correct joining. (Score very strictly).

(c) Motor co-ordination. Head outline—outline of head without obviously unintentional irregularities. Simple ellipse not credited.

(d) Motor co-ordination. Trunk outline—as for (c).

(e) Motor co-ordination. Arms and legs without irregularities and without tendency to narrowing at junction with body. Arms and legs in 2 dimensions.

(f) Motor co-ordination. Features symmetrical in all respects— eyes, nose, mouth in two dimensions. Score strictly. More likely to be plus if profile rather than full-face.

15. (a) Ears present—one or two according to profile or full-face. Any clear method.

(b) Ears present in correct position and proportion—vertical measurement must be greater than horizontal—in profile some detail for aural canal. Within middle of 2/3 of head.

16. (a) Eye detail—brow, lashes or both shown. Any clear method.

(b) Eye detail—pupil shown—dot with curved line above not credited as dot represents eye itself and is credited in 7(a).

(c) Eye detail—Proportion—horizontal measurement of eye must be greater than vertical.

(d) Eye detail—Glance—face must be in profile—eye shown either in perspective or, if almond form, pupil must be placed toward front of eye rather than in centre.

17. (a) Both chin and forehead shown—eyes and mouth present, sufficient space left for chin and forehead. Score rather leniently.

(b) Projection of chin shown; chin clearly differentiated from lower lip.

18. (a) Head, trunk and feet shown in profile without error. One only of these errors allowed: bodily transparency, legs not in

profile, arms attached to outline of back and extending forward.

(b) Figure shown in true profile, without error or bodily transparency, except that shape of eye may be ignored.

Each point credited is the equivalent of a quarter of a year. To calculate the mental age, count the total number of points scored and divide this by 4. Add 3 to the result. This gives the mental age in years (3 years is credited as this is immediately below the age level at which the scoring begins). 40 points gives a mental age of 13 years. The scale is not valid beyond this, although the maximum score on the test is 51 points (Goodenough, 1926 and *Figures 64 (a)* and (b).

Observing a child's drawing of a house reveals his awareness of spatial relationships and of perspective. Free drawings, especially if accompanied by discussion with the child, provide much information about conceptual and emotional development which is beyond the scope of this volume. The interested reader is referred to the considerable literature on this subject*.

Writing

Pencil and paper skills culminate in the act of writing. This complex skill requires an appreciation of the individual symbols and their sequence and an ability to reproduce them accurately, precisely and quickly. Over the years children have been taught various methods of writing. Each method has its merits. Some emphasize clarity of reproduction, others neatness and regularity, others an easy flowing style, and so forth. So many factors affect a child's writing ability that it is often difficult for even an experienced teacher to say whether a particular sample is abnormal or not. Nevertheless it is useful for the developmental paediatrician to have some guide as to what to expect at different ages and those shown in *Figures 45 (a–f)* have proved quite useful in this respect.

Tea-set play

Doll's tea-set play reveals the development of a young child's manipulative ability particularly well. This is a fascinating task for a 2 to 5-year-old child and is seldom associated with any difficulties of administration. Horton and Rosenbloom (1971) used this technique to study

*Bender L. (1938). *A Visual Motor Gestalt Test and its Clinical Use,* New York: American Orthopsychology Association.

Harris, D. B. (1963). *Children's Drawings as Measures of Intellectual Maturity,* New York: Brace and World Inc.

Di Leo, J. H. (1967). *Young Children and their Drawings,* London: Constable.

manipulative skill in young children. They analysed the movements and efforts involved in the task. It is worthwhile consulting their original paper for a full description of their findings. Whilst children play with the tea set observations are concentrated upon the teapot and note is

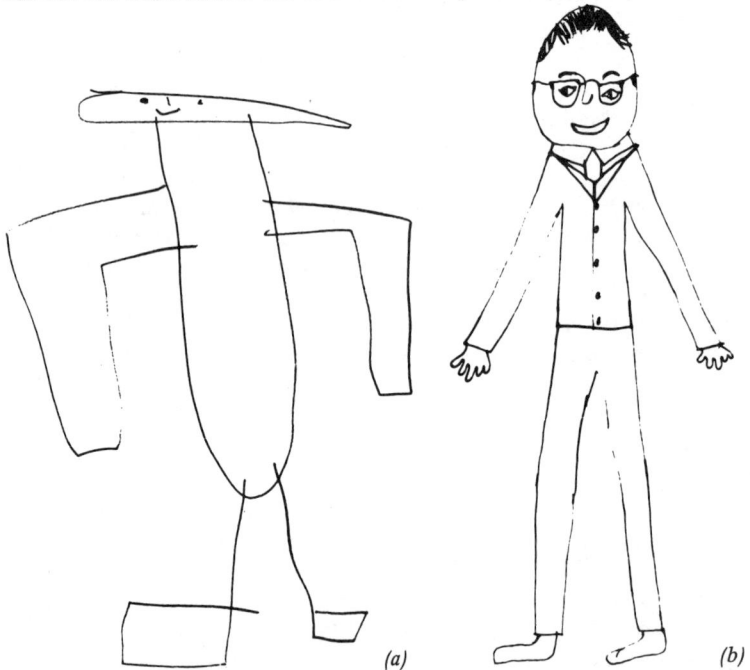

(a)   *(b)*

Figure 64. Goodenough Draw a Man Test: (a) drawing by boy aged 7 years with a mental age of 7 years; (b) drawing by boy aged 8 years with a mental age of 11½ years

made of how the child holds and controls the teapot in pouring, the adjustment of height of pouring, appreciation of degree of filling of the cup and overall precision and freedom from spilling. This method is not a standardized test, but a definite sequence occurs in the development of skill in handling the teapot and it is possible to indicate approximate age levels for the different stages, as follows:

(a)   Holds teapot handle with a cylindrical grip and may steady it with other hand; attempts to pour without lifting teapot or only lifting part way; frequently spilling occurs—around 2½–3 years of age (*Figure 65 (a)*).

(b)   Holds teapot handle with a cylindrical grip; raises teapot to pour, but height and position in relation to cup may be ill judged and frequent spilling occurs—around 3–3½ years of age (*Figure 65 (b)*).

(c) Holds teapot handle with a cylindrical grip and with hand rotated so as to permit control of the teapot by radio-ulnar movement at the wrist; much better judgement of distances and of filling of cup; little spilling occurs—around 3½–4 years of age (*Figure 65 (c)*).

(d) Teapot handle held with a cylindrical grip as before and also with thumb on spine of handle to give better control in pouring which is now more precise and there is no spilling—around 4–4½ years of age (*Figure 65 (d)*).

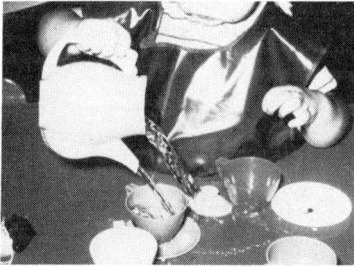

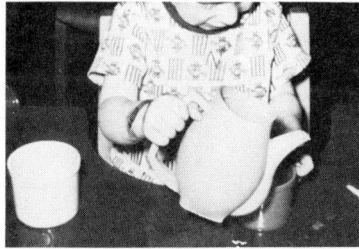

(a)

(b)

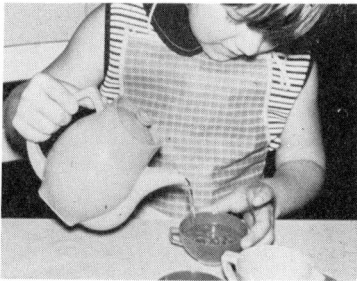

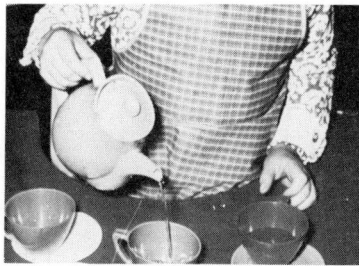

(c)

(d)

Figure 65. Dolls tea-set play. Handling teapot: (a) early stage, cylindrical grip, poor positioning and spilling; (b) positioning still imprecise; (c) hand rotated to give better control; (d) precise positioning and pouring

Pegs and cup manipulation

Some years age I described a simple test of manipulation which has proved very useful in clinical practice (Holt, 1965). It also shows neatly the maturation of motor skills. A child of one year can pick up a small peg and drop it into a cup. The task is already understood at this early age, but performance is very imperfect. Performance improves steadily with age, as is shown by the ability to carry out the task more and more quickly, but the maximum speed is not obtained for several years. It takes all this time to perfect all the neuromuscular components concerned in this skill. Up to 10 years of age the relationship between speed and age is virtually linear, so it is possible to devise tests based upon age norms.

In the tests the child is asked to pick up pegs one at a time and to drop them into a cup as quickly as he can. The best score in three tries over a set time—usually 30 seconds—is noted. The child is then asked to take up pegs one at a time and to place them in a peg board.

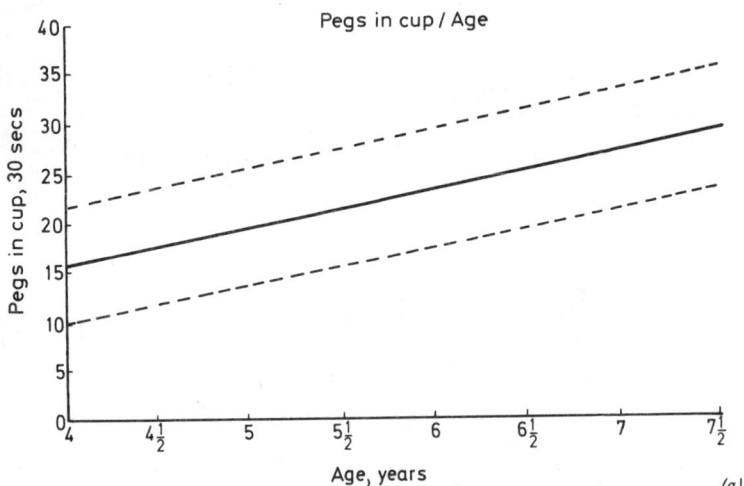

(a)

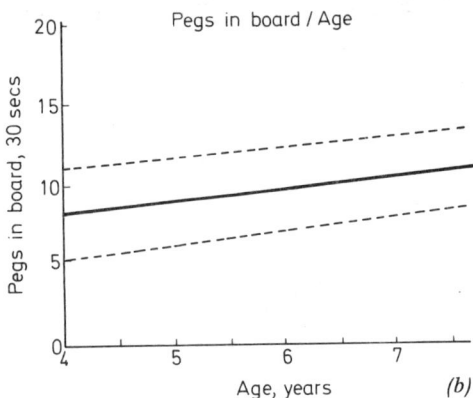

(b)

Pegs in cup–in board / Age

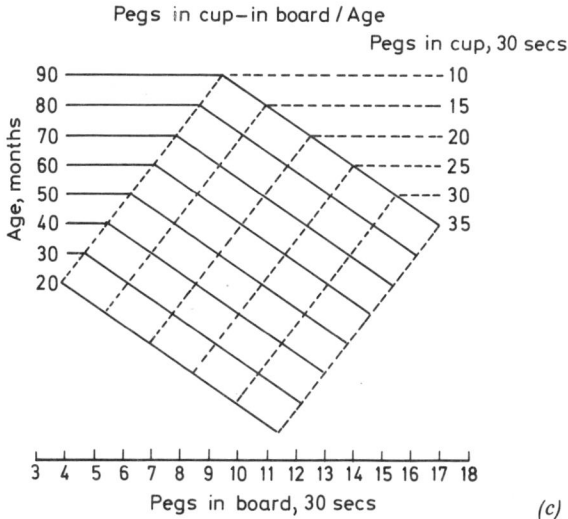

Figure 66. Manipulation tests–pegs and cup: (a) relationship
between number of pegs in cup in 30 seconds and age; (b)
relationship between number of pegs in board in 30 seconds
and age; (c) prediction of score on board test from age and
score in cup test

The best score in three tries in a set time—usually 30 seconds—is noted.
The results in both these tests are related to age. The score on the
second test is directly dependent upon the score of the first test, so
knowing the child's age and score on the first test, it is possible to
predict the score which should be obtained on the second test
(*Figure 66(a–c)*). If the actual score is appreciably below that pre-
dicted, this is a clear indication of impairment of manipulation. This
test enables one to examine manipulative ability without confusion
from intellectual influences.

This, and other tests of manipulative function are described more
fully elsewhere (Holt, 1965).

Ball skills

A child's behaviour with a ball reveals much more manipulative ability,
and in addition shows the importance of timing and perceptual awareness of the task. Kay's (1970) description of all the events involved in
catching a ball is particularly lucid and should be read by all who study
this subject. The 50 per cent levels (i.e. the age at which 50 per cent of

children are able to achieve that level of performance) for various ball abilities are shown in Table 16 (McCaskill and Willman, 1938).

TABLE 16

Fifty Per Cent Age Levels for Certain Ball Skills of Children

Bounce along with one hand a distance of:	3 feet	2 years
	5 feet	3½ years
Catch with arms straight		3 years
Catch with arms bent		4 years
Throw with one hand a distance of:	5 feet	2½ years
	10 feet	4 years
	15 feet	5½ years

Ball throwing skill varies greatly between children. At each age there is a wide range on either side of the mean, and there are also marked sex differences, as shown in Table 17 (Keogh, 1965).

TABLE 17

Variability of Ball Throwing Skill According to Age and Sex

	Age and sex			
	5 years		10 years	
	Male	Female	Male	Female
Distance thrown in feet, mean	34	19	94	49
2 Standard deviations mean (assumed as the minimal acceptable normal level)	22	4	52	13

LOCOMOTION AND GROSS MOTOR SKILLS

Gesell and Amatruda (1947) described the cephalocaudal progression of early gross motor development. The biological value of this observed sequence is obvious. The early stabilization of the head greatly facilitates survival by making feeding easier, and also enables the child to become aware of the world around through the use of his eyes and ears. The features of early motor development have been described many times. They are best considered as they occur in the supine, prone and upright postures as summarized in Table 18.

TABLE 18

Features of Early Motor Development in Supine, Prone, and Upright Postures

Posture	Requirements for progress	Advantages	Disadvantages
Supine	Head flexion & stability; Symmetry; Ability to support trunk upright	Hands free early facilitating early play & hand-eye co-ordination	A static posture apart from babies who shuffle
Prone	Head extension & stability; Control of symmetrical tonic neck reflex; Symmetry	Leads to early mobility by hauling or crawling	Hands occupied
Upright	Stability of head & trunk against gravity; Balance and fine control of distribution of body weight	Socially acceptable and effective mobility; Hands free	Time taken to acquire anti-gravity postural control

As the baby is raised to the sitting position from the initial supine posture the head becomes increasingly stable on the shoulders. Then the head is raised in anticipation of being pulled to sitting, and it also becomes sufficiently stable on the shoulders for the infant to be able to be placed in a supported sitting position. As independent sitting develops the back becomes more erect, and the widespread legs provide a broad base. The appearance of the upper arm protective reflexes at this stage increases stability in the sitting position, because if the infant topples forwards or sidewards the arms spontaneously extend and so help to restore the original position. As confidence develops many children enjoy the sitting position because it leaves their hands free for play and exploration. This is usually a static position and many infants appear happy to sit as unmoving masters of their little play area. A few infants, however, move by shuffling on their bottoms. Robson (1970) claims that there is a familial tendency to bottom-shuffling. Bottom-shufflers, without any other apparent abnormality acquire independent walking later than other children. From sitting some infants fall forwards to assume a crawl position and some lean forwards to hold on to a firm object and then contrive to pull themselves to standing.

The first feature of gross motor development in the prone posture is head stabilization which is achieved by some degree of extension of the neck, and not with flexion of the neck as occurs with head stabilization in the supine posture. Ability to support the chest on first the forearms and then the hands develops next. At this stage the baby in prone posture is much more proficient above the waist than below so far as motor skills are concerned. There are two interesting associa-tions: firstly, some babies who are very familiar with the prone posture acquire an ability to pull themselves forwards or push themselves backwards with their arms. This is called *hauling* or *scooting*. Secondly, an infant will be seen from time to time in whom this motor discrepancy between the upper and lower parts of the body persists. This often presents a diagnostic problem, but in many cases locomotor develop-ment does ultimately occur although it is likely to be later than usual. (Hagberg & Lundberg, 1969). The prone posture is particularly adapted to movement. Movement involving both arms and legs and with the trunk on the floor is known in Britain as *creeping*, and it usually occurs before *crawling* in which the trunk is held off the floor and is supported by the four limbs. Crawling can be a most effective means of movement, but if the infant wants to use his hands he must stop and fall back to a sitting position. From a crawl position some infants are able to pull themselves to standing.

The upright posture is so much an anti-gravity posture that infants have to be held supported in this position in their early months. Initially a stepping reflex may be elicited. This is not true walking because there is no pelvic stability. The reflex is suppressed, and at about 6 months of age is replaced by a positive supporting reflex in which the lower limb muscles contract and turn the legs into. very good supporting pillars. In this way the infant is helped to acquire a sense of anti-gravity balance, and to learn to maintain an upright posture with less and less muscle effort. Increasing confidence when standing with support or holding on to a firm object enables the infant to make movements of the legs which lead to *cruising*. From this point the infant progresses to independent standing and to taking his first steps on his own. Both cruising and pulling to standing are important actions for they promote strength and stability of the hip musculature. From standing an infant can drop to sitting or crawling postures, but, in most instances, once a child is on his feet he wants to be off walking and exploring.

In normal individuals development in the different postures, prone, supine and upright, occurs simultaneously and the child is able to change from one posture to another very easily. Early motor development in normal infants shows an easy flexible interchange between the different postures. This flexible interchange between postures does not occur in some neurologically impaired children, and studies of their motor development have revealed the features of development in the different postural pathways as described above. Motor development as observed consists of a combination of motor abilities in each of these postural pathways, as illustrated in *Figure 67*. Progression to a new ability, it is suggested, probably occurs as a result of progression from a previous motor activity in the same posture and not necessarily as a result of a previously exhibited motor skill in a different posture. For example, shuffling develops as a progression from earlier activities in the supine posture, and not because of a previous ability to scoot, nor does shuffling prepare a child for a future ability to crawl.

The fact that a motor skill arising from one posture does not necessarily prepare for the development of a motor skill based upon another posture is further supported by a consideration of the muscles involved and the kinaesthetic stimuli arising from the different actions. For example, compare the sitting posture at 9 months with the crawl posture at the same age. In the former posture the short hip extensor muscles are relaxed and only contract briefly if they are required for postural support. In the latter posture, however, they have to be prepared to contract alternately to extend the thigh at the hip whenever crawling is attempted. The muscles are used quite differently, and the kinaesthetic stimuli are different in the two situations. Recognition that early motor development is composed of progress in the supine, prone and upright postures, makes it easier to understand (and to accept) the facts that the pattern of motor development may vary from child to child, and that some features of motor development may be omitted altogether even in perfectly normal children. All children do not have to go through all the stages of sitting—crawling—standing in a strict order. Nor does there seem to be any justification for forcing a child to do so because it is thought, erroneously, that failure to follow a set pattern accounts for some disability at a later age. The

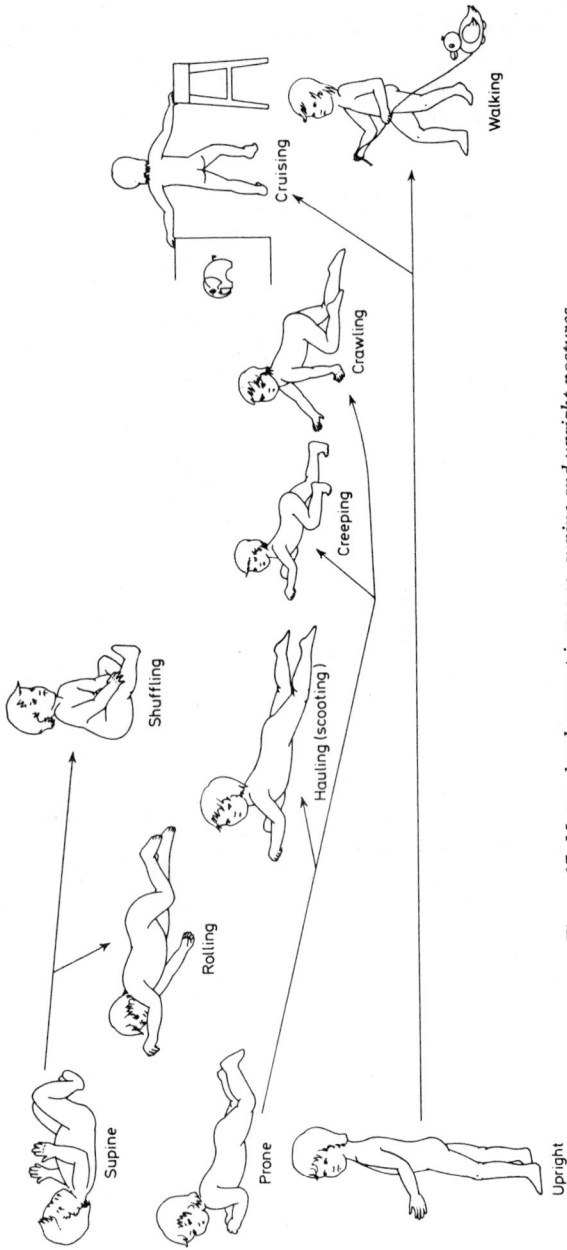

Figure 67. Motor development in prone, supine and upright postures

evolution of motor development in the different postures is illustrated in *Figure 67*.

Most children follow a fairly similar pattern of early motor development. Those who follow a less common pattern should be examined carefully because there is a greater incidence of motor abnormalities in this group. Nevertheless, some who show deviant motor patterns are perfectly normal and the recognition of this can save much parental anxiety and distress. Normal variations of early motor development have been studied very fruitfully by Robson (1970, 1975) and he has now described the ages at which children exhibiting these variations acquire the important abilities of standing and walking alone. These are shown in Table 19.

TABLE 19

The Influence of Early Motor Patterns on Ages for Sitting, Crawling, Standing and Walking (Robson, 1975)

Motor activity	Predominant pattern of motor development				
	'Crawler'	'Roller'	'Creeper'	'Shuffler'	'Just stands and walks'
Sitting alone	5−7−9	6−8−10	6−9−12	7−12−15	5−7−11
Crawling	6−9−12	11−14−17	12−15−19	−	−
Shuffling	−	−	−	7−12−16	−
Getting to Standing	7−10−13	12−15−20	11−19−24	10−18−26	8−10−13
Walking	11−13−15	14−18−26	15−20−27	12−19−28	8−11−14

The figures refer to the ages in months. They are given in the order: initial−mean−limited ages. (*see* Chapter 11)

Gross motor development is directed towards two ends: the attainment of stable positions, especially against gravity as described above, and the achievement of movement. For most children movement opens up many avenues of development (Table 20). For those for whom it does not, movement does at least provide some personal stimulation and gratification, as in the rhythmical rocking which is exhibited by some children. Most children however, get full value from their mobility. It is only necessary to contrast the activities of a normal two-year-old making full use of his mobility with those of an immobile child to realize the great advantages of mobility to a developing child. Such consideration inevitably leads to speculation about an immobile child: how can one maintain and stimulate his physical development?; how can he learn about the world around him if he cannot explore; and what happens to his emotional development when he cannot run over to his mother and fling his arms around her neck, or hide from his brothers and sisters?

TABLE 20

Advantages of Mobility in Infancy

Physical	(a)	Enhanced physique—circulatory effects, increased muscle strength etc.
	(b)	Practice in development of skills—sensory, motor co-ordination, balance etc.
Intellectual	(a)	Exploration—spatial awareness, promotion of audio-visual development, increased learning opportunities etc.
	(b)	Communication—more effective, wider scope etc.
Emotional	(a)	Internal stimulation and enjoyment
	(b)	Interpersonal relationships enhanced and controlled.

When studying the motor development of children it is useful to know the advantages and disadvantages of the various movements and to note the use the child makes of his ability to move.

Rolling

The great limitation of this movement is that it is not possible to look in the direction of movement or at the object the child is moving towards all the time, whereas in other forms of movement the child is able to do so. For most children, therefore, rolling is an early transient form of movement which may occur accidentally or be indulged in for pleasure. It might be used occasionally for the purpose of moving to another point or to reach an object. Some disabled children have to use this as their only means of movement, and in these cases its limitations, and therefore their difficulties in making this a functionally useful movement, must be kept in mind.

Scooting, creeping and crawling

All these actions involve the active use of the legs and arms. Consequently, although they can become very effective means of movement, their usefulness is limited by the fact that the hands are not free. It is difficult for a child to carry anything with him as he crawls, and if he wishes to use his hands for exploration, he has to stop and often change to another position.

Pulling to standing, cruising and walking

Pulling to standing requires considerable strength, especially in the hip extensors, and difficulty here may provide a useful clinical clue to isolated weakness of this muscle group. The hands are occupied in pulling to standing and cruising. It is not always realized that cruising requires a somewhat unique side-stepping ability which needs good control of the pelvis. Walking, of course, is the one action parents wait for and acclaim with great joy. The prospects opened up by the development of independent walking are considerable. It is a mature and socially accepted means of progression; considerable distances can be explored; the hands are free for manipulation and carrying; progress is visually directed and controlled without difficulty; and it leads to other skills such as running, jumping, hopping etc.

Other motor skills

After the first year many other motor skills appear and then become increasingly developed as shown by increased speed and precision and

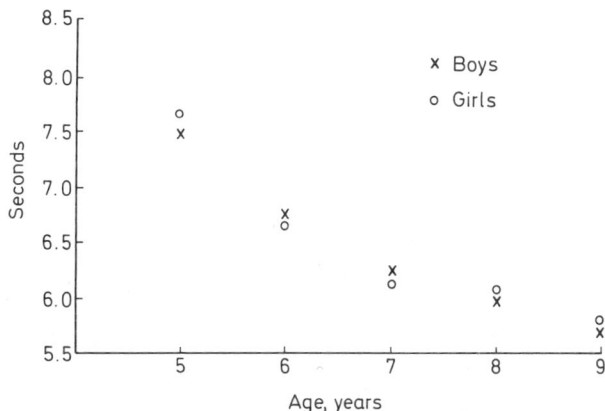

Figure 68. Development of proficiency in running—30 yard
dash, mean scores, age 5 to 9 (Keogh, 1965)

decreased effort in performance. Some skills show a similar pattern of development and proficiency in both boys and girls (e.g. a short run, *Figure 68*). Boys tend to be superior even from the early years in skills involving strength e.g. throwing a ball (Table 17), whereas girls are superior in skills involving precision (e.g. mat hopping test (*Figure 69*).

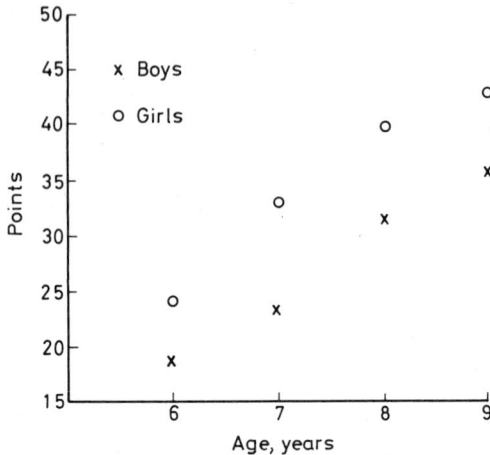

Figure 69. Girls' superiority over boys in precision skill—mat hopping test, mean scores, age 6 to 9 (Keogh, 1965)

An overall pattern of the development of motor skills is shown below.

A Selection of Motor Skills in Childhood

Unless stated otherwise age levels refer to the age when 50 per cent of normal children show the particular ability.

Walking

First independent steps appear at about 1 year of age. Upper acceptable limit, 18 months (Frankenberg *et al*., 1971; Neligan & Prudham, 1969). At 18 months many children walk well, and some can walk backwards.
   Walking on tip toe: 2½ years
   Walking along a straight line (1 inch wide, 10 feet long):
      not more than 3 steps off: 2½ years
      no steps of: 3 years

Walking along a circular line (1 inch wide, 4 feet diameter):
not more than 3 steps off: 3 years
no steps off: 4 years (McCaskill and Willman, 1938)
Walking heel-toe: this ability appears early in the fourth year and is shown by 90 per cent of children by 5 years of age.

Running

This skill develops during the second year and is usually well established by 2 years.

By 5 years of age all children should be able to run 30 yards in under 10 seconds; and by 9 years in under 7 seconds (Keogh, 1965).

Timed standards for a 40 yard sprint are shown in Table 21 (Arnheim and Pestolesi, 1973).

TABLE 21

Timed Standards for 40 Yards Sprint (in seconds)

% level	Age, years				
	5	6	7	8	9
50%	8.4	8.3	8.2	7.8	7.4
5% (assumed limit of acceptable normal)	9.7	9.5	9.4	9.2	8.9

Negotiating steps

There is very wide variation in acquiring this ability depending upon support, method adopted and experience.

Going up, without support, alternating feet: 2½ years
Going down, without support, alternating feet: 4 years (McCaskill and Wellman, 1938)

One-leg skills

The ability to stand on one leg appears at about 3 years of age. Mean duration of maintenance of this posture is as follows:

3½ years: 2 seconds
4 years: 4–8 seconds
5 years: over 8 seconds
Hopping on the spot: 5 times, 4 years
                      10 times, 5 years (McCaskill & Willman, 1938)
Hopping forwards: at 5 years mean time for 50 feet, 10.5 seconds
                      at 10 years mean time for 50 feet, 4.8 seconds
                      (Keogh, 1965)

Kicking

Ability to kick a ball forwards develops in the second year and is possessed by 90 per cent of children by 2 years of age (Frankenberg *et al.* 1971).

Jumping

The first efforts at 'jumping' often consist of stepping down or dropping from a step. Such early jumping down a small distance is greatly affected by confidence. Most children learn to lead with one foot at first and only later jump with both feet together. The 50 per cent age levels are as follows (McCaskill and Willman, 1935):

Depth	*One foot leading*	*Both feet together*
12 inches	2 years	3 years
18 inches	2½ years	3 years

The standing jump is a complicated manoeuvre which begins with the child standing with his feet together and requires a sudden co-ordinated effort to spring with both feet together to project the body forwards. Children acquire considerable ability as shown by the distances they cover. In the later school years, boys do much better than girls so the standards in these later years are shown separately for the two sexes in Table 22 (Arnheim and Pestolesi, 1973).

The minimal acceptable distance (i.e. 2SD below mean) for a standing jump is 20 inches at 5 years and 43 inches at 10 years (Keogh, 1965).

TABLE 22

Fifty Per Cent and 5 Per Cent Levels for Standing Jump (in inches)

	Age, years				
% level	*5*	*6*	*7*	*8*	*9*
50%	37 inches	40 inches	43 inches	47 inches	53 inches
5%	26 inches	29 inches	32 inches	36 inches	40 inches
	10	*11*	*12*	*13*	*14*
50% (girls/boys)	55/60	58/62	60/66	60/70	63/76
5% (girls/boys)	42/48	45/48	45/48	45/53	46/59

Clumsiness

Clumsiness refers to poor performance in motor skills. Developmental paediatricians are frequently concerned with clumsy children whose difficulties are brought to their attention by parents or teachers. Behind the comment that the child is clumsy may be concern because he is not as good as his fellows either in what he is able to do, or in the speed of his actions; or complaints occur because he is always bumping into things, or dropping things, or is untidy and messy, or has poor hand-writing; or anxieties arise because he is not participating, e.g. with others in games and sports.

In some cases the child is not clumsy at all. His motor skills are perfectly reasonable for his age, but his parents or school may be expecting above average performances from him. This occurs particularly with the sons of very skilful parents, and with children attending schools where great store is set upon games and athletic prowess.

In other cases the child's inferior performance in motor skills will be confirmed, but this may not be due to pathological causes. There is a very wide range of motor skills in childhood. Some selected items are listed in Table 23. A ten-year-old girl who can throw a ball only 20 feet may seem decidedly feeble, especially as almost all 5-year-old boys will be able to do better, but her performance is well within the 'normal' range for her age and sex. Lack of interest and opportunities may have accentuated her limitations, and she might show improvement with training. Drawing excessive attention to her poor performance and labelling her as clumsy will undoubtedly increase both her difficulties and her reactions to them.

TABLE 23

The Wide Range of Motor Skills in Childhood: Some Selected Items

Item	Poorest (2 SD)	Average	Best (+ 2 SD)
5-year-old girls running 30 yards	6.25 seconds	7.67 seconds	9.09 seconds
5-year-olds hopping 50 feet	31% boys) unable 19% girls)to do it	10.4 seconds	
7-year-old boys' grip strength	11.5 lbs	26.3 lbs	41.1 lbs
8-year-olds' standing jump	41.6 inches	55.2 inches	68.8 inches
9-year olds' beam balance	16.6 seconds	40 seconds	63.4 seconds
10-year-olds' beam walk	15.7 steps	24.3 steps	32.9 steps
10-year-old boys' ball throw	52 feet	94 feet	136 feet
10-year-old girls' ball throw.	16.4 feet	49 feet	81.6 feet

The medical management of clumsy children requires considerable skill. Very often an impetuous search for a neurological lesion or 'minimal brain damage' and a desire to apply a diagnostic label is often the most detrimental step possible so far as the child's overall development is concerned. The handling of these situations requires considerable expertise and appreciation of developmental needs by the doctor.

Sometimes, however, a child may be clumsy as a result of a pathological cause. This may be revealed by finding that the motor skills are outside the normal range and that other abnormal features are present. For example, an experienced clinician will notice when excessive movements or unusual postures occur in performing a particular skill and will also be on the look out for grimacing, tremors, ataxia and the presence of mirror movements. The Fog tests are useful in this connection (Fog and Fog, 1963):

(a) The child is asked to stand on the lateral borders of his feet with his feet turned inwards. In young children this action causes supination of the arms in most cases, and pronation or extension in others. With increasing age the arm movement is seen less often, and is seldom seen after 10 years of age. The presence of such a reaction over this age is, therefore, an indication of probable abnormality.

(b) The child is asked to open a spring clip with the fingers of one hand. In the young there is associated movement of the other hand, but this diminishes with increasing age and is not seen very often after 14 years provided that the clip is not excessively strong. The presence of such a reaction over this age is, therefore, an indication of possible abnormality.

There is no satisfactory test for clumsiness or for motor skill. This statement will not seem surprising after what has been said already about the many factors affecting motor development. Several tests of motor proficiency have been described, notably the Oseretsky and Stott tests (Oseretsky, 1923; Stott, 1966), which help to identify a clumsy child but do not untangle the various factors involved. Furthermore, both tests include items which are largely dependent upon motor perceptual ability rather than the other components of motor skill and so add to the difficulties of analysing the results.

Rather than trying to solve this situation by tests, the clinical approach recommended is as follows. In the case of a child already labelled as clumsy:

(a) to determine if there really is impairment of motor skills.
(b) to determine the extent of this impairment and the ways it is affecting the child.
(c) to determine if there is a pathological cause for the clumsiness. It is important to do this because if it can be shown that there is a definite cause for the clumsiness the child cannot be blamed for it. It also helps decide whether training will help or only frustrate, and it gives a guide to future ability. It may further provide some insight into, or forewarning about, associated learning problems.

(d)   the clumsiness should be analysed to find which components are at fault, e.g. speed, strength, precision, co-ordination and endurance, in order to determine the best ways to overcome the difficulty.

In the case of a child who has not already been labelled as clumsy, but who is found to be so in the course of examination, the above steps should be followed, but caution should be exercised before applying a diagnostic label. On the whole, more harm than help arises from the indiscriminant labelling of children as clumsy.

Recommended Additional Reading

Morris P. R. and Whiting, HTA. (1971). *Motor Impairment and Compensatory Education.* London: Bell and Sons
Cratty B. J. (1967). *Movement Behaviour and Motor Learning.* 2nd Edn. London: Kempton

REFERENCES

Arnheim, D. D., and Pestolesi, R. A. (1973). *Developing Motor Behaviour in Children.* St. Louis: C. V. Mosby
Barsley, M. (1966). *The Left-handed Book.* London: Pan Books, Cox & Wyman
Bayley, N. (1965). *Bayley Infant Scales of Development (revised) Mental and Motor.* New York: Psychological Corporation
Benton, A. L. (1959). *Right-left Discrimination and Finger Localisation.* New York: Hoeber
Buchler, C. and Hetzer, H. (1935). *Testing Children's Development from Birth to School Age.* London: Allen and Unwin
Fog, E. and Fog, M. (1963). Cerebral inhibition examined by associated movements, *Clinics Devl. Med. 10,* 52. London: Heinemann
Frankenberg, W. K., Camp, B. W., van Natta, P. A., Demersseman, J. A. and Voor Lees, S. F. (1971). Reliability and stability of the Denver Developmental Screening Test. *Child Dev.* 42, 1315
Gesell, A. and Amatruda, C. S. (1947). *Developmental Diagnosis of Normal and Abnormal Child Development.* New York: Hoeber
Goodenough, F. L. (1926). *Measurement of Intelligence by Drawings.* New York: Brace and World
Griffiths, R. (1954). *The Abilities of Babies.* London: University Press
Hagberg, B. and Lundberg, A. (1969). Dissociated motor development simulating cerebral palsy, *Neuropaediat.* 1, 187
Holt, K. S. (1965). *The Assessment of Cerebral Palsy.* London: Lloyd Luke
Horton, M. E. and Rosenbloom, L. (1971). The maturation of fine prehension in young children, *Devl. Med. Child Neurol.* 13, 3
Illingworth, R. S. (1966). Development of the Infant and Young Child; Normal and Abnormal, 3rd Edn. Edinburgh: Livingstone

Kay, H. (1970). Analysing motor skill performance. In *Mechanisms of Motor Skill Development*. Ed. K. J. Connolly. p. 139. London: Academic Press

Keogh, J. (1965). *Motor Performance of Elementary School Children*. Berkeley: Department of Physical Education, University of California

McCaskill, C. L. & Wellman, B. L. (1938). A study of common motor achievements at the preschool ages. *Child Dev*. 9, 141

Neligan, G. and Prudham, D. (1969). Norms for four standard developmental milestones by sex, social class and place in family. *Devl Med. Child Neurol.* 11, 423

Oseretsky, N. (1948). Metric scale for studying the motor capacity of children, *J. consult. Psychol.* (1948), 12, 37.

Robson, P. (1970). Shuffling, hitching, scooting or sliding; some observations on 30 otherwise normal children, *Devl Med. Child Neurol.* 12, 608

– (1975). Personal communication

Sheridan, M. D. (1960). *The Developmental Progress of Infants and Young Children*, London: H.M.S.O.

Slosson. (1963). *Slosson Intelligence Test for Children and Adults*. New York: Slosson Education Publications

Stott, D. H. (1966). A general test of motor-impairment for children, *Devl Med. Child Neurol.* 8, 523

Stutsman, R. (1948). *Mental Measurement of Preschool Children*. New York: Harcourt Brace & World

Terman, L. M. and Merrill, M. A. (1937). *Measuring Intelligence*. Boston: Houghton Mifflin

Touwen, B. C. L. (1972). Laterality and dominance, *Devl Med. Child Neurol.* 14, 747

Valentine, C. W. (1958). *Intelligence Tests for Children*, 6th edn. London: Methuen

CHAPTER 9

The Development of Language : Importance of Cerebral Processes

Human behaviour consists of the responses to internal and external stimuli. During the course of development the child becomes aware of many stimuli; he acquires abilities to interpret and understand these stimuli, to select the important and useful ones, and to suppress or reject others. At the same time as the child responds to various stimuli he notes the results of such responses. As development proceeds his abilities to receive and to respond become more complex and more effective. Between these two aspects—the reception of stimuli and the performance of actions—are interposed the all important cerebral mechanisms, rather like the meat in a sandwich. The cerebral mechanisms are alerted to receive various stimuli, to interpret and memorize the incoming sensations, and then to select an appropriate response and initiate the action (*Figure 70*). An understanding of this central cerebral mechanism is essential for all who would seek to comprehend the basis of child development. The role of the central mechanisms is most clearly seen in relation to the development of language (*Figure 71*), which is considered in this chapter.

To continue the analogy of a sandwich with respect to language development, the top and bottom layers are represented by the receptive and expressive aspects, and both these aspects can be observed and measured. Between the two layers lie the all important central cerebral processes. If these central processes do not function properly quite serious disorders of language development ensue. The 'meat' in the sandwich is all important. The central language processes are not as directly observable as are the receptive and expressive aspects. They can be revealed, however, by specially designed tests and by study of language disorders in children.

204

RECEPTIVE　　　　　CENTRAL CEREBRAL PROCESSES　　　　　EXPRESSIVE

Auditory
Visual
Tactile
Other external
and internal
sensations

INPUT

INTELLECTUAL

Comprehension
Interpretation
Correlation
Memorization

Response selection
and organization
especially appropriateness
sequence, intensity
and timing

EMOTIONAL

FEEDBACK

Internal effects:
Hormonal
Circulatory
Emotional

OUTFLOW

External actions:
Movements
Vocalizations

Adjustment of attention
and alertness

Monitoring of responses

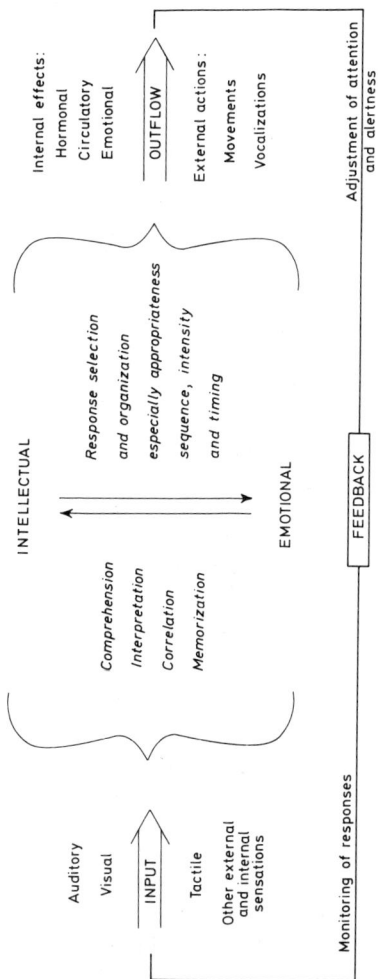

Figure 70. The central cerebral processes concerned with language

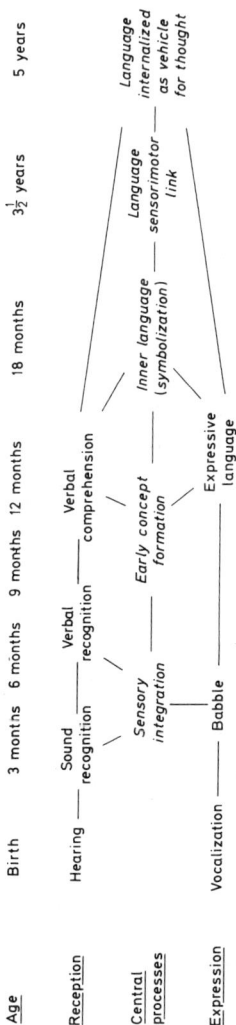

Age	Birth	3 months	6 months	9 months	12 months	18 months	3½ years	5 years

Reception: Hearing — Sound recognition — Verbal recognition — Verbal comprehension

Central processes: Sensory integration — Early concept formation — Inner language (symbolization) — Language sensorimotor link — Language internalized as vehicle for thought

Expression: Vocalization — Babble — Expressive language

Figure 71. Diagrammatic representation of language development (Reynell, 1969)

The receptive aspect of language consists of the reception, selection and recognition of sounds, verbal recognition and verbal comprehension. The expressive aspect consists of vocalization, verbalization and expressive language. A further consideration of the components of these two sides of the sandwich will reveal the importance of the central mechanisms.

Much of the receptive aspect of language has been described already in Chapter 5. Infants are exposed to sounds which they hear. Certain sounds come to mean more to them than others. These are the sounds which occur most frequently, are distinct from other sounds, and are associated with other sensations, especially pleasurable ones. Infants learn to recognize sounds with these characteristics, to give them more attention when they occur, and to listen to them and for them. Infants who do not have opportunities for hearing sounds, or who are exposed to a noisy environment from which it is difficult to identify particular sounds, do not develop sound recognition skills as easily or as early as other babies.

In the course of normal development, sound recognition, having been acquired at about 3 months of age, is followed a few months later by verbal recognition. Familiar words are recognized. Then this leads to verbal comprehension when the meaning and significance of words are recognized.

These features of the development of verbal comprehension from sound recognition can be seen, heard, and recorded. The fact that they occur indicates that essential central processes have been at work. The development of these progressive steps depends upon sensory integration and concept formation. The infant has to link the sounds he hears with the sight of the sound-producing objects and with the objects identified by particular words. The observation and testing of these features of language reception provide an insight into the activity and functioning of the central processes.

The other side of the 'sandwich', namely expressive language, also shows observable and audible signs of progressive development which reflect the activity of the central cerebral processes. Thus, the early vocalizations become a repetitive babble and then recognizable syllables and words are produced, at first in imitation, and later with purpose and meaning. The two external aspects of language, reception and expression, reinforce one another and in this way promote the development of the central processes. For example, as the infant develops sound recognition he also acquires the ability to babble and his practise of his new-found skill reinforces his interest in sounds and their recognition.

From these early stages the central processes develop rapidly and extensively. The progression from the early simple concept formations to symbolization represents big forward strides. The inner language so created becomes a tool for the control and direction of actions and a basis for intellectual development.

The various aspects of expressive language and of symbolization are considered more fully in the following paragraphs.

Expression

Expression may take many forms. It may arise spontaneously, in response to internal or external stimuli, or may be initiated for a specific purpose. Consider the smiling of infants. A baby asleep in his pram may smile. Is this occurring spontaneously or in response to an internal stimulus such as a dream or wind? There is clearly no intention of affecting the environment, but if the baby's mother is watching just at that moment, she may well be influenced by the smile. The same baby when awake will smile upon seeing his mother coming towards his pram, an expression occurring in response to an external stimulus. On another occasion he might deliberately smile at someone in order to attract them towards his pram, an internally initiated expression with the set purpose of influencing his environment.

Some expressions have an immediate effect upon the environment, for example knocking over a tower of cubes in a moment of temper, but other expressions are only effective if they are received, accepted and interpreted by another person. This is the basis of interpersonal communication. Expressions may be divided into those which are (a) deliberately communicative, (b) coincidentally communicative and (c) non-communicative.

The process of communication can be extremely complex and sophisticated, according to the subtlety of the expressions and the ingenuity and sensitivity of the observer. Expressions based upon various movements and actions are often fairly crude, but facial expressions and eye movements can be used to convey a wide range of meanings. Indeed, a glance between two people may convey a world of meaning which could not be communicated as effectively in any other way. An astounding degree of communication is sometimes achieved between severely disabled children and their mothers. Other attendants may find the same child completely unresponsive because, (a) they do not create an environment which encourages attempts at expression and communication by the handicapped child,

(b) they do not recognize the expressions used by the child for communication, and (c) they do not have the mental preparedness to accept and interpret the expressions. In these circumstances communication never begins or soon fails through lack of reinforcement.

Some individuals communicate by expressions known only to themselves. Twins, for example, often appear to anticipate each others wishes and actions by means of expressions to which they are particularly sensitive, but which are seldom apparent to others.

All the above examples of communication consist of non-vocal expressions. Expressions can be divided into vocal and non-vocal groups. Vocal expressions can cover a wide range of situations and may be used for many purposes. They are particularly useful for communication at a distance. An extension and elaboration of vocal expression is available to humans in the form of verbal expression. Expressive language consists of the externalization of inner language produced by the central cerebral processes (the meat in the sandwich!). Vocalization and verbalization are considered more fully in the following paragraphs.

Vocalization

Humans are exceptionally gifted in possessing a voice which equips them with a range of vocal expressions, and which, when linked with the all-essential central processes enables the development of verbalization and expressive language.

Ability to vocalize is present at birth, and vocalization is the only means of voice expression in the early months of life. Verbalization develops later and then becomes the principal means of voiced expression, but vocalization is not lost and it remains effective throughout life. For example, it is used as a means of attracting attention by shouting; expressing emotion by roaring with anger, and sighing with pleasure; and communicating by cooing to soothe.

Crying

Crying is one form of vocalization. The cry of a newborn infant is quite distinctive. Mothers often claim to be able to recognize the cry of their own baby. A trained observer with a keen ear will recognize both variations in the cries of normal babies which express different emotions, and also abnormal cries. Wasz-Höckert, Lind, Vuorenkoski, Partanen and Valanné (1968) studied these differences in infants' cries spectrographically, and were able to show that crying is purposive.

THE DEVELOPMENT OF LANGUAGE209

They distinguished the cries of the baby in pain, the baby who is
hungry, the contented baby, and the birth cry.

The cry pattern changes markedly during the first two years of
life. The changes appear to follow a definite pattern and presumably
occur as a result of changes in the size and configuration of the oral
structures, neuromuscular characteristics and posture of the infant.
Karelitz, Karelitz and Rosenfelt (1960) drew attention to these developmental changes.

The first cry is probably the result of the anoxic stimulus following
severing of the umbilical cord. In the early days the cry is of very short
duration. It seems staccato. If produced by a stimulus such as pinching
the cry rises in crescendo with the stimulus, but then fades, so the
stimulus has to be repeated. In consequence the cry seems very repetitive.

As development proceeds the duration of each cry lengthens thereby
slowing the tempo and reducing the sense of urgency imparted by the
early cry. The rhythmic pattern persists, but is less noticeable because
there are more syllables and the pitch is more variable. The inflections
seem to be more plaintive and meaningful.

By 2 to 3 months, cooing and gurgling sounds are heard. These
consist of simple sounds at first, but as more sounds are added babbling
begins to appear. An expressive 'Ah-Ha' is added to the cry in the later
months.

Appreciation of the cry characteristics at different ages enables one
to recognize abnormality and immaturity. Such skill is an invaluable
asset to every clinician concerned with babies and infants.

Non-crying vocalizations

The early non-crying vocalizations are variously described as *cooing* and
gurgling. They are pleasant musical sounds made with the mouth open.
The repertoire is increased later by sounds made with the lips at the
front of the mouth, often called *buzzing*. It is said that all babies throughout the world produce the same range of these sounds in their early
vocalizations although they will later learn to speak very different
languages.

The earliest sounds appear to be produced spontaneously, often to
the apparent surprise and pleasure of the child. Within a few months,
however, a repetitive element appears in the vocalizations which is
called *babbling*. Congenitally deaf infants seem to vocalize normally at
first but this does not persist, and failure of babbling to appear or to
continue is one of the early features which alerts a developmental
paediatrician to the possibility of deafness.

A great advance occurs in the second half of the first year, when the infant begins to imitate sounds. To be able to do this, he must have been exposed to a number of sounds and been able to hear them; to have selected particular ones—perhaps those which were most distinctive, or most frequently heard, and to have modified his own vocalizations to match those he had heard. At this stage interesting little vocal games can be played with infants.

Babies use their crying and non-crying vocalizations as expressions of their present state, crying when wet and uncomfortable or hungry, and gurgling when happy and playful. Perceptive mothers come to recognize the meaning of certain vocalizations. For example, a certain pattern of grunts may mean that the nappy is about to be filled. Some use their vocalizations as a means of communication, especially to get attention. The greater the astuteness of the child, the greater the use he can make of vocalizations. If verbalization does not develop then much use may be made of vocalizations in communication. Any child who has to rely upon vocalizations should not be condemned as severely retarded, infantile, or animal-like until careful study has been made of all aspects of his development.

Verbalization

Verbalization develops when vocalizations are modified to reproduce word sounds. An ability to select and imitate sounds is important for verbalization to develop, An infant will learn to reproduce the sound of a word if he hears it frequently and clearly, and if it is associated with other pleasurable sensations and means something to him. Frequent close contacts between a mother and her infant are essential in this connection. For example, when he sits on her lap he hears her pleasant and familiar voice clearly because she is so near. Each recurring interaction reinforces verbal awareness. Each occasion is a new learning opportunity which the mother should utilize. She cannot give verbal stimulation once and hope that that will do. The spoken word, unlike the written word, is gone once it has been uttered and cannot be referred back to. Constant repetition is necessary. It has been estimated that infants are usually exposed to 500 to 600 repetitions of a word before they reproduce it.

Even so, the imitative reproduction of familiar speech sounds does not at first constitute expressive language. It has to be linked with the recognition of the objects being named and the realization that they can be identified by a sound, a word, a name. The central processes which bring about this recognition and realization are normally developing while the infant is learning to be aware of sounds and to imitate them.

The processes involved in the development of speech will be better understood by considering a particular example, for instance, an infant learning to recognize, identify and name his own cup (Table 24). Several times a day, as he sits on his mother's lap or in his high chair with her nearby, he will be given pleasurable drinks from the same

TABLE 24

Processes Involved in Learning to Recognize a Cup

Child sees the cup on the table or in his mother's hand, begins to recognize shape.

Child touches the cup, lifts it and bangs it, begins to recognize the feel of it.

Child hears his mother say 'cup' as she holds it or gives him a drink from it, begins to associate sound with object

Child enjoys drink from cup, begins to associate pleasurable experience with object and sound of word 'cup'.

container. He will many times hear his mother refer to his 'cup', and will learn to associate this word with the object from which he has pleasurable drinks. The close proximity of his mother, the constant repetition at appropriate moments of the word 'cup', the recognition of his own cup and his ability to see it, touch it and take it to his mouth, all reinforce his learning of the word 'cup'. At first he may confuse the word for the container 'cup', with that for the contents 'milk'. Later on he will learn that there are other cups in addition to his own, and that cups are identifiable by their shape and the use to which they are put. This Table shows the importance in the early development of language of close mother–child verbal stimulation, and of such a simple thing as the child having his own cup. Most infants receive adequate verbal stimulation but some do not. Some of the results of a study by Rheingold (1960) shown in Table 25 show how infants in an institutional nursery suffered as a result of inadequate verbal stimulation.

Children may develop an ability to imitate speech without acquiring the associated verbal concepts (and some alas are even trained to do so.) At this early stage in the development of language the acquisition of verbalization without the basic concepts has disastrous consequences.

The problem is seen principally in children with cerebral disorders. Some retarded children who have not acquired this all important central understanding of the meaning of the words they reproduce show repetitive word imitation (echolalia) without making any progress in language development. Echolalia continues for years in some cases.

TABLE 25

Verbal Stimulation in an Institutional Nursery as Compared with Home (Rheingold, 1960)

Item	Mean Score	
	Home	Institution
Looks at infant's face	140	28
Talks to infant	166	17
Holds infant	285	46
Infant out of own room	304	43
1 or more adults within 6 ft	524	217
Bottle in mouth	54	299

Difficulties in the accurate reproduction of word sounds, despite the acquisition of the appropriate concepts occur quite commonly and are not usually serious. For example, one little girl had very clear concepts of her sister and her name 'Alison', but could not reproduce this exactly and called her 'Ice-on'. This was a temporary phase, however. Such discrepancies between concept readiness and quality of expressive language often occur in bright children whose thoughts seem to run ahead of their articulatory skills. This effect is sometimes seen even more markedly a year or two later when a child produces a long stream of unintelligible speech which often represents the outflow of many active ideas. The term *jargon* is used to describe unintelligible speech of this nature. In the situation quoted the jargon was meaningful in that there were sensible ideas behind it, but sometimes jargon is meaningless.

Once verbalization has begun, it usually proceeds rapidly. In consequence the average number of words produced at different ages increases sharply as is shown in Table 26. The ability to identify an object which he can see and touch (a so-called concrete object) with a verbal label is a great achievement, and is one which the child applies to everything he encounters. This normally occurs during his second year, and as a result he adds many nouns to his vocabulary. He then begins to learn the verbal labels for actions he performs, such as drinking, sitting, walking, etc. His vocabulary then expands to include verbs of action. The process of conceptualization and naming continues and his vocabulary expands rapidly. Because the child is becoming more aware of himself and of his relationships to others there are frequent confusions of expression between 'I', 'me' and 'you', but these resolve in time. Later still he develops an ability to conceptualize abstract subjects and to name them. The great increase of expressive vocabulary with its sequence of nouns, verbs, personal pronouns, and adjectives, is an outward manifestation of the increase in understanding which is occurring in the brain.

TABLE 26

Size and Type of Vocabulary According to Age (Duffy & Irwin, 1951)

Item	Age, years				
	1	2	3	4	5
Number of words	1−2	20−100	900	1500	> 2000
Type or words: nouns	+	+	+	+	+
verbs		±	+	+	+
pronouns		±	+	+	+
adjectives			±	+	+
Sentence length		2−3 words	3−4 words		> 5 words
Intelligibility		66%	90%		100%

A big step forward occurs when the child becomes able to link concepts together. This is seen in the linking of words. For example, 'Daddy gone' represents two clear concepts. 'Me ride it' indicates three concepts. A phrase like 'All gone', however, does not represent an advance. Although we see it as two distinct words and appreciate the meaning of 'all', to the young child the concept of 'all' is too abstract for him to understand as yet, and the phrase is really a double-syllabic single-concept phrase which represents no major advance upon 'gone' so far as language is concerned.

Symbolization

So far the discussion of the development of language has been concerned with the acquisition of vocabulary and the demonstration of the importance of the central processes of concept formation and association. There is another major process involved in the development of language, namely symbolization. Reynell (1969) described the development of symbolization very clearly. Symbolization is a process by which objects, persons, actions, and states are represented by some means which can be recognized intellectually by others. The simplest symbols are models or pictures of the real object. Verbal symbols are the spoken or written words which represent and identify the object.

A communication is symbolic when the content of the message is coded into symbols. Reynell defines language as *any* symbolic communication, and verbal language as communication by verbal symbols, i.e. words.

The linking of a name to the concept of an object is an early example of verbal symbolization. It should be clear how this phenomenon of verbal symbolization greatly facilitates the development of both language and the acquisition of vocabulary. Not only does the process of symbolization promote the development of verbal language, it also facilitates the integration of the central processes concerned with reception and expression. For example, a cup may be represented symbolically by a model, picture, word or sign (*Figure 72*). The use of such symbols facilitates the integration of the visual, auditory and tactile impressions which arise from them. Through symbolization a child can take a picture, model, sign or other representation and not only recognize it, as representing the real thing, but do to it what he might do to the real thing. Thus, a child might take a doll and play with it as if it were a baby, trying to feed, bathe and dress it. Much of a child's symbolic understanding is best seen in his play, and play observation forms an essential part of the evaluation of language development.

Observation of play is necessary for another purpose, namely, to observe the use of language in the direction of play. Young children often talk as they play. They are directing their own actions in this way until these actions have been fully internalized. Language plays an important part in the pre-school years when children use this skill to organize and integrate their actions. At this stage they can be helped by being guided in the sequencing of their actions.

Communication

Communication has been discussed in the earlier section on expression. For communication to take place between two individuals one must

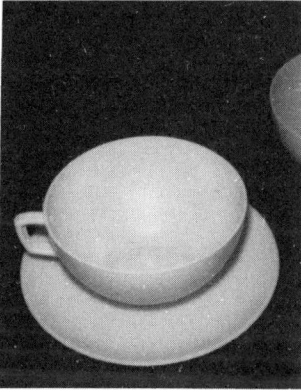
A model

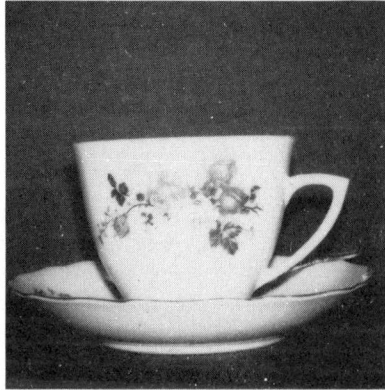
Photograph of actual cup

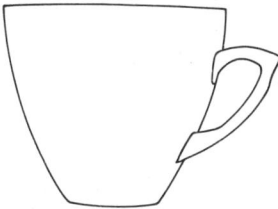

Drawing

a cup

A CUP

Writing

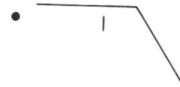

Shorthand

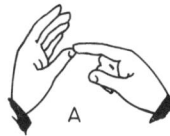
A

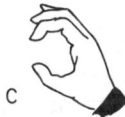
C

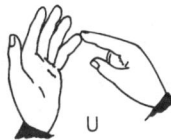
U

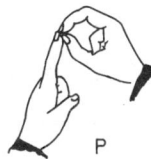
P

Sign language

Figure 72. Symbolization: representation of 'a cup'

initiate some expressive action, however simple it may be (e.g. moving closer, looking towards the other person), and the second individual must make some response if the communication is to continue. The acquisition of language in childhood greatly enriches the possibilities of communication. Through language the extent and complexity of communications is increased, and so also is the range of communication between two or more individuals.

Language should be seen in this context of communication, because language disorders may impair communication and communication errors may affect language development or simulate language disorders. For example, a lack of desire to communicate, or the using of non-verbal expressive actions may cause failures of expressive language development.

The acquisition of language in childhood enables a child to understand many of the events in the word around him, and it also gives him an effective means of communication. This review of language development shows clearly the importance of the central processes—the meat in the sandwich. Language assessment, described in the next section, reveals and tests some of the central processes.

LANGUAGE ASSESSMENT

This is one of the most difficult areas of clinical assessment because there are many features which have to be examined, and also because there is considerable variation between individuals.

The many features which have to be examined include the following:

    ability to hear
    desire to listen
    ability to discriminate word sounds
    verbal comprehension of increasing complexity
    ability to attach verbal labels to objects
    ability to form verbal concepts
    ability to link verbal concepts
    ability to formulate verbal responses
    ability to organize expressive language
    ability to articulate verbal expressions.

There are several reasons for the variations in language development which occur between individuals. Genetic influences play some part. Variations also reflect differences in basic cerebral endowment. Overall, girls show more advanced language development in the early years than boys. Environmental factors play a very considerable part by influencing the pattern and frequency of language exposure, and by stimulating or inhibiting the child's desires to communicate and to express himself verbally.

It is not surprising, therefore, that delays and deviations of speech and language development in the early years occur frequently, and must be taken seriously as they may be the presenting signs of a wide range of serious conditions including deafness, retardation, emotional disturbances, and social deprivation.

Developmental paediatricians must be familiar with the various aspects of language development at different ages so that whenever they encounter a child they are sensitive to any abnormality or deficiency of verbal comprehension, expressive language and the pattern of communication. They also have to be able to satisfy themselves about the adequacy of language development in children having developmental examinations; to be able to carry out screening examinations at selected ages, e.g. at 3 years; and to determine whether a child who presents with complaints suggestive of a language disorder, e.g. not talking at 3½ years of age, really does have such a disorder. In the study in depth of the language development of any child, and in the diagnosis and assessment of those with possible language disorders, paediatricians find it invaluable to work with suitably experienced psychologists and speech therapists.

In addition to knowledge and technical skills the evaluation of language development requires two other assets, namely skill in dealing with young children and a suitable setting for the examination.

All too often doctors attempting this work find that if they are able to elicit any responses at all these are usually only monosyllabic responses from a tense child. Most young children are intimidated by adults in strange surroundings and they must be put at ease. Paediatricians must first establish rapport with the child and then present the test material in such a way as to stimulate co-operation and speech.

The usual hospital ward and out-patients department are just about the worst possible places for this type of examination, although they need not be so. The examination should be carried out in a comfortably furnished room of appropriate size, neither so small that the child feels trapped, nor so large that he feels lost. It should be quiet so that he can hear, and be heard. There should be sufficient suitable toys to hold his interest, but too many toys (and sounds, and adults) should be avoided. A play situation is often very suitable for exploring a child's language development.

Quick Checks and Alerting Signs

There is no quick way for evaluating all the aspects of language development, and nothing written in this section should be construed as being a test of language. It is however extremely important to detect any delays and deviations as soon as possible so whenever he sees a child the developmental paediatrician should enquire about the child's understanding and production of speech, and should observe the child's response to his speech, and should listen to the child's speech. A few quietly spoken words, and requests to point to two or three familiar objects and to carry out commands of increasing length and number of concepts, soon show if the child hears, listens, discriminates word sounds, understands verbal requests, and the number of verbal concepts with which he can deal. Then a request to name some objects, and to say what they see in a picture elicits expressive language which can be analysed for its clarity, word content, subject appropriateness, sentence structure and length. Observation and listening during spontaneous play will reveal how the child uses objects—level of symbolic understanding—and also the features of expressive language.

The paediatrician will be alerted to the need for further investigation when:

(a)   the parents make definite complaints about some aspect of language development;

(b)   child appears not to hear or does not attempt to listen;

(c)   child by 12 months of age not responding to his name, or not understanding 'No', or making at least one response to a clue word such as 'shoe' (e.g. 'Where's baby's shoe?');

(d)   a child by 18 months of age not producing at least one or two words;

(e)   a child by 2 years of age not showing any appreciation of symbolic representation (e.g. a doll, spoon, cup are not recognized for what they are);

(f)   a child by 3 years of age not listening to a story, who cannot carry out verbal requests, who does not understand positional prepositions such as 'inside', 'underneath' and 'beside', and who does not use phrases of 2 or 3 words;

(g)   a child of 3 years of age or more producing a flow of speech which is not related to the situation.

Screening Tests

There is not, so far as I am aware, a wholly satisfactory screening technique for the detection of language disorders. Most of the techniques are an extension of the quick checks described above. They serve to identify those children who need further investigation, and such investigation is necessary to determine the cause and significance of the deviations detected.

Dr P. Zinkin (1975) and colleagues in my department have been following the development of young children in a clinical setting and used the items shown in Table 27 in their examination.

TABLE 27

Hearing, Speech and Language Items from the Developmental Schedules of the 'Hounslow' Study (Zinkin, 1975)

at 2 years

Comprehension

Identifies:	ball, brush, cup, doll, car, spoon
Obeys:	Put the spoon in the cup
	Put the brush in the box
	Put the lid on the box

Expression

Names:	ball, brush, cup, doll, car, spoon
Spontaneous speech:	simple words, phrases

Symbolization

Spontaneous play:	
Guided play:	Give dolly a drink

at 3 years

Comprehension

Identifies:	what we sit on, drink from, cut with, write with, eat with, ride in
Obeys:	Show me the biggest baloon
	Put the penny underneath the cup

Expression

Spontaneous sentences heard

Dr M. Pollak (1972) carried out a study of the development of 3-year-old children in South London which highlighted the serious language deficits of the West Indian children. She used a book (*'I see a lot of things'*, Dean Hay, 1966) containing attractive full-page colour photographs of everyday objects. There were 25 objects altogether which the three-year-old children were asked to identify, and they were also asked the purpose of some of them. She asked each child to recite a nursery rhyme and asked several questions about personal identity such as 'What is your name?' Several familiar objects were given to the children who were asked to name them and say how they were used. The children were asked to perform simple actions to show their comprehension of adverbs and to repeat three digits. Throughout the test their spontaneous speech was noted. Pollak awarded one point for each of 14 items which she expected the 3-year-old children to pass. The mean score of 3-year-old children in English families was 12.04 showing that most normal 3-year-olds reared in English families were able to pass most of the test items. The 14 items are shown in Table 28.

TABLE 28

Pollak's Items for Testing the Language Attainment of Three-Year-Old Children. (One point is awarded for each item passed by the child.)

Can name 22 out of 25 pictures	1
Can give purpose of 7 out of 8 objects	1
Recites most of one nursery rhyme	1
Sings a song	1
Knows his full name	1
Names his mother	1
Names doctor	1
Is heard to use sentences of three or more words	1
Calls himself 'I'	1
Names 6 out of 7 objects	1
Correctly answers 6 out of 7 questions about everyday objects	1
Knows meaning of two adverbs	1
Can repeat three sets of three digits	1

Dr J. Cash (1975) devised a language screening test for 3-year-old children while studying at The Wolfson Centre. His scheme was based upon Reynell's work, and is shown in *Figure 73*. Cash's test includes

```
SURNAME .......................  FORENAME(S) ...................................
D.O.B.  ...................  PARENT S/E GROUP ..............................................
DELIVERY ........................................................................
PARENT-GUARDIAN'S LANGUAGE .......................................
```

1) Time available for play with parents   good/av/poor
   "   "   "   "   "   siblings   good/av/poor
   "   "   "   "   "   friends   good/av/poor
   Attends play group   yes/no
   Is the home isolated?   yes/no

2) Has hearing been tested? if Yes - is it satisfactory?   yes/no/satis

3) _____
   object: what is it: what is it for/it do/is she

table			Table
cup			cuP
teapot			teapot
car			Car
CHair			CHair
spoon			SpooN
dog			DoG
chair			chair
doll			doLL
cat			cat
bath			Bath
baby			babY

4) Show me which we drink out of   right/wrong
   "   "   "   "   sit on   right/wrong
   "   "   "   "   drive in   right/wrong

5) Give me the red chair   right/wrong

6) Put the spoon in the cup   right/wrong
   Pour Mummy a cup of tea   right/wrong

7) Make dolly push the car   right/wrong
   Now make the car push dolly   right/wrong
   Now you tell Mummy "dolly pushing car"   puSHiNG

8) Put the cat on the chair   right/wrong
   Put the dog under the table   right/wrong

9) What are these? (2 chairs for pleurals)   chairZ   right/wrong

10) What colour is this chair?   Red

11) Say "he put the milk in the fridge"   He put the
                                                      Milk in
                                                      the friDGe

12) Count my fingers (1-5)   One tWO
                                                      THree Four
                                                      fiVe

13) Opinion of child's verbal stimulation   good/av/poor
14) What is your name?   right/wrong
15) Are you a little boy or a little girl?   right/wrong
16) Ask what is happening when you - (write full answer)
    (a) place baby in the bath _____
    (b) put the dog on the chair _____

                    Total number of consonants incorrectly articulated ....

Any comments:-
                                                      Fig. 73

Figure 73. A language screening scale for 3-year-old children. (Cash, 1975)

items pertinent to each stage of language comprehension and expression. For example.

Opportunity to experience verbal stimulation:	items 1, 13
Ability to hear:	item 2
Ability to understand what is heard:	items 3, 4
Ability to form language concepts:	items 3, 4, 5, 6, 7, 8, 9
Ability to assemble expressive language:	items 3, 9
Ability to articulate correctly:	items 3, 9, 10, 11, 12
Opportunity for verbal expression:	items 1, 13

Investigation and Evaluation Procedures
(Lenneberg, 1966; Berry, 1969; Irwin, Moore and Rampp, 1972)

In the case of children with language disorders the following investigations are carried out.

(a)   Tests of peripheral hearing including audiometry (*see* Chapter 7).

(b)   Tests of auditory discrimination—word and sentence discrimination, parts of the Stycar hearing tests and the Michael Reed picture tests (*see* Chapter 7). Other tests which have been devised include the Sound Discrimination Tests of Templin (1957), Auditory Discrimination Test of Wepman (1958).

(c)   Tests of verbal comprehensions—The Reynell Developmental Language Scales (*see below*), The Peabody Picture Vocabulary Test (Dunn, 1965) and the verbal items of general intelligence tests such as the W.I.S.C. (*see* Chapter 10).

(d)   Tests to analyse central language processes: Illinois Test of Psycholinguistic Abilities (McCarthy and Kirk, 1961).

(e)   Test of expressive language—The Reynell Developmental Language Scales (*see below*).

(f)   Attainment tests of articulation—The Renfrew Articulation Test (1966), and The Edinburgh Articulation Test (Anthony, Boyle, Ingram and McIsaac, 1971).

The Stycar Language Test (Sheridan, 1975)

Sheridan bases her test upon four codes of communication. The principal one is the *verbal code*. The others are the *pictorial code*; the *mimed*

TABLE I
Outline of expected ages and stages in development of spoken language

Ages	Manifestations	Stages
4½mths.	Reception	Pays obvious attention to nearby meaningful sounds, particularly familiar voices.
	Expression	Vocalises responsively when spoken to face-to-face; chuckles and squeals. Babbles to self and others using sing-song intonation and single or double 'syllables'. Cries loudly when hungry, annoyed or uncomfortable.
7mths.	Reception	Immediately attends to and localises nearby everyday meaningful sounds, particularly human voices. Beginning to respond discriminatively to emotional overtones in speech of familiar adults (e.g. soothing, prohibitive).
	Expression	Babbles continuously to self and others in long, tuneful repetitive strings of syllables with wide range of pitch, combining open vowels and (usually) single consonant sounds. Beginning to imitate adults' playful vocalisations in face-to-face situations.
14mths.	Reception	Responds appropriately to quiet meaningful everyday sounds within 3 or 4 metres. Recognises own and family names and words for several common objects and activities. Sensitive to expressive cadences in speech of familiars.
	Expression	Jabbers continuously to self and others employing loud, prosodic tuneful jargon. Emergence of first single words used correctly, consistently and spontaneously (i.e. not imitatively) but usually comprehensible, even to familiars, only in situational context. Ekes out articulatory difficulties with urgent intonations and finger pointings.
21mths.	Reception	Shows clearly by correct response to spoken communications that he hears and understands many more words than he can utter.
	Expression	Speaks 20 or 50+ single words and is beginning to join two or three words in meaningful sentences of agent-action-object type. Refers to self by name. Owing to numerous infantilisms, speech sometimes unintelligible to familiars and almost always to strangers. Echoes final or stressed word in sentences addressed to him. Shows brief imitative rôle-play alone or with friendly adult. Beginning to play meaningfully with miniature toys, accompanied by occasional spoken words.
3yrs.	Reception	Comprehends literal meanings of words and beginning to appreciate common semantic variations.
	Expression	Echolalia persists. Vocabulary rapidly enlarging. Uses sentences of three to five words, personal pronouns and most prepositions. Talks continuously to self at play. Infantilisms of articulation and grammar gradually diminishing. Intelligible even to strangers. Asks many questions of who? what? type. Engages in simple make-believe play alone or with one or two others. Plays meaningfully with miniature toys, providing simultaneous running commentary.
4½yrs.	Reception	Competent for most everyday situations provided sentences are not longer than six or seven words and vocabulary employed reflects child's experience.
	Expression	Uses large vocabulary with conventional grammar and syntax. Articulation still shows residual infantilisms, chiefly involving r-l-w-y, t-k, and s-f-th consonant groups, but speech (usually) intelligible even to strangers. Narrates long stories. Asks numerous questions of when? why? how? type, and meanings of words. Engages in elaborate make-believe play with group of three to six peers. Draws 'pictures' (usually) of people, houses, transport and flowers.
6½yrs.	Reception	Completely competent for all home, school and neighbourhood situations.
	Expression	Spoken language fully intelligible, grammatical and fluent. Engages in elaborate make-believe play and win/lose team games with chosen friends, explaining rules and objectives lucidly. Draws more elaborate 'pictures' showing people and objects in all sorts of everyday situations. Interested in learning to read, write and calculate.

Figure 74. Outline of expected ages and stages in development of spoken language (Sheridan, 1975)

code both improvized and systematized forms; and the *model representative code*. The development of these codes, especially the verbal and pictorial codes, as summarized by Sheridan is shown in *Figure 74*. This *Figure* shows the evolution of spoken language and is concerned principally with the verbal code, but the importance of the pictorial code is shown in the child's interest in pictures and his use of drawings of people and everyday situations. The mimed code appears early when pointing is used to reinforce verbal expression (14 months), and the model representative code applies in the play situations with miniature toys.

The test consists of three overlapping procedures: The Common Objects Test (1–2 years); The Miniature Toys Test (21 months–4½ years); and The Picture Book Test (2½–7 years). Sheridan emphasizes that the Stycar Language Test is neither a screening test nor a pass/fail type of test. Rather, it is intended to provide a descriptive profile for clinical assessment and must be used by examiners with sound experienced clinical judgement.

The Reynell Developmental Language Scales (Reynell, 1969)

These were created for the assessment of the two most important central language processes, verbal comprehension and expressive language. Each scale consists of sections arranged in developmental sequence and increasing complexity. During the test a child will pass some of the early items and then reach a point beyond which he cannot pass. The score of the items passed indicates the developmental level.

The sections of the verbal comprehension scale are as follows:
(1) Verbal preconcepts.
    (a) Response (e.g. change of facial expression) to familiar vocalization.
    (b) Association of particular vocalization with a particular situation (e.g. turning to door in response to 'Daddy coming').
    (c) Word pattern associated with particular object or person in a single context (e.g. 'Where's your shoe?' evokes looking at shoe only when it is on the foot).
(2) Verbal labelling of familiar objects (e.g. 'cup', 'ball', 'doll').
(3) Internalized verbal concepts (a particular word is applied to all objects and models having similar features, e.g. 'dog' applied to all dogs).

(4)   Relation of two verbal concepts (e.g. put the *spoon* in the *cup*).

(5)   Interpretation of question into subjective action related to the perceived object (e.g. 'Which one do we sweep the floor with?'— child has to identify the brush).

(6,7,8)   Increasing elaboration of intellectualization of language processes (e.g. 'Which one cooks the dinner?'; 'Put the penny underneath the cup'; 'Put all the pigs in the box and give me a brown horse').

(9)   Recreation of situations and their solution (e.g. 'This little boy has spilt his dinner. What must he do?').

The sections of the expressive language scale are as follows:
(1)   Language structure.
    (a)   Vocalization.
    (b)   Single-syllable sounds.
    (c)   Two different sounds.
    (d)   Four different sounds.
    (e)   Double-syllable babble (e.g. 'mum-mum').
    (f)   One definite word.
    (g)   Expressive jargon (defined as patterned vocalization simulating speech).
    (h)   Estimate of number of words produced.
    (i)   Word combination.
    (j)   Sentences of 4 or more syllables.
    (k)   Words other than nouns or verbs.
    (l)   Correct use of pronouns, prepositions, questions.
    (m) Correct order of words in sentence with no omission.
    (n)   Use of complex sentences.
(2)   Vocabulary.
    (a)   Elicited with objects.
    (b)   Elicited with pictures.
    (c)   Elicited with words.
(3)   Language content.

Conclusion

This brief review shows the features and complexities of language development, the importance of the central cerebral processes—the 'meat in the sandwich'—and describes the strategies employed in unravelling developmental language disorders. It is far too brief a review, however, to do full justice to the subject and the reader is encouraged to refer to the references and to engage in further reading from the considerable literature on the subject.

REFERENCES

Anthony, A., Boyle, D., Ingram, T. T. S. and McIsaac, M. W. (1971). *The Edinburgh Articulation Test*. Edinburgh: E. & S. Livingstone

Berry, M. F. (1969). *Language Disorders of Children*. New York: Appleton Century Crofts

Cash, J. (1975). A screening test of language development of three year olds. Dissertation, The Wolfson Centre, Institure of Child Health, University of London.

Duffy, J. K. and Irwin, J. V. (1951). *Speech and Hearing Hurdles*. Columbus, USA: School Service

Dunn, L. (1965). *Peabody Picture Vocabulary Test*. Minneapolis, USA: American Guidance Service

Irwin, J. V., Moore, J. M. and Rampp, D. L. (1972). Non-medical diagnosis and evaluation. In *Principles of Childhood Language Disabilities*, Irwin, J. V., Marge, M. New York: Appleton Century Crofts

Karelitz, S., Karelitz, R. and Rosenfelt, L. (1960). Infant Vocalisations and their Significance. In *Mental Retardation*, Eds Bowman, P. and Mautner, H. New York: Grune & Stratton

Lenneberg, E. (1966). The natural history of language. In *The Genesis of Language*, Eds. Smith, F. and Miller, G. Cambridge, Massachusetts: M. I. T. Press

McCarthy, J. and Kirk, S. (1961). *Illinois Test of Psycholinguistic Abilities*. Urbana, Illinois: University of Illinois

Pollak, M. (1972). *Today's Three Year Olds in London* London: Heinemann

Renfrew, C. (1966). *Renfrew Articulation Attainment Test*. Abingdon: Abbey Press

Reynell, J. K. (1969). A developmental approach to language disorders. *Br. Jl Disord. Commun.* **4**, 33

Reynell, J. (1969). *Reynell Developmental Language Scales*. Windsor: N.F.E.R.

Rheingold, H. L. (1960). The measurement of maternal care. *Child Dev* **31**, 565

Sheridan, M. D. (1975). The Stycar Language Test. *Devl. Med. Child Neurol.* **17**, 164

Templin, M. (1957). *Certain Language Skills in Children*. Minneapolis, USA: University of Minnesota Press

Wasz-Höckert, O., Lind, J., Vuorenkoski, V., Partanen, T. and Valanne, E. (1968). The infant cry. *Clinics. Devl Med. 29*. London: Heinemann

Wepman, J. P. (1958). *Auditory Discrimination Test*. Chicago

Zinkin, P. (1975). Personal communication

CHAPTER 10

Integration of Developmental Activities :'It All Hangs Together'

Children grow up and are adults before their parents know what is happening. They make tremendous advances with little apparent effort on their part or help from without. Even in adverse circumstances children seem to have considerable resources for development. What is really impressive about normal development is its magnitude, especially in contrast to the apparent effortlessness with which it occurs. It could be the ease and inevitability of development which causes many people to take it for granted and so give it little attention or assistance.

A major process contributing to the apparent ease with which child development occurs is the integration of the various activities. Links develop between the various receptive channels; between the different expressive channels; and also between both of these groups. In addition each new skill normally appears at the most appropriate time to make use of information coming in at that time; to carry out actions required at that time; and to prepare the way for the next stage of development. This sequential pattern is often distorted, however, when there are delays and abnormalities of development, and the breakdown of developmental integration produces further problems for young disabled and handicapped children. A study of the characteristics produced by breakdowns in development seen in young handicapped children provides considerable insight into the mechanisms of normal development. In this chapter various examples of developmental integration and the effects of its distortion will be presented.

Advantages of Developmental Integration

The many advantages of efficient developmental integration have been described already, and they can be summarized as follows:

(a)   Developmental integration increases the scope of any one of the receptive channels by linking it with other receptive channels, and the effectiveness of any action is increased by links with other means of expressive response.

(b)   Developmental integration increases the potential for learning and for effective action.

(c)   Developmental integration promotes the smoothness of the developmental pattern.

(d)   Developmental integration creates a possibility of utilizing alternative means for acquiring information and carrying out actions. The possession of alternative means to achieve a particular goal is biologically most important, because if one route is blocked then compensatory mechanisms can be evoked. The importance of this is seen in the case of many handicapped children.

RECEPTIVE INTEGRATION

In Chapter 7 the development of a child's awareness of the outside world was described, and indications were given there of some of the integrative links between sensory functions. The full range of sensory-receptive links is shown in *Figure 75*. There are 10 dual combinations, all of which can be demonstrated to occur during the course of normal development. Some links become so established that they are accepted as one entity. For example, smell and taste are so intertwined that many people consider the two as one entity all the time. Some links, such as those between tactile sensation and smell and taste are of little importance compared to others. The most important links are those between the auditory, visual and tactile sensory channels as shown by the thicker lines in *Figure 75*. These three modalities become associated during the course of normal development until any one, or combination of two, or all three can be brought into use whenever necessary. An important 'critical' period for the development of these links is the second six months of the first year. At this stage the infant is very receptive to all types of stimuli, but much of the information conveyed is new and strange to him. In order to be receptive to the information conveyed by way of these sensory channels, and not just a passive recipient of stimuli, the infant has to apply considerable intellectual effort, especially concentration upon the one sensory channel and inhibition of other activities and interests. Infants show this selective concentration. Visual, tactile and auditory preoccupation are terms which frequently occur and recur in descriptions of child development between 6 and 12 months. Such preoccupation makes it difficult to examine infants. For example, failure to respond to sounds may not be due to deafness, but to intense visual or tactile preoccupation. Such normal infants seem to prefer one of these channels

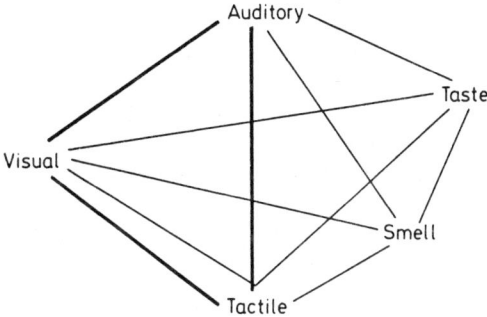

Figure 75. Diagram of sensory-receptive links

to the others and they present as predominantly visually-interested babies, or auditorily-or tactilely-interested. However, marked preference for one channel compared with the others should always lead to a careful check upon the intactness of the other channels.

Emergence From Simple Sensory Preoccupation

Most infants show increasing ability to switch from one input channel to another. The succeeding steps can be summarized as follows:

    (a)   preoccupation with one sensory input at a time;

    (b)   increased flexibility to switch from channel to channel;

    (c)   comprehension of the nature of objects as perceived auditorily, visually and tactilely;

    (d)   ability to associate different sensory impressions about the same object received consecutively;

    (e)   ability to associate different sensory impressions about the same object received apparently simultaneously;

    (f)   ability to receive simultaneous sensory impressions from different objects.

During the examination of infants it is useful to notice how they deal with multiple sensory stimuli. The observations can alert the developmental paediatrician to otherwise unsuspected abnormalities, and they give an indication of the maturity of development. It is highly probable that further study of this subject could lead to a fruitful means of early prediction of future potential.

Auditory-Visual and Auditory-Tactile Integration

The development of the location of sounds by normal infants is a good example of audiovisual integration. The processes involved are summarized in *Figure 50*. A blind child cannot make this link and appears to be insecure as he searches for more tangible accompaniments to the sounds heard. In normal circumstances an auditory-tactile sensory link does not play a large part in development and an appreciation of the association between vibratory tactile sensations and sounds may not occur until quite late. For a blind child, however, such associations are important from an early stage. The tactile ability to distinguish points a small distance apart is made use of in the construction of the Braille alphabet for the blind, but the method is of use only if the tactile sensations are linked with auditory-language concepts.

Visual-Tactile Integration

The integration of visual and tactile sensory functions is important for child development because even fully developed visual sensation does not provide all the available information about an observed object. It reveals size, shape and colour, but not weight, texture, consistency or temperature. These latter features can be learnt only by tactile exploration. So it is essential to have a visuotactile link if the maximum amount of information is to be learnt about the surrounding world. One remarkable case illustrated the limitations of experience which occur when tactile sensation is not available. The child concerned was severely handicapped by cerebral palsy and was completely unaware of the difference between sand and water. He had seen both flowing downwards from buckets as he watched children playing nearby in sandpits and pools, but because he had never had the tactile sensations, he was unaware of the dry grittiness of the sand and the smooth wetness of the water.

Visuotactile sensory links develop early in life as a result of action by the nervous system. The asymmetrical tonic neck reflex appears normally between 1 to 3 months of age. It extends the arm on the side to which the head is turned just at the time that visual fixation upon nearby objects is developing.

The first tactile contact with the object the child is looking at is probably accidental knocking of the object by the extended arm. After this accidental contact has occurred a few times, the infant may contrive for it to occur again until gradually a voluntary element is introduced into the action. From this beginning the infant rapidly builds up an ability to reach out, touch and even to take hold of the object he sees. Having served its purpose, the ATN reflex fades and so permits the next stage of development to occur. Once the reflex ceases to dominate upper-limb posture, the hands can be brought together in the mid-line. This means that the infant can now look at an object, reach out towards it, take hold of it and then bring it into the mid-line closer to himself, so permitting a fuller examination of the object by mouthing, close visual inspection, and a little later, tactile exploration by the other hand. This is a neat example of developmental integration. The linking of visuotactile sensations with appropriate motor actions leads to the acquisition of eye-hand co-ordination, which then develops rapidly and extensively from these early stages. Eye-hand co-ordination then becomes an essential part of the human motor skills and daily life activities. For example, a tennis player is able to see his opponent deliver a service, to judge the flight and speed of the ball, to place his racket in the correct position at the precise moment to ensure a good return shot, having either glanced momentarily just before the shot to correct his positioning if there was time to do so, or else not needing to do so because of his proficiency. And all this had to be done in about a tenth of a second! Such considerable skill develops out of developmental integration in the early months of life.

EXPRESSIVE INTEGRATION

The fact that sensory impressions are received through several different channels, and that it is advantageous to link these receptive functions is easily understood and widely accepted. That a comparable situation exists on the expressive side is not so widely appreciated. At first sight there appear to be only two channels of response—motor actions and vocalizations; but these attributes are used so diversely that a very effective expressive repertoire is created (*Figure 76*).

From the expressive point of view motor actions fall into three main categories, as follows.

(a)   Movement of the body i.e. displacement, as when the child moves towards or away from a particular stimulus. The inhibition of movement is also important and can be considered in the same category. The ability to stand still is a valuable asset, for example, when listening.

(b)   Movement of various parts of the body, especially the face, eyes and arms in ways which come to convey meaning. The value of gestures and facial expressions in everyday life is well appreciated by everyone.

(c)   Manipulation, which can take many forms; and, of course, modelling, drawing and writing are sophisticated forms of expression through manipulation.

The other major channel of expression is through vocalization. Vocalization may be non-verbal or verbal. Non-verbal vocalizations such as shouting and crying and coo-ing can be very effective means of expression, often with a high emotional content. The great richness and effectiveness of verbal expressions needs little additional comment as it is so much part of all our lives.

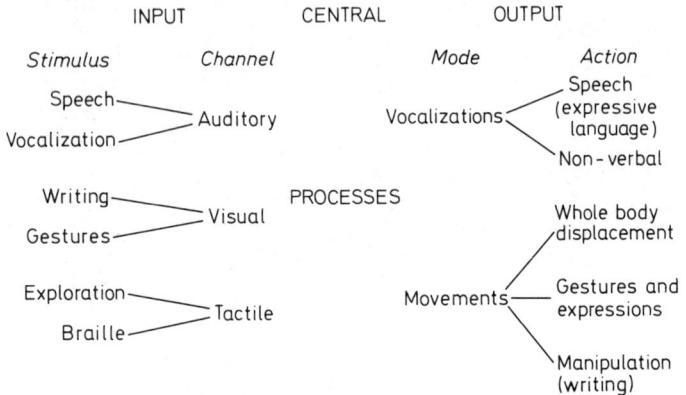

Figure 76. Receptive and expressive functions which can be associated by sensorimotor integration

The important aspect of development with respect to expressive functions is the acquisition of selection and control of the responses. Some integration of actions is present from the beginning. The example of the young child who is frustrated and cross and who as a result cries, stamps his feet, waves his arms, runs away and crossly denounces everyone is familiar to everyone. As development occurs control over the integrated actions is achieved and responses are modified accordingly.

RECEPTIVE–EXPRESSIVE INTEGRATION

Essential to child development are the integrative links which occur between receptive and expressive functions. The range of these functions is shown in *Figure 76*. The central neurological processes play an all-important role in creating and maintaining this integration as has been described already in Chapter 9. Developmental paediatricians must consider the links between receptive and expressive functions with regard to both their contributions to the child's development and the effects of their absence.

Auditory-Vocal Integration

Children receive by the auditory channel many sounds which include non-verbal and verbal vocalizations from others and from themselves. The range of their own vocalizations depends upon the frequency, richness and clarity of the input received from others and when such input is missing, as in the case of a severely deprived child or a deaf child, the expressive side does not develop. The normal pattern is for children to understand what they hear before they are able to reproduce it themselves. If the imperfect utterances of a young child are played back to him he is usually irritated because he is used to hearing and understanding much clearer speech than he can produce himself. The internal auditory feedback mechanism constantly monitors the vocal expressions from an early age and this monitoring ensures that what is expressed is what was intended to be expressed. A delay in auditory feedback of even less than a second produces confusion and frustration and inhibits the free flow of expressive language.

Auditory-Motor Integration

Auditory reception is enhanced by motor activity. The ability to turn the head helps to locate sounds; abilities to move to the source of sounds and to produce sounds by using the hands for clapping and plucking a musical instrument increase the awareness of, and interest in, sounds. To be able to stop movement helps the child to concentrate on 'listening'. However, if the movements do not correspond with the requirements of auditory reception then difficulties arise and development is disrupted. For example, young children receive auditory stimuli at 'knee level' as they sit on their mother's lap and she speaks to them with her mouth only a few inches from the child's ear. When the child can slip off the knee and crawl or walk across the room he immediately extends the distance between himself and his mother's voice. If he is ready for this move he retains auditory awareness and receptivity at the greater distance, but if he is not ready he moves out of the zone of verbal stimulation and an arrest occurs in language development. This phenomenon is seen in some mobile, mentally handicapped children as shown in *Figure 77*.

Normally mobility occurs at just the right stage, and the greater number of personal contacts and opportunities for exploration enjoyed by the mobile child increases his vocabulary and language. In this respect motor activity and auditory reception work together to promote

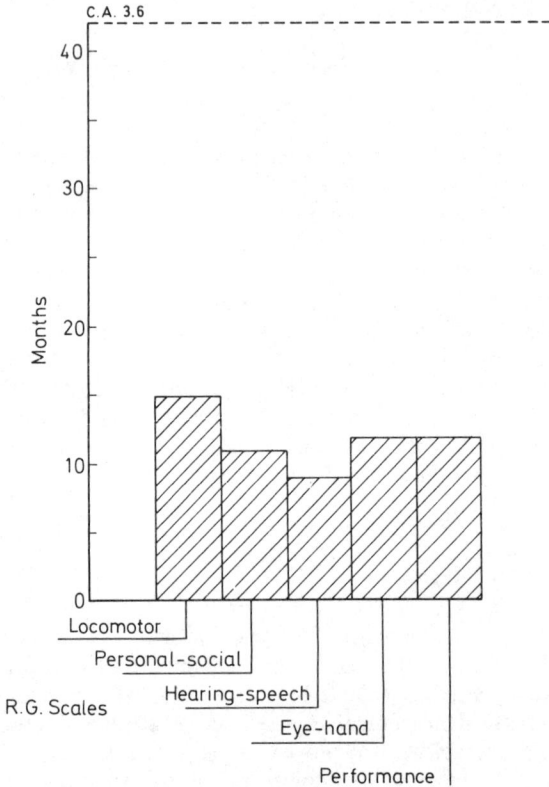

Figure 77. *Arrest of language development in a mobile, mentally handicapped child*

development. In contrast a child who cannot move about has to wait until others come near for him to hear what they say and for them to hear what he says. This can be a very stultifying experience and adversely affects the child's development.

Visual-Vocal Integration

Reading aloud is a ready example of visual-vocal integration. The visual input is interpreted centrally, formulated into auditory language and then expressed vocally. Vocalizations express reactions to visual events such as a gasp of delight at a particularly beautiful scene. Verbal ability is used to describe what is seen, and this skill can be used to communicate with others and to direct one's own actions. In these ways visual-vocal integration plays a frequent and important role in development and failure of this integration leads to serious consequences, most important perhaps being various reading disabilities.

Visual-Motor Integration

Visual reception and perception provide information about the size, shape and colour of objects, their position and relationship with one another, and their movements. This applies to both external objects and to one's own body. Motor activities enable one to move about oneself and also to move other objects. This reinforces visual perception and leads to the development of awareness of spatial dimensions, movement and speed. The ability to move oneself whether this be of the whole body or a fine manipulative movement, and the ability to move other things, enhance visual perception and learning, and without these motor experiences development suffers. In a widely known experiment described by Held and Hein (1963) two kittens were placed at either end of a roundabout. One was harnessed to the roundabout and provided the motor activity to turn it. The other was a passive passenger positioned on the end of the roundabout arm. The active kitten of each experimental pair responded better than the passive kitten in subsequent tests indicating that self-produced movement with concurrent visual feedback is necessary for the development of visually-guided behaviour.

The integration of visual reception with motor activity in the development of eye-hand co-ordination has been described already.

Tactile-Vocal Integration

Tactile sensations can provoke vocalizations especially if they are particularly extreme. The information obtained by tactile exploration is enhanced by verbal labelling and description. Braille reading is an example of sophisticated tactile information being interpreted and understood and then reproduced as expressive language.

Tactile-Motor Integration

Motor activities increase the range and scope of tactile exploration. Children who do not possess arms utilize whatever means they have to obtain tactile information. This might be by using their feet or their mouth. Tactile sensations frequently provide the information for motor action. For example, touching a hot plate leads to rapid withdrawal of the hand.

CONCLUSION

The associations described above are important for child development and can assume especially great importance in certain circumstances. As one studies child development, it is necessary to examine each function and to consider whether or not attempts are being made to integrate this with other functions; whether this integration is proceeding appropriately and adequately; whether it is so efficient that it has been internalized; or so deficient that problems are arising and special help is needed. Much of the developmental guidance programmes for handicapped children is concerned with stimulation of the associative processes.

REFERENCES

Held, R., and Hein, A. (1963). Movement-producing stimulation in the development of visually guided behaviour. *J. comp. physiol. Psychol.* **56,** 872

CHAPTER 11

Developmental Diagnosis and Psychological Tests

Both developmental paediatricians and psychologists are concerned with child development and its variations. Confusion, and sometimes even conflict, exists over who does what. This is regrettable and unnecessary. Both have important rôles which complement rather than conflict with each other, and both gain considerably by working closely together. What is much more important is that the children benefit from such mutual collaboration. The purpose of this chapter is to examine the rôle of the developmental paediatrician, the methods he uses and the assistance he obtains from psychological test procedures.

Parents are not confused about the rôle of the developmental paediatrician. He is a doctor, and as such they turn to him for reassurance that their child is all right, or, if this is not the case, for an explanation of what is wrong, to learn what can be done, and to learn what the future holds both for this child and any others they may have. This situation prevails at the very first contact between parents and paediatricians, which thus becomes a potential therapeutic situation whatever its primary purpose. Although concerned with developmental problems, a developmental paediatrician should never forget that as a children's medical specialist he must be competent to recognize and to deal with the full range of the medical problems of children.

Consideration has to be given to four types of situation which involve the developmental paediatrician:

(1) The routine examination of supposedly healthy and normal infants and children. In addition to satisfying himself about the normality of growth and nutrition and the absence of sensory disabilities, the developmental paediatrician must ensure that there is no serious error of development and that the child is receiving adequate developmental opportunities and stimulation. Time is usually limited, so he has

to rely upon history, casual observation, and a few selected tests, particularly 'limit' tests (*see later*).

(2)   The examination of ill children. Obviously attention to the illness predominates in this situation, but the paediatrician must be alert to the presence of any associated abnormalities and developmental deviations, despite limitations imposed by time and circumstances.

(3)   The examination of children with symptoms and signs which indicate, or might be the consequence of, abnormal development. In these circumstances the developmental paediatrician must ensure that he has sufficient time to arrive at a sound conclusion and, depending upon the supporting facilities which are available, he must be prepared to carry out planned observation studies, or more detailed tests, or both of these.

(4)   The examination of children with established defects and disabilities both initially and on routine surveillance. This requires a wide range of competence and special experience. It usually requires the performance of test procedures which, if supporting psychological services are not available, may have to be done by the paediatrician.

When psychologists are asked to examine supposedly normal healthy children in group (1) above, they will usually require longer time than is available to the developmental paediatrician because their task is to measure the children's intellectual functioning as precisely as is possible in order to give sound educational guidance.

Psychologists contribute greatly to the diagnostic exploration of children in groups (3) and (4) above. Here their rôle is much more than that of a psychometrist. They possess a wide range of exploratory test procedures which help to define the type of disorder and to expose possible therapeutic channels. Close collaboration between psychologist and developmental paediatrician is invaluable in these circumstances.

The paediatrician's approach to the evaluation of a child's development, and in particular a child with suspected developmental problems, must include information gathered from the history, observation, age level attainment and quality of performance.

The History

It is common knowledge that the history may be misleading and erroneous. Memories are uncertain and sometimes the history given is tailored to the enquirer's expectations. Nevertheless the history often provides valuable clues to the etiology of the developmental disturbance, its progress to date, confirmation of the findings of the examination, indications of how the disorder has affected the child and parents, and how it has been dealt with and with what results.

Experience soon teaches the paediatrician to be alert to certain situations. Every comment by parents should be taken seriously. It is surprising, for example, how many mothers report that they thought (and rightly) that their baby was deaf, but that this was not accepted at the time by the doctor. Also, recurrent complaints about apparently trivial symptoms may reveal a need to discuss a more serious problem which they cannot express directly. Not uncommonly an apparently trivial comment made during the history-taking provides a useful lead to the alert clinician.

Developmental paediatricians are aware of the limitations of a history, but nevertheless find that it is an essential part of their evaluation and would never do without it. Information about a child's abilities obtained from the reports of parents or other attendants is always recorded. It is advisable to record it separately from information about a child's performance actually observed by the paediatrician because different weight is attached to the two types of information in the final analysis. In contrast, some schemes for the psychological evaluation of children do not take account of the history.

The history-taking period is also of value as a time when doctor, patient and parents get to know each other and establish a comfortable relationship.

Observation

Casual observation

Casual observation requires familiarity with child development combined with clinical alertness so that the observer is instantly aware of discrepancies in behaviour and performance. This skill, which is acquired only as a result of training and experience, is especially useful on developmental ward rounds in nurseries and schools (as described in Chapter 12). All doctors should receive sufficient training as undergraduates to acquaint them with the essential features of child development. Those who continue to train to be developmental paediatricians have further opportunities to acquire the experience to make them efficient observers of development.

Planned observation

Planned observation studies provide valuable additional diagnostic techniques for both physiologists and paediatricians. They are described in detail elsewhere (Holt and Reynell, 1967) and are summarized here.

Planned observation techniques require time, but not as much time as might be imagined, and, as they are sometimes the only methods available to provide reliable information, this time is very well spent. The circumstances in which they are particularly useful include the following.

(a)   In the evaluation of children who will not co-operate in any other form of examination or test. By this means it is possible to obtain some objective information in even the most difficult cases.

(b)   As a supplement to conventional examinations and tests when these do not provide all the information which is required, e.g. observation of strategies used by a child to deal with difficult tasks.

(c)   In the evaluation of some particular aspect of behaviour for which there is no other form of test, e.g. attention, co-operation.

(d)   In the study of children's reactions to situations, e.g. behaviour in a group situation.

The observation techniques which are useful in developmental paediatric practice are the following.

(i)   Descriptive techniques—diary or specimen.
(ii)   Sampling techniques—time or event.
(iii)   Rating techniques of specified traits.

In addition, the above techniques can be combined into a scheme called a *field unit analysis*. For example, it might be decided to observe the behaviour of five children playing together. During the observation the situation will change from time to time such as when one child leaves the group or when the teacher joins the group. The time of each change is noted and the observation period is divided into units at these times. The composition and situation of the group is homogeneous during each unit of observation. The observations in each unit will consist of specimen descriptions, and time and event samplings as appropriate, and ratings may be applied to particular traits.

Descriptive techniques These are precisely what the name suggests. They consist of carefully recorded descriptions of everything done by and to the child. Such observations may be carried out at regular intervals over a long period, the so-called diary description technique, which was used so effectively by Piaget; or they may cover a particular section of the child's activities, the specimen description.

A quantitative element is introduced into observations by using sampling techniques.

Event sampling   This consists of recording the time of occurrence and the circumstances associated with some preselected aspect of behaviour as it occurs during a period of observation. For example, it may be decided to study a child's aggressive behaviour by event sampling during a 30-minute observation period. The time and the circumstances of each aggressive act during this period are noted. This information gives a quantitative measure of the frequency of aggressive acts, and a qualitative description of the circumstances from which it might be possible to deduce the cause of the aggression. This method is both quantitative and qualitative.

Time sampling   This consists of recording whether or not a particular type of behaviour is occurring at regular time intervals during the observation period. The observation period is divided into appropriate intervals—say 10 seconds—and at each interval a note is made as to whether or not the child is performing the particular action being studied. For example, this method can be used to determine the frequency of use of a hemiplegic hand during a 10-minute play session. To know that the frequency of use of a hemiplegic hand increased from 5 per cent to 30 per cent after a period of therapy is a more satisfying basis for clinical work than simply recording 'He is using his hand more'. This method provides information about the frequency of occurrence of the behaviour being observed. It is almost wholly a quantitative method.

Further precision is introduced into observations by grading the behaviour observed. This is known as trait rating.

Trait rating   A range of 3, 4 or 5 grades is usually chosen stretching from absence of the particular behaviour to its most florid presentation. This method provides a measure of the severity or intensity of the particular behaviour being observed. For example, attention, an important part of a child's behaviour, might be rated as follows.

(i)   Attention cannot be obtained by any means.

(ii)   Attention obtained on considerably less than half of the occasions and usually only after several attempts.

(iii)   Attention obtained on about half the occasions and usually on the first or second attempt.

(iv)   Attention obtained easily on considerably more than half of the occasions, but not on all of them.

(v)   Attention obtained promptly every time.

242

TABLE 29
Dangers of Inference (Holt and Reynell, 1967)

Actual observation	Observer biased towards 'autism'	Observer biased towards deafness
2.45. Pulling a chair around the floor. Snatches at B's pram. Desists when his mother says quietly 'No, Robin'. Spins a wheeled-chair. Goes back to ordinary chair, pulls it around and spins it. Spins himself. Spins wheeled-chair. Champing jaw movements all the time. Spins all chairs in turn, flaps hands.	2.45. Pulling a chair around the floor. Interested only in the furniture and not people. Takes B's pram just as an object with wheels, spinning everything. Takes no notice of people. Does not go to his mother or look at her when she speaks to him.	2.45. Pulling chairs around. Does not respond to the sounds of the other children, or to his mother's voice calling him.
2.50. Sitting on the floor gazing at a red square. Champing jaws. Spins a chair. Climbs onto a chair and off again. His mother goes out of the room, and his behaviour does not alter. Sits on the floor. Spins a chair. Hand flapping. Quiet, monotonous vocalization.	2.50. Mesmerized by the colour red on the floor. Still spinning chairs. Does not notice his mother leaving the room.	2.50. Sitting on the floor. Visually absorbed. Climbs onto a chair. Does not hear his mother go out of the room. Monotonous vocalization, just like a deaf child.
2.55. Still spinning chairs and champing jaws. Vocalizes a loud 'er'. Rests his face on a chair, then lies on the ground. Gets up again and spins chair. His mother goes out. Pokes his eye. Spins a chair. Screams when his mother comes in and picks him up. She takes him to the toilet where he continues to scream.	2.55. Still obsessed by his spinning activities. Then tries to retreat from the world by hiding his face on a chair and then on the ground. Objects to the interruption of his activity when his mother takes him to the toilet. Panics at the strange surroundings.	2.55. Still the same monotonous vocalization. Lies down for a rest. Does not hear his mother go out again. Does not hear her come up to him, so he screams when she picks him up. She cannot explain to him about the toilet, because he cannot hear words, so he continues to scream.

These different techniques may be used in combination according to the requirements of the situation. Although these methods are easy to describe and to understand, considerable practice is required before reliable observations can be made. They require an ability to record precisely what is observed without any inference. This is not at all easy at first. The extract in Table 29 (Holt and Reynell, 1967) shows how personal bias and inference can lead to very dangerous false conclusions, against which the developmental paediatrician must always be on guard.

INITIAL, KEY, LIMIT AND MEAN AGES

Many developmental paediatricians value the concept of the various 'ages' which have been described by different workers because of the help they provide both to the understanding of developmental problems and in the performance of practical work.

'Key Ages'

The idea of 'key ages' originated with Gesell and Amatruda (1969). These are empirically chosen ages. A characteristic developmental picture can be described for each key age. On the basis of their experience Gesell and Amatruda selected as key ages, 4, 16, 28 and 40 weeks and 12, 18, 24 and 36 months. Their cross-sectional studies of child development at these ages give a clear picture of typical behaviour at these times. A particular item of developmental behaviour will be seen first at one of these ages, which is then said to be the key age for that particular behaviour. In this respect there is a link between key ages and initial ages which are discribed below.

The description of development in Chapters 3, 4 and 5 are based upon key ages of 6 weeks, 3, 6, 9, 12 and 18 months, and 2, 3, 4, 5, 7, 9, 12 and 14 years. Egan, Illingworth and MacKeith (1969) base their developmental examination procedures upon this concept of key ages and use the ages of 6 weeks, 6, 10 and 18 months, and 2, 3 and 4½ years.

Anyone who is thoroughly conversant with the developmental picture at the key ages is able to give an approximate estimate of a child's performance—for example, 'fairly typical of 40 weeks' or 'somewhere between 40 and 52 weeks'. This is not a developmental diagnosis of course, but it does enable the examiner to select the age to concentrate upon in further examinations, when he will look at many more items of behaviour at that age level.

TABLE 30

Developmental Screening Examination at 7 Months (Starte, 1972)

Test	Grade of response				
	1	2	3	4	5
Brick (cube)	No grasp	Palmar grasp	Mouthing	Transferring	Finger manipulation
Smartie (coloured sweet)	No interest	Whole hand scrabble, No pick-up	Whole hand scrabble and pick-up	Fingers and thumb pick-up	Index finger and thumb pick-up
Rattle	No interest	Transient interest and manipulation	Prolonged interest and manipulation	Manipulation and eventual imitation	Immediate imitation
Bell	No interest	Transient interest and manipulation	Prolonged interest and manipulation	Manipulation and eventual imitation	Immediate imitation
	3/4 inch	1/2 inch	1/4 inch	3/16 inch	1/8 inch

		difference between 2 sides	4–5 sounds	4–5 sounds	6 sounds
Prone	Head up not sustained	Head up, weight on forearms	Head up, shoulders up, weight on hands	Head and shoulders up, knee up	Crawls
Sitting	No sitting stability Hyper-or hypotonic	Sits briefly with support then unstable, back hypotonic	Sits upright, needs Examiner's hand on back	Sits upright steadily, unsupported	Reaches to each side without toppling
Standing	No weight-bearing	Stands with support, full weight not taken	Full weight taken on legs	Shifts weight from one leg to the other	Walks supported
Babbling	Silence or purposeless noise	Occasional purposeful babble	Frequent purposeful babble	Two-syllable babble	Recognizable word

TABLE 31

Developmental Screening Examination at 2 Years (Starte, 1972)

Test	Grade of response				
	1	2	3	4	5
Bricks (tower)	1–3	4–5	6–7	8–9	10 or more
Screws	1	2	3	4	5
Form-board (3 shapes)	0–1 in board	2 in board	3 in board	3 in reversed board eventually	3 in reversed board immediately
Comprehension	0–2 recognized	3–4 recognized	5–6 recognized and 'spoon in cup'	'Ball to Mummy' and 'doll with spoon'	'Car on top of brick' and 'brick under cup'

Vocabulary (words)	0–2	3–5	6–12	13–20	21 or more
Sentence (length)	None	Occasional connected words only	3–4	5–6	7 or more
Rolling balls (Stycar)	1/4 inch or larger	3/16 inch	1/8 inch	3/16 inch right and left separately	1/8 inch right and left separately
Throwing ball	No throw	Throws with poor direction and force	Good try but fails to get ball in box	Gets ball in box from 2 feet	Gets ball in box from 4 feet
Kicking ball	No kicking attempted	No kick, tries but runs into ball	Kicks ball, occasional miss or stumble	Strong kick with poor direction	Strong kick with good direction

The study and testing of child development in this cross-sectional way is valuable, but there are potential dangers. Too rigid adherence to 'key ages' introduces too rigid an approach to the study of child development, and too quantitative a bias in the evaluation of observations. Continued appreciation by the examiner of the flowing continuity of development, and attention to the quality of the child's performance in every examination will safeguard against these dangers.

A good example of the use of key ages is the screening examination which has been devised by Starte (1972). He examines supposedly normal children, and is concerned with the detection of any abnormality. His screening tests therefore consist of tests of development and tests for sensory impairment. He chose the key ages of 7 months and 2 years; decided which were the important features at these ages and then based his examination upon the *quality* of performance of these items which he scores from 1 to 5 according to whether the performance is inferior (1), average (3) or superior (5). His scales for these two key ages are shown in Tables 30 and 31. Similar tests have been devised by Starte and his general practitioner colleagues (the Ashford Child Development Group) to cover the additional ages of 1, 3 and 4½ years.

'Initial Age', 'Limited Age' and 'Mean Age'

Children's abilities do not appear at a precise age. In any group of normal children each individual ability appears over an age range as illustrated in *Figure 78*. The duration of this range varies considerably

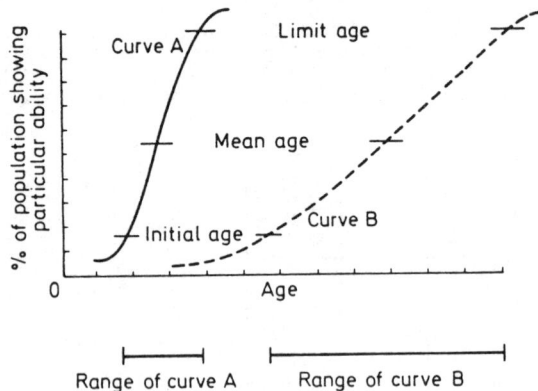

Figure 78. Diagrammatic illustration of acquisition of abilities showing initial, mean and limit ages, and range of abilities

with different abilities. In some cases the range is quite small. In other words only a short time elapses between the first appearance of the particular ability in a few children and its manifestation by all children (curve A in *Figure 78*). In other cases the range may be much longer (curve B). In the case of each ability, the age at which a few children first show that particular ability can be called the 'initial age'. The age at which the majority of children show the ability is the 'limit age'. The 'mean age' is the age at which 50 per cent of the normal population manifest the particular ability.

These terms are used in the following way:

'Initial Age'

It is possible to use the concept of an 'initial age' to say of a child, when he shows a particular ability, that his performance is comparable to the 'initial age' level, at least, however old he actually is. This gives a minimal developmental age level. For example, suppose that a particular ability has an initial age of 5 months, a mean age of 7 months and a limit age of 9 months: when that ability is observed it is possible to say that the child's developmental level is *at least* 5 months.

This method is especially useful in the examination of handicapped children. It may not be possible to carry out a full examination and the clinical picture may be dominated by the child's limited abilities, but it may be possible to note a few items which can be given a minimum 'initial age' level.

A list of 'initial ages' for various abilities has been compiled mostly from the writings of Gesell and Amatruda (1969) and Griffiths (1967) (Table 32). This is not a complete list, but could provide a basis for a paediatrician's own personal list which he will tend to build up automatically as he becomes more experienced in developmental work.

'Limit Age'

The concept of 'limit ages' is used most often in developmental screening programmes in which many normal children are examined with the aim of detecting a few who may not be normal and who require fuller examination. In these circumstances any child who is not showing abilities when beyond the limit age for those abilities (i.e. beyond the age when the majority of children show the particular ability) should be identified and examined more fully. Unlike the concept of 'initial ages' which can be applied to both what Gesell and Amatruda called

TABLE 32

Initial Ages for Various Childhood Abilities

Age	Ability, observation of which indicates a minimum developmental age level	Age	Ability, observation of which indicates a minimum developmental age level
1 month	Regards object in line of vision and follows for short distances. Immobilizes to nearby sound and social approach. Prone, raises head just clear of table.	1 year	Gives a toy; releases cube into cup. Co-operates with dressing. Walks one hand held. Responds to 'No' and 'Give it'.
4 months	Very slight head lag when pulled to sitting. Almost complete head stability in sitting. Prompt visual regard. Holds ring, reaches for it with free hand and takes it to mouth.	1½ years	Sits down on chair. Builds tower of 4–5 cubes. Spontaneous scribble. Looks at picture book and may name or point to one picture. Carries doll or teddy and hugs it. Obeys simple directions.
6 months	Immediate reach for object and retention in radial palmar grasp. Transfers object (cube) from hand to hand. Sits momentarily on a firm surface. Takes feet to mouth. Discriminates strangers.	2 years	Towers 6–7 cubes. Imitates vertical stroke and circle. Names pictures (2 or 3). Kicks ball. Follows directions. Walks up and down stairs.
9 months	Index finger approach to small objects. Early pincer grasp. Shakes bell. Pulls objects towards himself with string. Pulls to standing. Pat-a-cakes (claps hands) and waves 'Bye bye'. Imitates sounds and uses 'Mama', 'Dada' with meaning.	3 years	With book turns pages singly and names pictures. With crayon early tripod grip, copies circle and names drawing. Asks questions: may answer one or two. Knows name and sex. Repeats up to 3 digits. Matches 3 colours.

TABLE 33

Limit Ages for Various Childhood Abilities

Age in months	Ability which should be shown by stated age (if absent or doubtful further examination is indicated)
1	Some indication of attention.
2	Attention to objects. Some response to nearby voices and everyday noises.
3	Head held erect.
4	Hands not fisted. Shows ordinary interest in people and playthings.
5	Reaches for object.
6	ATNR not present or producible. Visual fixation and following established. Turns to sounds.
7	Holds objects in hands.
9	Gives attention to gestures.
10	Sits independently on firm surfaces. Uses tuneful babble to self and others. Bears most of weight on legs. Chews lumpy food.
12	Attends to words.
15	Releases held object.
18	Walks alone. No casting, mouthing, drooling.
21	Kicks when standing. Says single words with meaning.
27	Puts 2–3 words together into a phrase.
3 years	Can stand on one leg. Talks in sentences.
4 years	Uses fully intelligible speech.

'permanent' and 'temporary' abilities, the concept of limit ages can be applied in developmental diagnosis only to permanent abilities.

Gesell and Amatruda had something similar to 'limit age' tests in mind when they presented their list of the latest ages for acceptable appearance of certain abilities. Egan *et al.* (1969) and Sheridan (1973), in describing the developmental examination of the young child, listed several items at each age of examination the absence of which made it mandatory to investigate further. Neligan and Prudham (1969) also introduced the idea of upper age limits for certain simple items which members of a primary medical care team—health visitor and general practitioner—could use in order to pick out those children in need of further examination. From these and various other sources a list of limit tests has been devised (Table 33). It must be emphasized that this concept of 'limit' tests is a clinical one to assist developmental paediatricians when there is only a little time available for the examination. Not all children selected for further examination in this way will be abnormal; examples can be quoted of children who were remarkably late in various skills and yet turned out to be normal (*see* Illingworth, 1972), and conversely some of the individuals not selected by 'limit age' tests will be abnormal and these children will be detected in most cases by observing an abnormal or poor quality of performance.

As an illustration of the application of initial and limit ages, we may consider the case of a 20-month-old child who is taken to see a paediatrician because of failure to walk. This is beyond the limit age for walking (18 months), and must be fully investigated and considered to be abnormal until proven otherwise. If the child is responsive to simple commands and will give a cube to the examiner on request the developmental level is at least 12 months because this is the initial age for these items. This child therefore requires an exploration of developmental abilities between 12 and 18 months.

'Mean Age'

The 'mean age' is used in most psychological tests as the age level basis for scoring the test. The use of standard deviations along with the 'mean age' is useful. The initial age corresponds to approximately 2SD below the mean age and the limit age to approximately 2SD above.

Quality of Performance

Paediatricians obtain many useful clues from noting the quality of performance of children as they carry out various tasks during a developmental examination. The information obtained in this way enables them to detect a number of children with developmental problems who would otherwise not be noted until much later. The paediatricians' medical, especially neurological, training is invaluable to them in this respect.

The items noted by an alert paediatrician include the following:

the child's composure;
the ease and smoothness of the child's movements;
the normality of his posture in standing and sitting;
his attentiveness and concentration;
the promptness of his comprehension and responsiveness;
the presence of tremor or ataxia especially during manipulative tasks;
unusual posturing of the hands when carrying out a task;
evidence of excessive muscle action;
the presence of mirror movements;
difficulties brought to light when the child is asked to increase the speed or accuracy of performance;
poor eye-hand co-ordination;
the use of trick movements.

PSYCHOLOGICAL TESTS AND DEVELOPMENTAL SCALES

Paediatricians must be conversant with the various tests which are used by psychologists. A vast number of psychological tests have been devised and are available. It is not possible, or necessary, to refer to all of these. The reader who wishes to delve more deeply into psychological tests and testing should refer to the many books on the subject. He could start with *Psychological Testing* by Anastasi (1954).

Paediatricians need to know what is involved in the more frequently used tests in order to decide whether a test is appropriate for a particular child and a particular problem. For example, how long does it last; what is the child required to do; what age range does it cover; how will it be affected if the child has motor, visual, auditory or emotional difficulties; what does the information tell you about the child; how reliable are the results?

Paediatricians who are establishing developmental units may have to budget for the purchase of test material. The current cost (1976) is indicated with the specific tests as they are described below. Costs may change in the future and figures are quoted only as an approximate guide. Almost all tests are available from the National Foundation for Educational Research (N.F.E.R.).*

*Address: 2 Jennings Buildings, Thames Avenue, Windsor, Berks SL4 IQS

The Nature of Psychological Tests

Many psychological tests were devised during the last few decades. The earlier ones attempted to sample a wide range of intellectual functions and to produce a measure of general intellectual ability. The limitations of this approach were soon appreciated. Later tests are more analytical and explore specific areas of intellectual function. Considerable effort has gone into the preparation of such tests, and specialized training and experience are required to appreciate their advantages and limitations, and to administer and interpret them accurately.

The use of many psychological tests is restricted to adequately trained personnel, who are usually registered psychologists. The restriction is understandable and is an attempt to ensure the maintenance of reliable work and to prevent abuse of the tests. Other tests are available for use by paediatricians provided that they have been trained in their administration and interpretation. The over-confident physician who feels he can carry out the tests from the book does himself and his patients an ill-service and deserves all the condemnation he receives. Only in extreme circumstances would he consider performing a surgical operation from the book and without other training. The circumstances are not too dissimilar, because important and vital recommendations and decisions are just as often associated with psychological tests as with operations.

Most of the tests have been standardized on a large population, and, provided that the prescribed technique is adhered to, the results of the examination of an individual can be reliably compared to the distribution of scores of the standardization population. By such means it is possible to define the position of the individual's score in relation to the average for the whole population. Furthermore, the tests are so devised that comparable results may be expected from different examiners provided they adhere to the test techniques. Errors increase considerably when the tests are performed by untrained personnel, the prescribed techniques of administration are ignored, and only portions of the test are used.

Limitations of Psychological Tests

Psychological tests reveal much about both general and specific intellectual ability, but they do have limitations of which the developmental paediatrician must be aware.

The standardization may be unsatisfactory: the population chosen may be too small, of biased selection, of an earlier generation, or of a different culture. For example, one must interpret very carefully the results of an intellectual test involving general knowledge administered to a handicapped British child who has had few opportunities to obtain such knowledge, especially when the results are compared to standardizations carried out on American children 30 years ago. Most American standardized tests, however, do have a set of revised items to make them comparable and suitable for use with British children.

Some tests of general intelligence are biased in certain directions so that children with difficulties in that area score unfavourably. For example, the Stanford-Binet test is a particularly sound test relating well to educational capability, but it is biased in favour of verbal items, with the result that language-impaired children score unfavourably.

Sometimes the test items are too vague and so give rise to ambiguous results. For example, one item of the Griffiths test concerns the child's ability to sit alone. No mention is made, however, as to whether or not this means that the infant has to sit on a firm or soft surface, or with his legs flexed or extended. Sometimes an infant will fail this item not because he is developmentally retarded, but because he is suffering from cerebral palsy and the tight hamstrings disrupt his sitting posture. The developmental paediatrician must be alive to such anomalies.

Tests tend to be least reliable towards the extremes of the age range for which they were devised because at their floor and ceiling levels they discriminate less well between different children. Care must be taken, therefore, in the interpretation of results at these extremes. Almost all tests were devised for use with normal children and were standardized on an appropriate normal population. When severely handicapped children are tested it is not always easy to interpret the significance of the results. For example, it is our impression that when some very retarded children are given the Merrill–Palmer test, which contains a lot of motor performance items, their scores seem to be spuriously high as compared with their overall developmental level.

It is debatable whether it is permissible or desirable to abstract items from the test procedures. Although in some cases copyright regulations do not permit this to be done, in practice it is impossible completely to ignore what one knows about the test items. Let us take a simple example: presenting a two-year-old with a set of small cubes and observing him building them up one upon another. When the child succeeds in making a tower of 6 cubes, it seems reasonable for the paediatrician to conclude that this particular observation has not revealed any abnormality or developmental delay, especially as he knows that the Griffiths test specifies an ability to build a tower of 5 cubes as one of the 2-year-level items. It would, of course, be wrong to claim that he had done part of the Griffiths test and the developmental paediatrician has no intention to do so. He is making use of his knowledge of the Griffiths test items to add a little more information to that which he acquires from watching a child tower cubes. In fact, as well as noting the number of cubes the child succeeds in building into a tower, the developmental paediatrician will have enquired about the child's play experience in general, and whether he has used anything similar to the cubes before. He then notes the child's interest in the task, his spontaneous actions, visual awareness, his method of manipulating the cubes, and the presence of any tremor or unusual posturing of the hands.

Paediatricians should beware of merely checking off a number of items of the child's performance on a list without understanding the developmental background, since by doing so they are not really engaging in developmental paediatrics. They are performing neither a psychological test nor making an adequate study of child development.

Individual Tests

The following are some of the more frequently used psychological tests and developmental scales.

The Bayley Scales of Infant Development (Bayley, 1965)

Cost £123.78.   Time approximately 30 to 60 min.

These scales were prepared very thoroughly and carefully standardized. There are three complementary parts; the mental scale, the motor scale, and the infant behaviour record. Although devised in California, U.S.A., the scales are used extensively in the U.K. where comparative standardization procedures have been carried out (Francis-Williams and Yule, 1967).

Denver Developmental Scale (Frankenberg and Dodds, 1968)

Cost approximately £17.00.   Age range 1 month to 6 years.
                    Time approximately 15 min.

The Denver scale was devised for use by developmental paediatricians and it has been used by ancilliary personnel (Frankenberg *et al.* 1970)

It enables a record to be made fairly quickly of the development of young children. The chart (*Figure 37*), which is an essential part of the test material, shows the normal age range of appearance of various items. It is very easy to see when any of the items appear later than the upper age limit and hence call for further examination. In this respect these items of the Denver scale are similar to the 'limit age' tests. The scale does not distinguish between reported and observed items, but this can be introduced.

Gesell Developmental Schedules (Gesell and Amatruda, 1969)

Cost £163.68.   Age range 0 to 5 years.   Time approximately 30 min.

Designed for use by paediatricians who must, however, receive appropriate training.

These scales have a clinical diagnostic orientation, and, being more concerned with the diagnosis and evaluation of abnormalities than with the measurement of attainment, they are more satisfactorily applicable to handicapped children than are some of the other tests.

There is a bias upon motor items especially in the first 2 years. The results are presented in four areas—motor, adaptive, language and personal-social.

Griffiths Scales (Griffiths, 1967, 1970)

There are two consecutive scales which together cover the period 0 to 7 years.
(a) Cost £38.   Age range 0 to 2 years.   Time approximately 30 min.
(b) Cost £40. Age range 2 to 7 years. Time approximately 45 to 60 min.

These scales are designed for use by clinicans who have received appropriate training. They are attractive tests because of the strong developmental emphasis and the analysis of the observations being divided into five areas.

The first, the 'infant' scale, is widely used and well liked, but the more recently introduced extension scale is not yet so familiar. It is possibly not quite as good as some of the other tests available for this age range and rather too many of the performance items are timed tests.

Goodenough   Draw-a-Man   Test   (Harris,   1963)   *Goodenough-Harris Drawing Test*

Cost £12.75.   Age range 3 to 15 years.   Time approximately 15 min.
This is a simple, interesting and easily administered test, which the child usually enjoys. The child is presented with a crayon and paper and encouraged to draw a man. By showing the child what is required the test can be entirely independent of verbal instructions. Adequate manipulative skill is required. A score is derived from an analysis of the drawing and is converted to a mental age (*see* Chapter 8). The test material provided is slightly more sophisticated than the above description. The ease and speed of administration make this an attractive test but it is inadvisable to use it alone because it tests only part of the range of intellectual skills.

Illinois Test of Psycholinguistic Abilities (Kirk and Kirk, 1971)

Cost £86.00.   Age range 2 to 10 years.   Time 90 min. plus.

This is a lengthy and complex test which explores the communication pathways and provides information about auditory-vocal and auditory-motor functions, and the organization of both receptive and expressive language functions. It may appear to provide a more precise analysis than in fact it does; it has a cultural bias; and it may become tedious for the child, the examiner or both. Despite these criticisms it is a sophisticated investigative tool which, when used by experienced psychologists in correctly selected cases, yields valuable information.

Merrill–Palmer Scale of Mental Tests (Stutsman, 1948)

Cost £250.00.   Age range 18 months to 6 years.   Time approximately
30 min.
The material of this test is attractive. The test taps various abilities, but the results are not presented in sub-sections. Considerable reliance is placed upon speed by the inclusion of many timed items, and this makes the test less satisfactory for children with physical disabilities.

Peabody Picture Vocabulary Test (P.P.V.T.) (Dunn, 1965)

An American test, but an English version is available.
Cost £23.50.   Age range 2½ to 18 years.   Time approximately 15 min.

A simple attractive test which is easily and quickly administered. It provides a useful means of exploring the extent and nature of a child's verbal understanding without his needing to use expressive language. The test is limited if the child has not experienced the items illustrated. This test seems to be used quite often by teachers.

Raven's Progressive Matrices (Raven, 1939)

There are three types—advanced, standard and coloured, but only the last two concern us.
Standard: Cost on application to N.F.E.R. Age range 8½ years to adult. Time approximately 30 min.
Coloured: Cost on application to N.F.E.R. Age range 5 to 11 years. Time approximately 20 min.

These tests are very easy for a child to understand so there is seldom any difficulty in administration or scoring. Many examiners like the matrices because of their lack of cultural bias and the fact that they do not require language for their administration and completion. The matrices test provides a measure of intellectual capacity. It is often used in conjunction with the Mill Hill Vocabulary Scale, which indicates how well that capacity has been realized in a particular cultural environment.

Reynell Developmental Language Scales (R.D.L.S.) (Reynell, 1969)

Cost £48.50.   Age range 1 to 5 years.   Time approximately 30 min.

These scales analyse and separately assess verbal comprehension and expressive language. There is a separate verbal comprehension scale which can be used for children with physical difficulties. The developmental basis, clinical orientation and ready relation to therapeutic requirements make these particularly attractive scales. They are being used increasingly by psychologists, developmental paediatricians and speech therapists.

Stanford-Binet Intelligence Scale (Terman and Merrill, 1961)

Cost on application to N.F.E.R. Age range 2 years to adult. Time approximately 45 to 60 min.

This is a very well known test of general intelligence which is used extensively in the British education service. It correlates well with educational attainments. It has a verbal bias which renders it unsuitable for some children as a measure of their possible intellectual potential; for example those with language disorders, and immigrant children for whom English is not their mother tongue. There are a wide variety of test items, some of which could be made more interesting than they are.

Wechsler Intelligence Scales for Children (W.I.S.C.) (Wechsler, 1944)

Cost £27.00. Age range 5 to 15 years. Time approximately 45 to 60 min.

Wechsler Pre-School and Primary Scale of Intelligence (W.P.P.S.I.)

Cost £49.00. Age range 4 to 6½ years. Time approximately 45 to 60 min.

The W.I.S.C. and W.P.P.S.I. tests are very similar and together they cover the age range of 4 to 15 years.

The W.I.S.C. has been used very widely for many years and is relied upon a great deal. The W.P.P.S.I. is a more recent addition, designed to carry the W.I.S.C. down to a lower age range and to discriminate better between children aged 4 to 6 years. The distinctive feature of both scales is the separate examination of verbal and performance intelligence. Although this was an advance upon methods measuring general intelligence it may perhaps have led to too great a separation of these two aspects which are, in fact, interrelated in many ways. The tests rely upon the presentation of the same task in increasingly complex forms until the child's limit is reached. This method sometimes frustrates the child and leads to blocking.

REFERENCES

Anastasi, A. (1954). *Psychological Testing*. New York: Macmillan

Bayley, N. (1965). Comparisons of mental and motor test scores for ages 1–15 months by sex, birth order and race, geographical location and education of parents. *Child Dev.* **36**, 379

Dunn, L. (1965). *Peabody Picture Vocabulary Test*. Minneapolis: American Guidance Service

Egan, D., Illingworth, R. S., and MacKeith, R. C. (1969). Developmental screening 0–5 years. *Clinics Dev. Med. 30*, London: Heinemann

Francis-Williams, J., and Yule, W. (1967). The Bayley Infant Scales of Mental and Motor Development. *Devl. Med. Child Neurol.* **9**, 391

Frankenberg, W. K., and Dodds, J. B. (1968). *The Denver Developmental Screening Test*. Denver: University of Colorado Press

– Goldstein, A., Chabot, A., Camp, B. M., and Fitch, M. (1970). Training the indigenous professional: the screening technician. *J. Pediat.* **77,** 564

Gesell, A., and Amatruda, C. S. (1969). *Developmental Diagnosis.* New York: Harper & Row

Griffiths, R. (1967). *The Abilities of Babies.* 4th edn. London: University of London Press

– (1970). *The Abilities of Young Children.* Chard, Somerset: Young and Son

Harris, D. B. (1963). *Children's Drawings as Measures of Intellectual Maturity.* New York: Harcourt, Brace and World

Holt, K. S., and Reynell, J. K. (1967). *Observation of Children.* London: National Association for Mental Health

Illingworth, R. S. (1972). *The Development of the Infant and Young Child– Normal and Abnormal.* Edinburgh: Churchill Livingstone

Kirk, S. A., and Kirk, W. D. (1971). *Psycholinguistic Learning Difficulties, Diagnosis and Remediation.* Chicago: University of Illinois Press

Neligan, G., and Prudham, D. (1969). Potential value of four early developmental milestones in screening children for increased risk of later retardation. *Devl Med. Child Neurol.* **11,** 423

Raven, J. C. (1939). The R.E.C.I. series of perceptual tests: an experimental survey. *Br. J. med. Psychol.* **18,** 16

Reynell, J. (1969). *Reynell Developmental Language Scales.* Windsor: National Foundation For Educational Research

Sheridan, M. D. (1973). *Children's Developmental Progress.* Windsor: National Foundation for Educational Research

Starte, G. D. (1972). "Child's Play" or paediatric developmental assessment in general practice. *Practitioner* **209,** 84

Stutsman, R. (1948). *Mental Measurement of Pre-school Children.* New York: Harcourt, Brace and World

Terman, L. M., and Merrill, M. A. (1961). *Stanford Binet Intelligence Scale, 3rd revision, Form L. M.* London: Harrap

Wechsler, D. (1944). *The Measurement of Adult Intelligence.* 3rd edn, Baltimore: Williams and Wilkins

The Developmental Approach to Handicapped Children; Developmental Guidance and Training

Developmental paediatricians are concerned with the achievement of optimum development by all children. Consequently, when they encounter any child with abnormal development, or with any condition which might interfere with development, they strive to find out all they can about the conditions and then they try to promote the child's development. Their efforts are made along the following principal directions:

(a)   conveying an understanding of the child's development to all who are concerned with him;

(b)   reinforcing the child's most recently acquired abilities and ensuring that they are used most productively;

(c)   providing missed experiences;

(d)   making use of other skills possessed by the child to overcome his difficulties;

(e)   using external means, e.g. aids, appliances and toys, at an appropriate developmental level to overcome the child's difficulties.

Conveying an Understanding of a Child's Development

This is best done by example. If we show our understanding of a child's development by the way we do things with him and to him this will be noticed by parents and others, and then copied by them. To be able to do this it is necessary to be able to size up the child's developmental level quickly and to make approaches to him at that level. It is also

262

most essential to be sensitive to the child's reactions. The following extract from the discussion of child—stranger encounters by Tinbergen and Tinbergen (1972) reveals the clumsy insensitiveness of our usual contacts with children:

'When meeting a child . . . . the observer . . . . either smiles or simply looks at the child. Its responses are extremely varied. They can range from, on the one hand, definitely positive to, on the other, gaze aversion, and closing of the eyes, turning of the head, and even of the whole body, and snuggling up against the mother; . . . . . Between these extremes there are numerous intermediate reponse patterns, some of them extremely subtle— so subtle in fact that, although one can learn to recognise them at a glance, one has to make a quite intense analysis of one's own perception before one can make explicit what one has actually seen . . . . the child . . . . can show various types of friendly, socially positive behaviour; subtle expressions of the eyes and body stance which one learns to recognise as, for instance, interested, or friendly, etc.; very slight curving up of the corners of the mouth; continued eye contact etc. . . . . The initial, exploratory glance can on other occasions be followed by a negative response pattern. . . . . The mildest expression of a rejecting attitude is a certain expression of the eyes . . . . the response of the adult to this first stage of the child's behaviour has in turn a powerful communicative effect on the child. . . . . These sequences, very obvious once one has observed them, are often overlooked because, as a rule, this happens so quickly, and because most of us react unconsciously by looking away ourselves, and so see no more than the child's first response.'

Conveying an understanding of a child's development may take the form of explaining to his parents why a child behaves in the way he does. For example, parents may complain that their young child ignores them when they speak to him when he is playing at the further side of the room. They fear he may be deaf. Careful hearing tests show that there is no hearing impairment at all. At this stage they are usually 'reassured' and dismissed, but this does not solve the problem. Parents' worries cannot be dismissed as being due to fussiness and anxiety. They want to know why their child is behaving as he does. Perhaps in this particular case it was because he became mobile before he was quite ready to do so from the point of view of auditory development and he cannot yet maintain auditory awareness at a distance. Consequently, if the parents are encouraged to move nearer to him and get his attention before speaking they will find he will respond to them.

It is often necessary to explain the reason for certain recommendations. For example, it is unwise to separate a two-year-old child from his parents, especially his mother, if he has to be admitted to hospital. This is because he has no time concept and to be apart from his mother for even a short period may seem to him that she has gone altogether. Therefore, we always recommend that mother and baby stay together. And again, it may seem strange to recommend to a mother of a deaf and blind child that she wear the same perfume each day—what has this to do with medicine? In fact it is vitally important that such an afflicted child receive every possible clue to his surroundings. The perfume becomes for him a familiar and constant signal from the outside world.

It is important to convey an understanding of a child's development to his parents. Many parents feel themselves to be all at sea with completely normal healthy babies. This is especially so if it is their first baby, if they have not had much contact with babies, and if their own parents live a long way away. If there is anything different about their baby they are quite lost and just do not know what to expect. They need to know what to expect and what they can do with regard to handling their child and administering discipline and stimulation. We find that it is very useful to give parents a report of developmental progress each time their child is re-examined. Developmental guidance is given at this time, as illustrated by the following example.

Peter is a 3½ year-old physically well-developed boy who shows considerable delay in all his abilities and his 'developmental level' lies between 14 and 16 months. His parents do not realize the limitations of such a physically active child with whom they constantly have battles because he does not do what they expect him to be able to do. They bought him a small tricycle which he ignores, and many other toys as well such as model cars and stuffed animals, but he does not play with them for very long and he treats them roughly, often throwing them on the floor.

What should they expect and what should they do? Peter is mobile, but he has few abilities to make constructive use of this mobility. He will use his mobility to explore, but when he arrives at some point he is unlikely to find anything to hold his interest for long. He is likely to move about apparently aimlessly seeming to have a short span of attention and being easily distracted. If this situation continues he is likely to increase his mobility even further and could go on to the full picture of 'hyperactivity'. They should try to make his movements as interesting as possible and try to arrange that there is something to hold his attention, however briefly, at appropriate intervals. Even trying to hold his attention for a short spell will help to prevent the development of valueless hyperactivity.

Peter is not yet at the stage of development when he can understand symbolic representation. So his toys are all objects and he treats them accordingly. He is at the stage of exploring the inside and outside of objects, so for play materials he needs boxes with lids which he can open and empty out, and attractive cubes and similar objects which he can put into and take out of the boxes. He cannot yet make use of the more sophisticated toys he has been given, but he can be given more visual, auditory and tactile stimulation at his present level of play, e.g. boxes of different textures, and colours and designs, and some of them capable of producing sounds.

So far as language is concerned he is still at the stage of needing much input. This should consist of appropriate verbal stimulation nearby. But what does this mean? Just because he is moving about all the time and apparently showing little interest is no reason to stop talking to him. His parents are advised to move towards him, and to get his attention and then to speak to him as clearly as possible. Because his attention is short and he still only has concepts of concrete objects, the verbal stimulation should be short and concerned with definite objects which Peter should be able to see and touch. For example, 'Peter, ball; this is the ball; Peter have the ball'. Here his attention is first caught by calling his name, then he is immediately shown the ball so that he mentally focuses upon the object, then several short phrases are used in which the key word 'ball' is repeated frequently.

Discipline is not easy at this stage. Although Peter's parents may feel that at 3½ years of age he is a big boy and should behave better than he does, he is just not ready to do so. He is at a developmental stage in which periods of resistance and tantrums are quite common. The more his parents try to overcome this, the more tantrums they are likely to precipitate. Use should be made of his easy distractibility, and when he does some undesired action he should be distracted on to some other task.

All this may seem very obvious, but it is extremely difficult for parents to take a new look at their own child and to begin to appreciate his real level of functioning. These basic developmental issues may have to be discussed with them many times.

Reinforcing the Child's Recently Acquired Abilities and Facilitating Their Productive Use

Normal healthy children may often be seen practising their recently acquired abilities. It seems to give them considerable pleasure and satisfaction. This practice is most useful because it helps to improve the skill of performance and ensures its establishment in the child's repertoire of abilities. When development is delayed or distorted, however, such spontaneous practice and reinforcement does not seem to occur as frequently. Consequently, new abilities are often very frail and tenuous and there is a risk that they may not persist. If, in these circumstances the newest abilities are pointed out to parents they will be able to play often with the child to provide the necessary practice. The following is an example of this type of developmental guidance taken from one of the case records of a deaf child.

'He demonstrates good object-recognition by using everyday objects appropriately and is just beginning to get an understanding of symbols, therefore extend his communication range from his present 'direct' system to a simple (pre-language) symbol system for everyday events. For example, put the brush and some other object in front of him, gesture hair-brushing at the same time as saying the word, and reward appropriate responses. He now appreciates personal rewards such as a kiss or clapped hands'.

The reinforcement of the very earliest step in the development of symbolization described above is recommended in order to establish this ability and so enable the child to be able to use it for further steps forward.

Providing Missed Experiences

Disabled children frequently miss out on experiences and learning opportunities which they would otherwise enjoy. It is desirable and sometimes possible to provide such a child with additional experiences to offset his developmental limitations. For example, a child who lacks mobility after the first year is greatly limited. As he cannot move around to explore as he would do if he could go over to the cupboard and open drawers, it may be possible to arrange for him to be able to get things to go to him. A useful device for such an immobile child is a small chest on castors which he can pull towards him with a piece of string in order to explore its contents. (*Figure 79*)

One mother's account of the response to her daughter's first experience of independent mobility through an electric-powered chair vividly revealed the importance of the new experiences. Her daughter was 4 years of age and was severely disabled by athetoid cerebral palsy. Her intelligence was good, but she could not move about and so was totally dependent on others coming to her and moving her from place to place. Placed in a powered chair she soon mastered the controls and could move about as she wished. Her mother called her for lunch and she moved away down the garden path—the first display of normal impishness her mother had ever encountered. She played hide and seek

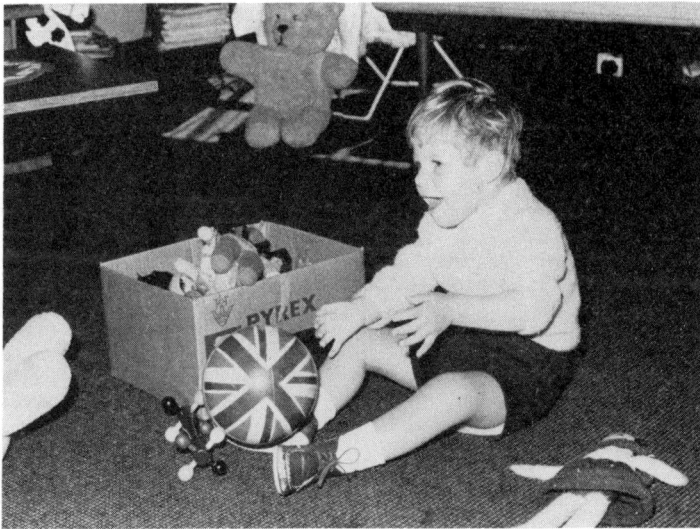

Figure 79. Overcoming immobility to get exploration experiences (this immobile child pulls the box of toys towards him with the attached string when he wants to play)

with her brothers and sisters in the garden. Even indoors she moved around in her chair and surprised her parents by her sudden appearances. Her joy with this sudden wealth of experiences showed how much she had been missing.

In various ways children who miss out on early learning experiences can be helped by being given comparable opportunities. Every child with developmental delay or distortion should be studied to determine what he is missing and what can be done to replace the lost experiences.

Making Use of Other Skills Possessed by the Child to Overcome His Difficulties

Sometimes it is possible to use one ability to help overcome difficulties due to the limitation of other abilities. Perhaps the best example of how a child might use one skill to assist another comes from those cases in which verbal abilities are fairly well developed and are used to assist a child's performance, and perhaps even to help him to overcome

TABLE 34

Uses of Play Materials in Early Childhood

Age group	Block and dramatic play	Big muscle equipment	Housekeeping
3-year-olds	Unit blocks wooden figures doll's house small doll, furniture	Walking board, rocking boat, doll wagon tricycle simple climbing equipment climbing equipment, climbing steps, hollow blocks, large wooden nesting boxes	Unbreakable d(simple doll clothes doll blankets doll-size bed & carriage, childsize furniture (such as: sink, table, refrigerator, stove, cupboar(pots and pans) ironing board, iron, wooden telephone, rocking chair, broom, dust pan, aprons
4-year-olds	Add: puppets puppet theater	Add: planks wheelbarrow scooter swings slide shovel, pail & rake, triangle set, coaster wagon	Add: chest of drawe: washbasin clothesline & basket, aprons, ties, et(childsize bed, cradle, carriage wardrobe
5-year-olds	Add: derrick		

TABLE 34 (cont.)

nsportation	Creative art and books	Classroom furnishings	Miscellaneous
cars and cks for ling and ng, cars trains pushing, lanes, tor and er	Easels paints brushes large crayons books records record- player	Bookcase clothing- lockers storage shelves, block cart, work and library tables and chairs	Soft ball wooden puzzles, portable screens (room dividers) cots plants
Add: ng train	**Add:** blunt scissors clay	**Add:** storage cart, work and library tables and chairs, chalk, peg and bulletin boards, sand and water play table, play tables and chairs	**Add:** aquarium pets
		Add: workhorse woodworking bench tool cabinet tools	**Add:** giant dominoes, construction set

visuomotor problems. The child is shown how to identify differences between objects and to verbalize these differences to help himself to carry out some action. He may have failed a formboard test, but succeeds when he has learnt to say to himself, 'This has a corner here and here and here and should fit into this hole.'

Using External Means at an Appropriate Developmental Level

The whole subject of the use of aids and appliances to assist handicapped children is beyond the scope of this present volume. One special group of aids, however, deserves special mention. These are toys. They are such a common part of child-rearing that they are all too often taken for granted. Table 34 is from a pamphlet entitled 'Criteria for selecting play equipment for early childhood education' published by 'Community Playthings' of Robertsbridge, Sussex. It shows the many uses of play material in the pre-school years.

By careful selection and use toys can be particularly useful for handicapped children. Highly expensive and 'special' toys are not necessary. The important thing is the proper selection and adequate use of existing toys. The following are examples of toys especially useful in the case of certain disabilities.

Toys for a Handicapped Child Unable to Move About (Vision and Hands Normal)

Mental age	*Requirements*
up to 6 months	Similar to a normal baby. Nearby toys to look at; to reach for and hold in palm; to explore with two hands; to take to mouth. Safety important.
6 to 12 months	Toys to stimulate developing skills of index-finger poking, finger-thumb grasp, grasp and release, squeezing. Toys are similar to those needed for normal child of this age, but, because the child is not mobile, various devices must be used to bring the toys into the child's range, e.g. trays, peg or magnetic boards fitted to side of pram or cot, hanging toys. Suggested toys: box to put things into and to take out, finger-flicking toys, wheels, squeezy toys, musical strings to pluck, paper, bendy toys.

1 to 3 years	A time when normal children are very active exploring and getting many new and recurring experiences. Needs: pictures and models to reinforce impressions, simple fitting toys, simple puzzling toys, e.g. boxes with different types of fastenings, adjacent locker, threading toys, different materials, e.g. clay, sand, simple building blocks.
3 to 5+ years	Similar to previous period but more advanced and more imitative of daily activities. Larger sizes. Not always toys but sometimes the real objects. Simple construction tasks lasting up to 10 to 15 minutes. Doll's house.

Toys as Walking Aids

Group 1

Solid firm objects which allow child to pull himself to standing.	Small, solid, fixed table and chairs, wall bars or frame.

Group 2

To provide support in walking.	Pushing toys must be sufficiently weighted not to tip, and be of adjustable height, with hand-holds of various types appropriate to the hand function.

Group 3

To motivate movement whether as crawling or walking.	Pushing, pulling, rolling and mechanical toys, e.g. balls, toys on wheels, skittles.

Toys to Stimulate Various Hand Functions

1. *Grasp (palmar)*: Small balls, squeezy toys, blocks, clay.
2. *Grasp (finger-thumb)*: Threading beads, peg board, small construction toys, chalk, pencils, small models, e.g. farms, doll's house, soldiers to pick up, pulling toys.

3. *Index finger use*: Pointing and pressing actions, cash register, telephone, finger-flicking toys, large clock.
4. *Supination of hand:* Carrying tray or large box, toys with large handles needing clockwise rotation for right hand and anticlockwise for left hand, large balls, toys working only on upward pressure with palm of hand.
5. *Bilateral hand use* (*both hands*): Large balls, large boxes, rolling pins, building jars, barrels, eggs, drums, xylophone (one holding), stirring, threading, winding, screwing toys, barrel organ.
6. *Individual finger use*: Sewing, knitting, piano, clay modelling, scissors.

Adjustments to Toys for the Child with Poor Vision

1. Avoid toys which are too small to be seen clearly and those with small parts and patterns.
2. Use toys which stimulate tactile impressions, e.g. different textures and shapes.

Adjustments to Toys for the Child with Poor Hearing

1. Use toys which produce a variety of different sounds.

Toys to Stimulate Space Perception

1. Toys consisting of simple shapes to fit together.
2. Toys fitting into one another.
3. Toys encouraging exploration of areas, e.g. toy sweeping brush, doll's furniture.
4. Toys needing hanging on hooks, etc.
5. Pouring from jars and buckets with water and sand.
6. Drawing and painting both on flat surfaces and of objects, e.g. wooden boxes.

Additional information about toys and developmental play is available from the Toy Libraries Association (Toynbee Hall, 28 Commercial Street, London E1 6LS).

THE DEVELOPMENTAL APPROACH TO CEREBRAL PALSY

The developmental approach to the management and training of handicapped children will be further illustrated by reference to one particular group of disabilities—namely cerebral palsy.

The first step in the developmental approach to cerebral palsy is to appreciate that abnormal interactions exist between mother and child. The mother is usually extremely anxious about her baby. Events during pregnancy or delivery such as episodes of bleeding, premature labour or severe asphyxia make her particularly sensitive about the progress of her baby. Many mothers are aware that all is not well with their baby some time before the diagnosis is established. The baby often appears to have been rendered especially sensitive and vulnerable as a result of the neurological lesion. These two aspects interact and reinforce each other. The tenseness and irritability of the baby makes the mother more anxious, and her greater anxiety is reflected in even more tenseness and irritability on the part of the baby. A vicious spiral effect results. These events are shown diagrammatically in *Figure 80*.

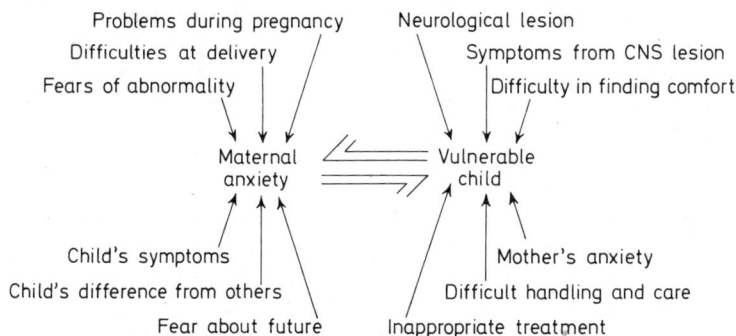

Figure 80. The initial mother–child interaction in cerebral palsy. What basis for future development?

Our experiences suggest that some of the clinical features observed in babies with cerebral palsy are due to this vicious spiral interaction effect. The first step therefore is to reduce and to reverse this spiral effect. This is done by showing an understanding of the child's problems and the mother's difficulties by discussing the symptoms and signs and showing how the baby can be examined and handled. As the mother loses a little of her anxiety she can be encouraged to carry out some of the everyday tasks which have been frightening her, such as picking up her baby, or feeding him. As she finds she can do this without the previous difficulties her confidence begins to return. In this way the vicious spiral of interaction is reversed. These initial steps need to be handled with great sensitivity. When this is done satisfactorily some of the infant's symptoms subside, his mother gains confidence and can actively contribute to the next developmental stages, and a firm basis is established for later treatment.

Too hasty action at this early stage, such as by simply attaching a diagnostic label and referring for therapy, aggravates the situation by confirming the mother's fears that her baby is abnormal, and her feeling of inadequacy because a professional worker now has to do things to her baby.

Although many problems and anxieties arise in the rearing of healthy babies there exist ready sources of interest and advice in friends, neighbours and relatives. Without this support mothers feel isolated and uncertain, and this is the situation with babies with developmental problems. The friends, neighbours and relatives cannot help because they feel uncertain and *their* babies were normal. A review of the everyday care of babies is essential in these situations.

The next step, therefore, is to make a very detailed review of the infant's care throughout each 24 hours. This review often reveals other maternal anxieties which may not otherwise have come to light. For example, did she buy the best cot for him?; does she keep the room temperature correct?; what should she do when he suddenly thrusts backwards? These items are discussed as they arise.

As the 24-hour review is carried out it is possible to indicate more effective ways of doing various things so as to cause less distress to the child and also to promote his progress and development. For example, the hip adductor muscles may be unusually tight and it is considered desirable to stretch them in order to safeguard the stability of the hip joints. This can be achieved by showing the mother how the baby can be carried with his legs spread either side of the mother's hip and ensuring that this position is adopted every time he is carried. In this way useful measures are incorporated quite simply and effectively into the everyday care of the child, whereas if this abduction of the hips were to be done in a special treatment session it would add to the day's work and disrupt normal routine.

Once the 24-hour routine is reviewed it is necessary to decide whether this will be sufficient or whether additional treatment programmes need to be included. Whichever decision is made all treatment, whether in special sessions or in the everyday routine, includes the following principles.

In most cases it is necessary to strive to overcome the persistence of early reflex activities. The persistence of these activities delays both general development and motor development; it may also lead to deformity; and it may become a self-perpetuating movement ritual. There are several good reasons, therefore, for attempting to reduce this excessive and persisting reflex activity. This is done by finding out the factors which precipitate the excessive activity and, if possible, eliminating them; by finding the postures which reduce the reflex activity, and here a treatment system such as that developed by the Bobaths (1957) can be useful (*Figure 81*); and by the judicious use of drugs such as diazepam (Valium) (*Figure 82*). In a few cases the early movement patterns can be used to enable the child to achieve a particular task.

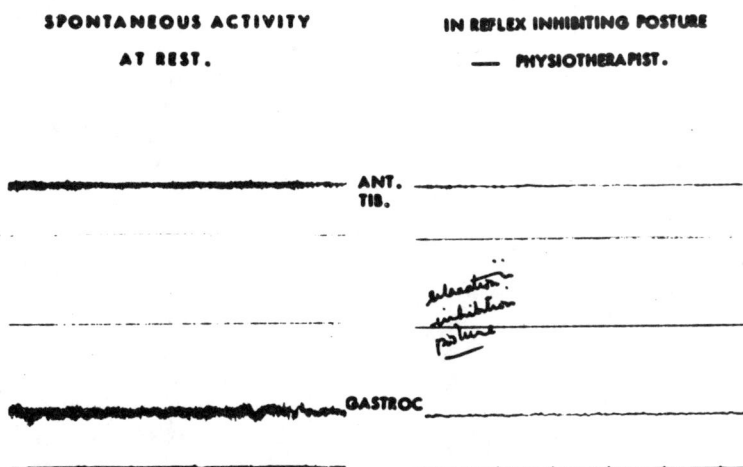

Figure 81. Inhibition of muscle activity (anterior tibial and gastrocnemius) by Bobath technique

As a result of the delay of motor development and the neurological abnormalities most children with cerebral palsy lie in one or two different postures. They find it particularly difficult to alter their posture and to get into and maintain any anti-gravity posture. There are several major consequences of these difficulties. The deformity-producing tendencies of cerebral palsy can exert their full effects. The

CASE G.C.　　　　　AGE 24 YRS　　　　ATHETOSIS

WITHOUT　　　　　　　　　　　　WITH VALIUM

RESTING ACTIVITY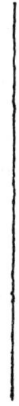

HELD UPRIGHT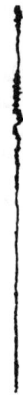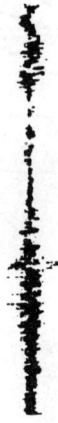

VENTRAL SUSPENSION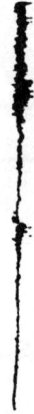

PLANTAR STIMULATION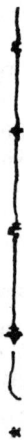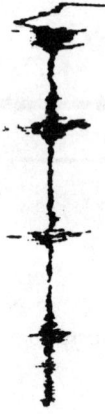

ALL RECORDS TAKE FROM ANTERIOR TIBIAL MUSCLE

＊ ONLY OBTAINED WITH LARGE DOSE OF VALIUM

Figure 82. Electromyograph record (surface) of effects of diazepam (valium) in cerebral palsy

failure to develop head control against gravity delays auditory localization and impedes visual exploration of the surroundings, and it also
makes feeding difficult. Impairment of head control and poor arm
movements delays the development of hand-eye co-ordination which is
so essential for the later development of many motor skills. So there are
a good number of reasons, many related to the child's developmental
needs, for ensuring that cerebral-palsied children are placed in many
different postures and are stimulated to acquire anti-gravity postures.
The components of early motor development are stimulated and
practised in several treatment systems (e.g. Hari, 1971; Cotton, 1974)
to enable the child to be moved, and to move into various postures
Figure 83). At the same time, while in these various postures, the
child is encouraged to make the fullest possible use of his learning
opportunities. For example, visual and auditory localization, eye-
hand co-ordination, and reaching are practised.

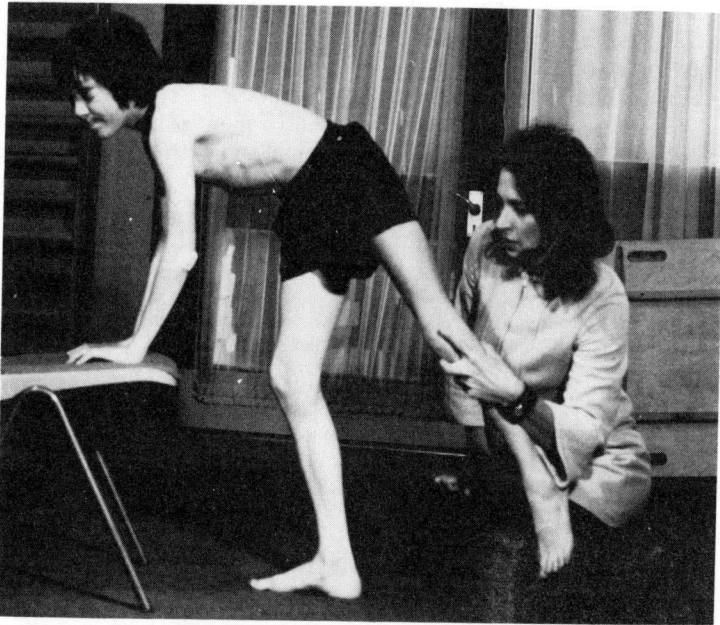

Figure 83. Therapy in cerebral palsy

Mobility is a most important aspect of early child development
(Holt, 1975). Children use movement for their own pleasure,
exploration, communication, and the elaboration of emotional

278 DEVELOPMENTAL APPROACH TO HANDICAPPED CHILDREN

relationships. For many children with cerebral palsy mobility does not develop at the appropriate time, so it is necessary to provide some form of movement, either passively or actively, and to overcome the detrimental effects of immobility such as deprivation of learning opportunities. To mention just one example, we have found, as mentioned previously, that electrically-powered chairs have opened up new worlds for quite young cerebral-palsied children.

It soon becomes necessary to promote mother–child emancipation. The mother's natural reaction to her handicapped child and all the extra things she does for him increases mother and child dependence in the early stages, but this situation cannot be allowed to continue too long. This severance does not occur spontaneously as in the course of normal development, but has to be managed. The immobile child cannot physically wean himself from his mother as a normal child does when he slips from her knee and crawls across the floor. If the early steps described above were achieved with full understanding the need to sever this bond will be appreciated by the mother. The handling of this situation is one of the most difficult, delicate and important tasks for anyone caring for the young cerebral-palsied child, and it requires much help and guidance.

The steps summarized above seem to follow sensibly once one begins to think in terms of the developmental approach to any disabling condition.

Bobath, B., and Bobath, K. (1957). Control of motor function in the treatment of cerebral palsy. *Physiotherapy, Lond.* October
Cotton, E. (1974). Improvement in motor function with the use of conductive education. *Devl. Med. Child Neurol.* **16**, 637
Hari, K. A. (1971). *Konduktiv Pedagogin*. Budapest: Tankönyukiado
Holt, K. S. (1975). Movement and child development. *Clinics Child Devl.* London: Heinemann
Tinbergen, E. A., and Tinbergen, N. (1972). *Early Childhood Autism–An Ethological Approach*. Berlin: Parey

CHAPTER 13

The Developmental Paediatrician: His Work and Equipment

The developmental paediatrician is primarily a paediatrician, that is, a physician who is specially trained and experienced in the problems and care of infants and children and who strives to promote their optimum health and development. He, or she, must be able to carry out a competent clinical examination and also be able to recognize abnormalities. It is just as important to be able to recognize the early signs of acute illness and to carry out an appropriate diagnostic examination, as it is to recognize and examine for developmental delay. Parents who consult a developmental paediatrician are usually anxious to know that their child is both healthy and normal. Experience in the diagnosis and treatment of acute illness in childhood therefore constitutes an essential requirement for developmental paediatricians.

Developmental paediatricians must have a sound understanding of the features of child development and of its underlying mechanisms. They must be fully competent to perform all the test procedures which might be necessary. These include the following:

Vision:	Stycar tests	Ophthalmoscopic examination
	Rolling balls test	Cover test
Hearing:	Stycar tests	Auroscopic examination
	Simple audiometry	

Motor and Manipulation: Tests of manipulation and motor skills

Behaviour and emotion: Tests and questionnaires to evaluate these items. Observation techniques applicable to clinical work

Language and communication: Reyness Developmental Language Scales. Clinical recording of expressive language. Observation of communication

Intelligence: Griffiths Scales Comprehension of other psychological tests, especially Stanford-Binet and W.I.S.C.

The work of developmental paediatricians includes the following.

(a)   The examination of apparently normal children and the administration of screening tests to detect defects and disabilities.

(b)   The offering of developmental advice and guidance in order to anticipate and to prevent developmental problems.

These two tasks can be performed by members of primary-health teams providing they receive adequate training and consultative support.

(c)   Some developmental paediatricians will be responsible for assessment and management of handicapped children. This requires much wider clinical experience and training which includes the specialities of neurology, psychiatry, orthopaedics, physical medicine, ophthalmology, audiology and rehabilitation. The developmental paediatricians will work with consultant colleagues in these specialities. In addition to the medical aspects, they require some training and experience in educational psychology and social work so as to be able to work with colleagues in those disciplines too.

Developmental paediatricians are sometimes criticized for their concern with child development, which may be considered to be the domain of the psychologist and teacher. This is an unnecessary criticism. Whilst acknowledging the considerable theoretical and practical contributions made to child development by other professions, it is indefensible to suggest that any one discipline has the sole right to work in this area. Knowledge and appreciation of the contributions of other disciplines is essential for paediatricians in obtaining a whole view of any one child which is their responsibility.

Paediatricians are very concerned with development, for various reasons. Their primary aim is to promote the health and development not of a restricted group, but of all children. They see many children in the course of their work, both in curative and preventive medicine, and have unique opportunities to detect the signs of developmental delay and abnormality. Children's illnesses may affect development if not dealt with correctly. Doctors are often consulted by parents and teachers because of children's problems which may be due to developmental abnormalities. Even in those cases in which the developmental problems appear to have little medical component, parents seek opportunities to discuss all the whys and wherefores of the problems with a doctor. Disabled children are likely to experience difficulties of development and doctors concerned with their habilitation need to be completely familiar with their developmental needs as well as their specific medical needs.

Difficulties do arise when doctors make developmental decisions and judgments beyond their training and experience and beyond the evidence available to them. Such actions are rightly criticized. The problem is best solved, I believe, by developmental paediatricians and psychologists and others concerned working more closely together in order to lead to a better understanding and integration of their respective contributions.

The Developmental Paediatrician's Bag

Developmental paediatricians are mobile. They see children on their visits to schools, nurseries, and homes as well as in hospitals and consulting rooms. A small, easily carried, bag or case containing their equipment is therefore an invaluable asset (*Figure 84*).

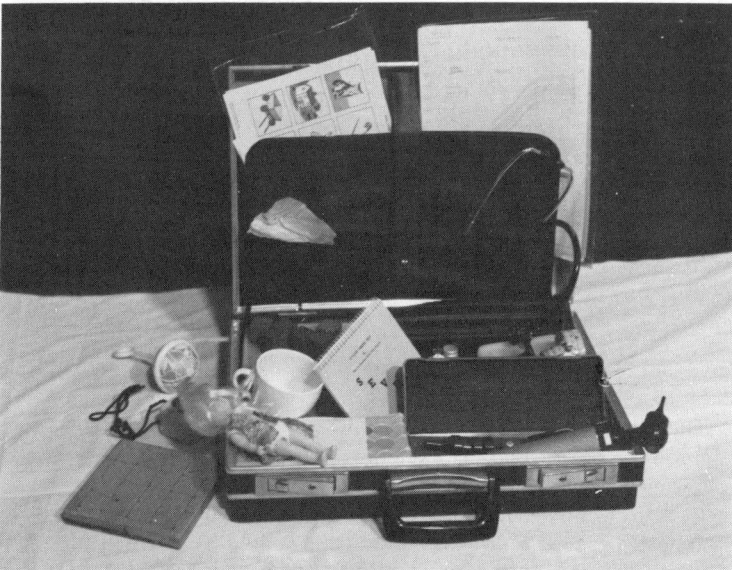

Figure 84. The developmental paediatrician's bag

Each paediatrician should select the contents for his own bag according to his particular experience and needs, so variations will be seen. However, the requirements will have much in common, and the following guide may be useful.

General medical equipment (*Figure 85*)

Stethoscope	Tendon reflex hammer
Ophthalmoscope	Tape measure
Auroscope	Spatula

These items of general medical equipment are essential for carrying out a full medical examination which should be linked always with any developmental examination.

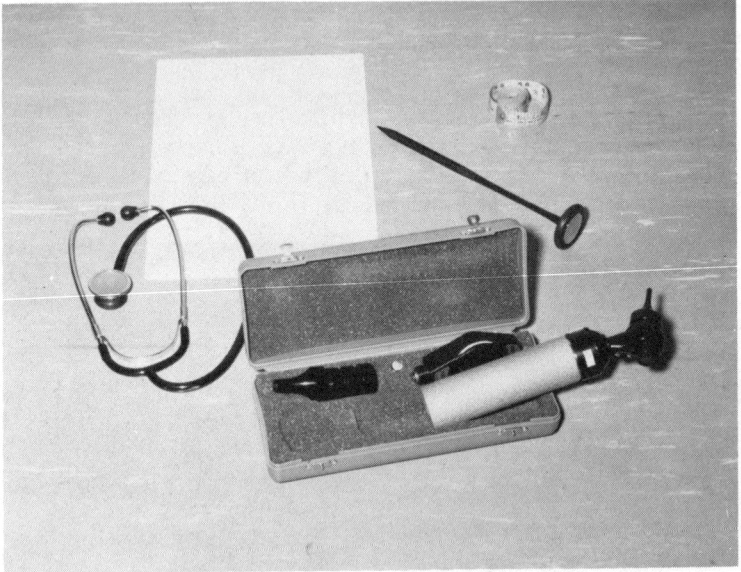

Figure 85. General medical equipment

The auroscope is a more versatile tool than is often realized. In addition to being used to examine the ears, it can be used in the following ways:

(i)   to examine the nose: the auroscope speculum is inserted into each nostril in turn whilst the child breathes through his mouth. A good view is obtained of the mucous membrane and discharge from the maxillary sinuses;

(ii)   to examine dermatoglyphics. The speculum is removed and the finger tip or other area to be examined are viewed through the magnifying lens of the auroscope.

(iii)   as a light to test visual following;

(iv)   to test the light reflex from the cornea;

(v) to test for nasopharyngeal competence. A game is played in which the child is encouraged to blow out the light. Nasal escape of air as the child blows is usually easily detected.

A thorough search of the retina is often necessary using the ophthalmoscope, but this is not easy. Sections of the retina are missed as the eye moves about and when the examiner forgets which parts he has seen. The best way to do this examination is to identify the optic disc, select one of the blood vessels which radiate outwards from the disc and to follow it to the periphery. Then to return to the disc and select the next vessel in clockwise rotation and follow this out to the periphery. This is repeated until the retina on either side of each blood vessel has been examined.

An illuminated spatula is an asset when examining the mouth, throat and teeth. By using it, one hand is freed for other tasks.

Some may wish to include material for sensory testing (cotton wool, pin, tuning fork, and test tubes for hot and cold water), but as this type of examination is very difficult on a young child, it is often better to reserve such testing for more formal occasions, such as in hospital or an assessment centre.

Paediatricians who combine their developmental work with general paediatrics may find it useful to include a few simple materials for collecting urine, blood and bacteriological specimens, and performing some simple tests.

Growth Charts (*Figures 86 (a) and (b)*)

The height/age and weight/age charts of Tanner, Whitehouse and Takaishi (1966) are useful and reliable. Those covering the period 0–5 years are essential, and if older children are also seen, the charts 0–19 years should be included in the bag.

Head circumference charts over a wide age-range are essential. Those showing mean and standard deviations such as the Nellhaus chart (*Figures 2 and 3*) (Nellhaus, 1968) are useful for general purposes, but for babies who might have abnormalities of head size and growth charts with a larger scale which extends into the antenatal period are more useful.

Ten 1-inch Wooden Cubes

These should be washable; painted safely, i.e. with non-poisonous paint; and of 4 assorted colours with at least 2 of each colour.

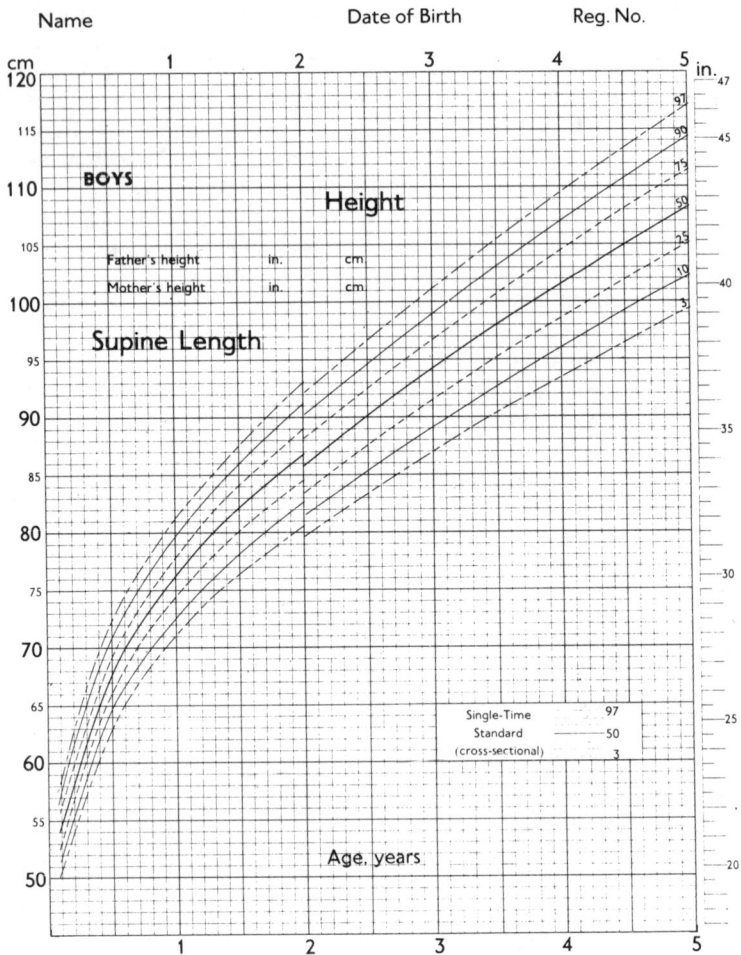

Name   Date of Birth   Reg. No.

BOYS

Height

Father's height   in.   cm
Mother's height   in.   cm

Supine Length

Single-Time   97
Standard ————— 50
(cross-sectional)   3

Age, years

Figure 86 (a) Height/age chart 0–5 years for boys

The cubes are used principally for testing manipulation. According to the age and ability of the child, they may be offered singly, or in a group. Note is taken of the child's grasp; his reaction to the offer of a second and third cube; what he does with the cubes, e.g. mouthing, banging table, releasing cube, searching for dropped cube, playing give and take, putting cube into and taking out of container (e.g. cup, *see later*), and seeking out hidden cube. The cubes are used to test the

Name _____ Date of Birth _____ Reg. No. _____

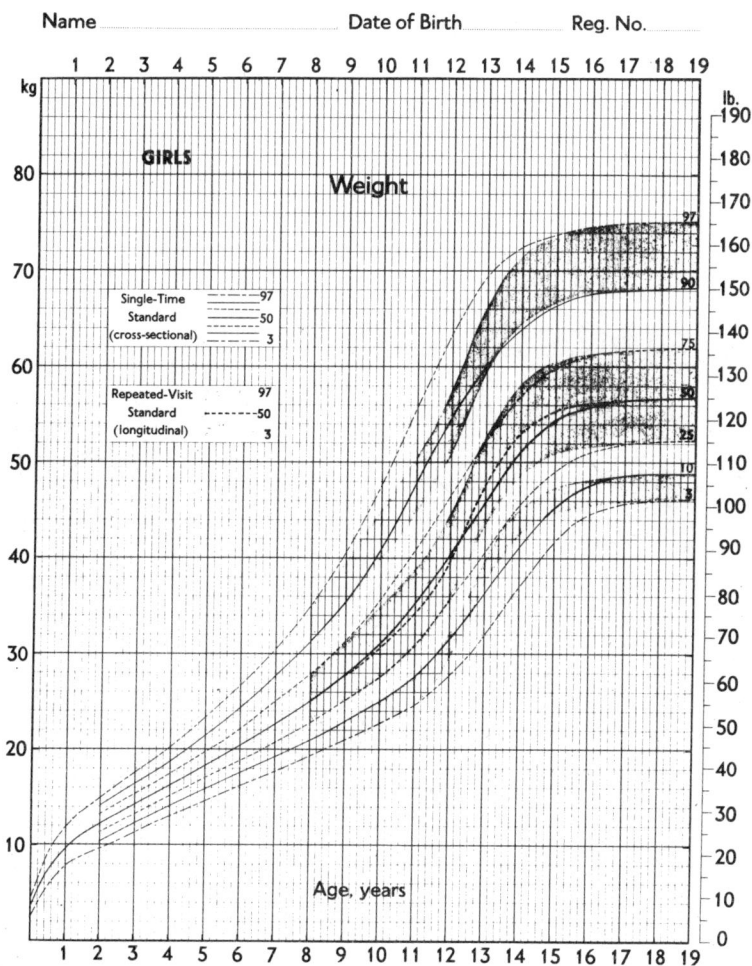

Figure 86 (b) Weight/age chart 0–19 years for girls

child's ability to construct a tower, train, bridge, gate and stairs. They are also used to check colour matching and counting. Two of them can be knocked together to produce a 'wooden' sound, so providing a useful addition to the hearing-test equipment.

Vision-Testing Equipment (*Figure 87*)

2-inch ball on a string	Stycar miniature toys
Small plastic container of small sweets, e.g. Smarties	Stycar 5-and 7-letter test
Small container of sugar pellets	Stycar instruction manual (vision)
Set of Stycar graded balls and rods	Snellen near-vision card

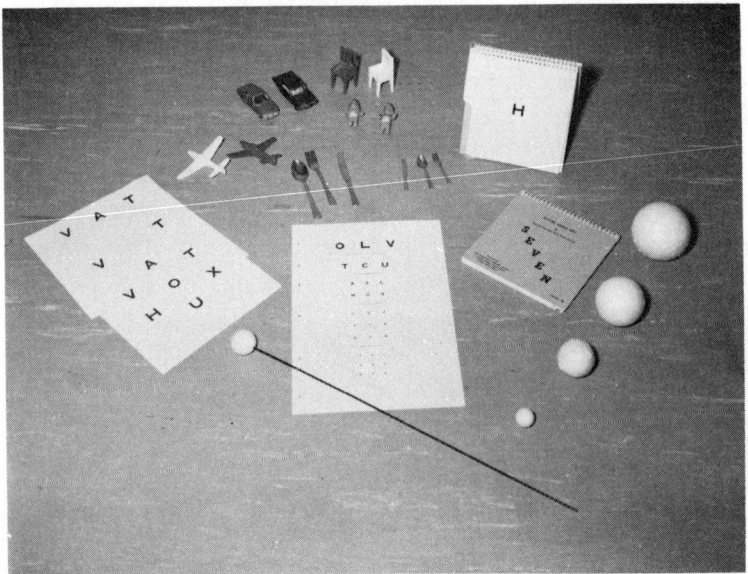

Figure 87. Vision-testing equipment

This material is used for vision examination. A red ring on a string is often said to be the ideal visual lure for babies, but we have found a 2-inch ball just as suitable and more versatile. A light-coloured plastic ball is best. This ball on a string is used to test visual fixation and following by babies, and the ability of children to follow the pendulum swing of the ball at different speeds (this examination often reveals abnormalities such as jerky saccadic movements). The ball and string also doubles as a test for infants since it can be noted if they can take hold of the string in order to pull the ball towards themselves. Smarties and small sugar pellets are used to test near vision in infants and also their ability to pick up these small objects. Both are safe if the child places them in his mouth. It is convenient to keep them in small plastic containers. If this is done, they rattle when shaken and can be added to the hearing-test equipment.

The Stycar graded balls are used in the rolling ball test of visual acuity and when mounted on rods can be used to test the fields of vision as well as acuity. For carrying in the bag the balls are best kept together in a plastic bag.

The Stycar matching miniature toys and the 5-and 7-letter tests are used according to the instruction manual. Near vision should always be tested. Apparatus to induce optokinetic nystagmus which might be used to estimate visual acuity in babies and severely handicapped children has not been included in this list because it is bulky and not everyone considers it to be reliable, but some paediatricians might wish to include it.

Hearing-Testing Equipment (*Figure 88*)

Rattles (limited intensity, various frequencies)	Stycar picture cards
Small bell	Stycar word and sentence lists

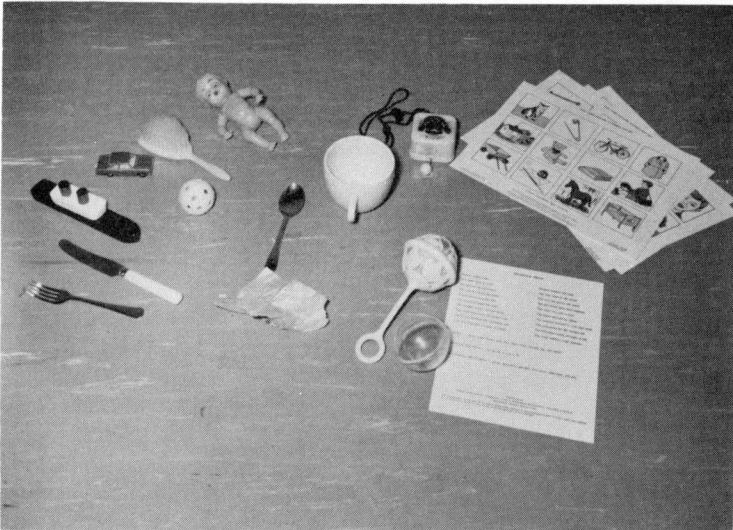

Figure 88 Hearing-testing equipment

Musical box   Stycar instruction manual
                                              (hearing)
Cup (china) and spoon (metal)

This material is for testing hearing. Some children respond only to a musical jingle so a musical box is useful in the examination bag. In addition to the items listed for producing free-field sounds, there are the sounds produced by knocking wooden cubes together, shaking the Smartie container, rustling some of the plastic bags used to contain the equipment, and also all the voiced sounds. The other material is used according to the instruction manual.

The 7 toys of the Stycar test have not been included because if these are needed, something suitable can be collected together from the other material in the case. Nor has a pure tone audiometer been included, but as quite small and light ones are now obtainable, anyone doing much testing of hearing might wish to include one.

In addition to being used in the hearing tests, the china cup is also used to hide the cubes as mentioned above, as well as in the pegboard test of manipulative skill.

Language and Play-Testing Equipment (*Figure 89*)

Dressed doll 8 to 10 inches tall   Miniature toys—table, 2 chairs,
Baby's hair brush   2 cups & saucers, teapot, jug, 2
Action pictures   spoons, bath, undressed baby
Ladybird books—'Baby's First   doll, cat, dog, aeroplane,
Book', 'Things We Like To Do'   dressed doll 2 inches tall

This is versatile material. It is particularly useful for an exploration of language function. The large doll excites and holds interest. The child can identify body parts and can demonstrate symbolic play. The other material is used to check verbal comprehension, symbolic play and appreciation of actions and their consequences. The material can also be used for the teapot test of manipulative skill.

Manipulation Testing Equipment

Paper and crayon   Pegboard and set of pegs in screw-
                                    topped bottle
Stopwatch (not essential)

Performance tasks are explored with this equipment. With the paper and crayon the maturity of handling the crayon is noted and the ability to draw and to imitate and copy various symbols. The Draw a Man test might also be tried with an older child. The child's ability to fold the paper can be studied. If desired, the addition of a small pair of scissors enables the performance of cutting to be seen. Ability

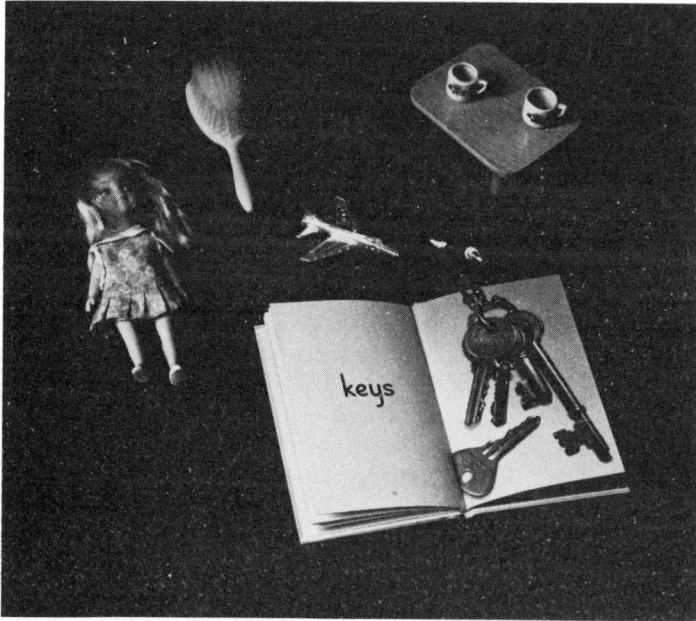

Figure 89 Language and play-testing equipment

to screw and unscrew is checked as the child opens the bottle containing the pegs for the pegboard test of manipulative skill (Holt, 1965). The stopwatch is used for timed actions, but it need not be included if the examiner has a watch with a good second hand.

Various other items might be included. For example, a piece of chalk is useful for drawing a line for the child to walk along as a test of motor skill. With constant use the developmental paediatrician will get his bag to the state he wishes, and it will then become a constant companion.

A VISIT TO A NURSERY FOR HANDICAPPED CHILDREN

The work of a developmental paediatrician will be understood most easily by considering some task he might perform such as a visit to a

290

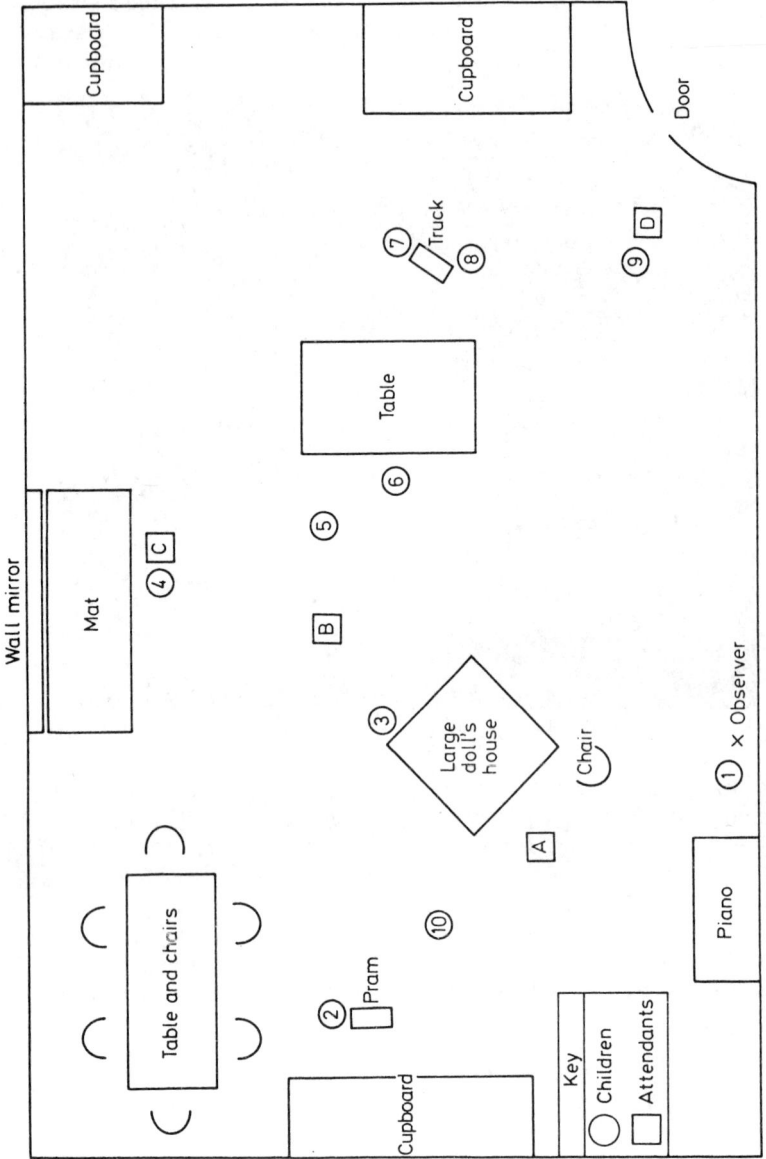

Figure 90 Distribution of children, attendants and furniture in nursery

nursery for handicapped children. The following is an account of an actual visit and is reported as it would be described to aspiring developmental paediatricians.

I went to the nursery on a routine visit and took with me a pair of special shoes for one of the children T (the letters refer to *Figure 90* and Table 35). The shoes were prescribed for her when she attended the regional assessment centre the week before.

TABLE 35
The ages and diagnoses of the children in the nursery

Identity	Age	Diagnosis
C	4.0	Not talking: social difficulties
J1	3.3	Not talking
G	2.9	Mongolism
D1	3.5	Mongolism
D2	2.11	Retardation
L	3.3	Specific language disorder
P	4.6	Albino: partially sighted
M	3.11	Cerebral palsy
D3	3.1	Hypothyroidism, delayed development
D4	3.5	Cerebral palsy-hemiplegia
D5	3.4	Mucopolysaccharidosis
J2	2.8	Retardation, ?chromosome defect
S	2.6	Delayed development, ?cerebral palsy
T	2.10	Cerebral palsy
D6	3.0	Retardation

While I was at the nursery these shoes were tried out and I discussed their use and purpose with the therapist and doctor.

On arrival at the nursery I was met by the senior nurse who explained that several of the children had just arrived by bus and one had been sick. We discussed the arrangements for seating in the bus and the route taken, hoping to find some way to make the journey easier and reduce the risk of sickness. We also considered the use of anti-emetics for travel sickness. Parents and staff are always anxious about giving even more drugs to handicapped children who may already be taking quite a lot, and for whom it may be difficult to find the correct dose. This question, therefore, had to be discussed carefully.

As I entered the main play area one of the children D2 opened the door for me, took my hand, and led me to the cupboards. As we walked this short distance she frequently turned and smiled and pointed to various objects. After we had explored the cupboard contents she sat on my knee for a while. This short spontaneous interlude provided me with a clear picture of her gait and manipulation, her behaviour, communication and interpersonal reactions—sufficient for me to feel surprised (and concerned) when I learnt that she had recently been admitted to the nursery from a hospital clinic with a label of 'retardation with autistic features'.

I then spent 15 to 20 minutes observing activities in the play area. The situation at one time during this period was as shown in *Figure 90*. The particular arrangement of the furniture and equipment in the room had been arrived at as a result of trial and error by the staff and had some features to commend it. For example, the large floor-standing doll's house was readily accessible to most of the children and attendant (A) could stimulate and guide constructive play. Attendant (C) was well positioned to assist the immobile children and put them into suitable postures on the mat, which was in a reasonably quiet and undisturbed position. Three children (2, 7 and 8) were very active and it would have been preferable for them to have a clear area to one side.

This period of observation was invaluable for noting the advantages and disadvantages of the room, furniture and equipment, and the success achieved by the attendants in communicating with the children in an appropriate way, getting them into good positions, and providing stimulating experiences.

Observations were made on a group of children using methods which have been described already elsewhere (Holt and Reynell, 1970). The technique of *event sampling* was used and the observations recorded as follows:

10.00   D2 comes over to me, plays with my tie, goes away.
         J and T lying together on floor.
         J gets up, does not look at T, goes to doll's house.
         D2 picked up by attendant.

J turns from doll's house and calls 'Hello' to attendant.

T lies passively on floor all the time.

10.02   J puts toy on top of doll's house.

Attendant lifts T and places her down on floor again—no communication between them.

J goes to attendant and taps her.

D2 brought by attendant to table and sat down, immediately gets up and runs off.

J sits on stool and calls out.

T squirms slowly towards cupboard.

C comes into group and stands by me quietly.

10.04   D2, J and C go to piano and tap keys. Attendant comes and closes lid.

T squirming on floor, ignored and stepped over by others.

C gives book to J says 'Here you are'.

C goes to D2 and says 'Hello'.

10.06   T on floor with toy alongside.

J goes to pram.

D2 picks up comic.

C takes book to D2.

G comes into group and pushes C—attendant stops him.

J comes over to me, looks at my notes and tries to speak to me.

10.08   D2 goes to cupboard, steps over T on floor, takes doll from cupboard to pram.

C takes book to attendant.

J comes to me and says 'Daddie, Daddie'.

T squirming on floor.

As a result of this 10-minute observation period, I was able to analyse the children's behaviour as follows, giving one point every time a particular item was recorded.

Activity	Child			
	D2	J	T	C
Movement between two points	6	9	1	6
Communication—non verbal	4	4	0	2
Communication—verbal	0	4	0	2
Symbolic play	0	0	0	4

These records show:

(1) the marked activity of D2, J and C, in contrast to T who perhaps would have been better out of the group;

(2) the two children attending the nursery as 'non talkers', J and C, actually communicated several times during the observation period, both non-verbally and verbally;

(3) only C showed any symbolic play.

The activity of the attendant was also analysed as follows:

Communication with child—non verbal	0
Communication with child—verbal	0
Initiation of activity for child	0
Control of child's activities	5

This attendant was clearly safeguarding and controlling the children, but did not communicate with them or initiate any activity for them either because she did not wish to do so, or, more likely, did not realize how she could do so. She will require help and training if the handicapped children are to be helped and the potential advantages of the nursery realized.

Later three children were seen with the physiotherapist in the treatment room. One was T, the unresponsive child who lay on the floor throughout the above brief observation. The therapist got T into a supported standing position from which T began to attempt to hand toys to a second child. There was constant communication between T and the therapist by gesture, expression, and eye pointing. T is an athetoid child with considerable drive and is not necessarily passive and unresponsive as she appeared to be in the group described above. The therapist was encouraged to show these to the attendant so that she might realize T's assets and abilities, and to show her how to position and stimulate T.

T was able to hold a rollator and to progress a few steps using an automatic stepping response. The developmental significance of the stepping response was discussed and it was suggested that as long as it persisted, independent walking would remain a distant possibility.

Another child observed during treatment had been referred from the regional assessment centre and had been attending the nursery for two weeks. He was still settling in and much of the time he was just a passive observer who was becoming familiar with the therapist and gaining confidence by watching the other children being treated. At his original assessment poor verbal communication was noted, the possibility of neurological involvement of the legs was queried, and a visual impediment was found to be fully corrected by his glasses. Already the staff of the nursery were able to report that he never wore his glasses and his parents never seemed to know where they were; that repeated examination by the therapist had not confirmed the suspected motor impairment of the legs; and that he was already losing his passivity and verbalizing a great deal. These valuable observations complemented the original assessment.

At the end of the morning all 15 children attending the nursery were discussed with the unit's doctor. Table 35 shows the wide variety of diagnoses in these cases. This discussion clarified and amplified some of the hospital reports about the children. Further investigations and observations were initiated for some of the children, suggestions were made about grouping the children for more effective training, and arrangements were made for further training of some of the staff of the unit.

The nursery 'ward round' ended informally with one of the senior staff describing a conference she had attended recently.

There are many small nurseries such as this one for handicapped children. They are full of children with complex medical and developmental problems. The developmental paediatrician has wonderful opportunities to do constructive work and gain experience in these nurseries which have been neglected for far too long.

DEVELOPMENTAL PAEDIATRICS AND REHABILITATION

As has been suggested already, the developmental paediatrician whose practice includes the care and management of handicapped children needs to be familiar with several medical specialities. He must know an appreciable amount about audiology, physical medicine, neurology, ophthalmology and orthopaedics. In this respect he is very akin to a rehabilitation specialist. However, no matter how broad and deep is his knowledge of these specialities, it is insufficient without the essential background of a sound understanding of all aspects of child development.

A rehabilitation specialist is concerned with the restoration of working and living capacity, whereas the developmental paediatrician is concerned with the creation of these capacities in children who usually have never possessed them and are not able to develop them unaided. They have to learn from the beginning. Habilitation would be a more appropriate term.

The developmental paediatrician or habilitation specialist enjoys rich and varied experiences as he does his rounds in schools for handicapped children. These situations call forth both his wide knowledge of other specialities and his understanding of child development. Consider if you will a fragment of reports of a visit to a school for physically handicapped children.

The visit began with a discussion of the management of children with muscular dystrophy in general, and with particular reference to several such children in the school. Many problems were considered; three were discussed at length, and these three between them show the range of knowledge required by the developmental paediatrician.

The first concerned the deformities developed by muscular dystrophy children. Do these arise as a result of primary muscle weakness, or secondary weakness due to disuse atrophy, or to unsuitable postures, or to other causes? The various mechanisms were discussed with the staff. How can the deformities be prevented? Are they inevitable? When should therapy, bracing and surgery be considered and what form should they take? These are obviously very difficult and specialized questions which need to be discussed with the staff on the spot so that they understand the reasons for the child's programme of treatment; they can then fit it into the general educational programme and be in a much better position to provide constructive help when they meet the child's parents.

The second issue arose from the first one. If the prevention of deformities requires the early introduction of therapy, how can this be done without alarming the parents about future problems and without disturbing the 'normalness' with which the child should be considered and treated? It is not easy for therapists to become involved in treating a pleasant normal-looking youngster whose only difficulties occur when trying to stand up or going upstairs, and to explain to parents that they do this in order to reduce the problems which will develop as he gets older. The therapists need to discuss these issues with the developmental paediatrician.

An older brother of one of the children had died as a result of muscular dystrophy. This situation introduced the third major topic of how to help a child who knows his grim future. The school staff, teachers and therapists, meet this problem every day with respect to the particular child. His school work is affected. He seeks to question teachers and therapists both directly and obliquely. The staff meet his parents frequently and the child's future is often discussed. The issues have to be dealt with on the spot when they arise. They cannot be solved by referral to a distant clinic. The developmental paediatrician must appreciate all that is involved and must provide ample time and opportunities for discussions with both child, parents, and staff.

An older child with quite severe ataxic cerebral palsy was seen and discussed because of increasing distress because he could not achieve independence in toilet care. The therapists had helped by showing him how to hold rails to steady himself whilst unfastening and fastening his trousers and standing to micturate, but they could not find out how to make him independent with defecation. He just could not manage to wipe himself. The difficulty turned out to be that he could not hold a rail with one hand and lean over and wipe himself from the side and behind without falling over. By advising him to wipe himself from in front between his legs he was able to control his posture better and became independent. This is the sort of major practical issue which the developmental paediatrician must help with if he is to assist the child as an individual.

The developmental paediatrician's competence neurologically was tested with the next child. This was a boy who had been diagnosed as having cerebral palsy, but who was not making the expected progress with therapy. In fact a review and re-examination cast doubt on the original diagnosis and raised the possibility of a degenerative lesion. Without a sound knowledge of neurology the doctor could easily have overlooked this child for a year or two until the deterioration became very marked.

The final child discussed on this 'ward round' suffered from epilepsy. His school work was deteriorating. The possible causes were time lost from school as a result of fits, deterioration of the cerebral lesion, or sedation and other side-effects from the anticonvulsant drugs. These are very common problems with epileptic children. It is much easier and more effective to unravel the difficulties and organize treatment on the spot than it is in a distant clinic.

These brief extracts illustrate the wide range of problems facing the developmental paediatrician and the rich contributions he can make provided he is adequately trained and conducts his ward rounds in the places where the children are living and working.

REFERENCES

Holt, K. S. (1965). *Assessment of Cerebral Palsy*. Vol. 1. London: Lloyd Luke
— and Reynell, J. K. (1970). *Observation of Children*. London: National Association for Mental Health

Nellhaus, G. (1968). Composite international and inter-racial graphs. *Pediatrics,* **41,** 106

Tanner, J. M., Whitehouse, R. H., and Takaishi. (1966). Standards from birth to maturity for height, weight, height velocity and weight velocity: British children, 1965. Part 1. *Archs Dis. Childh.* **41,** 454

Index

Abilities, 170
  application of, 88
Abnormal growth, 10, 11
Abnormalities,
  detection of, 68
    apathetic, 68, 69
    first year, in, 83
    hemi-syndrome, 68, 69
    hyperexcitable, 68, 69
    1 to 5 years, 102
    6 to 10 years, 120
    11 to 15 years, 125
  mechanism of, 142
  neurological, incidence at 2 to 4
    years, 69
Accommodation, 133
Activity, 170
  neonates, in, 64
Adolescence, 138
Age (*See also* under specific periods
    First year, Two years etc.)
  actions and, 171
  Babinski reflex and, 31
  ball skills and, 188
  brain growth and, 12
  criteria of neonatal maturity and,
    64, 65, 66, 67, 68
  electroencephalographic pattern
    and, 18
  fetal brain appearance and, 15
  grasp reflex and, 25
  increase of head size with, 9, 10, 11
  initial, 248, 249, 250

Age (*cont.*)
  key, 243
  limit, 248, 249, 251, 252, 257
  maturity and, in neonates, 64
  mean, 248, 252
  Moro reflex and, 20
  reflex changes with, 21, 34
  reflex response from light touch
    and, 23
  sitting, crawling, standing and
    walking, 193
  size of vocabulary and, 213
  spoken language and, 223
  support reflex and, 36
  tonic neck reflex and, 39
  variation in development and, 86
  psychic orientation changes at, 136
Alertness in neonates, 58
Anencephaly, 13
Anus, malformations, 55
Attainment tests of articulation,
    222
Apgar score, 54
Assimilation, 133
'At risk' registers, 3
Attention, 241
Audiometry, 156, 222
  puppet, 155
  telephone, 155
Auditory discrimination tests, 222
Auditory function, (*See* Hearing)
Auditory-motor integration, 233
Auditory orientating reflexes, 43, 45

Labyrinthine head righting, 44
Labyrinthine reflexes, tonic, 47
Labyrinthine stimuli, reflex response
  to, 44
Language, 134, 135
  assessment of, 216
    Cash test, 220
    equipment, 288
    features of, 216
    investigation and evaluation,
      222
    jargon, 94, 212
    quick checks and alerting signs,
      217
    Reynell Developmental Lan-
      guage Scales, 224, 259, 279
    screening examinations, 217,
      218
    Stycar Language Test, 222
  communication and, 216
  conceptualization, 213
  development of, 204–226
    cerebral mechanisms of, 204
    delay in, 218, 234
    1 to 5 years, during 93, 102
    18 months, at, 94
    2 years, at, 94
    3 years, at, 96
    5 years, at, 101
    6 to 10 years, 106, 109
  disorders of, investigations, 222
  expressive, 206, 207, 224
  Hounslow study of, 219
  play and, 214
  receptive aspect of, 206
  symbolization, 214, 215
  verbalization, 210
  vocabulary and age, 213
Lanugo, 66
Learning,
  disabilities, 120
  1 to 5 years, 102
  6 to 10 years, 112
Left-handed children, 178
Limit age, 248, 249, 251, 252, 257
Locomotion, development of, 189

Magnet (traction) reflex, 31, 33
Manipulation, 172–188, 232
  ball skills, 187
  cubes, of, 172, 174, 284

Manipulation (*cont.*)
  development,
    3 months, at, 172
    5 months, at, 172
    6 months, at, 172, 174
    8 months, at, 174
    9 months, at, 77, 79, 174
    first year, in, 70, 82
    1 to 5 years, during, 92, 102
    18 months, at, 94
    2 years, at, 175
    3 years, at, 98, 176
    5 years, at, 100, 176
    6 to 10 years, 108
    9 years, at, 112
  drawing, 180
  imitating and copying symbols, 179
  pegs and cup, 185
  pencil and paper, of, 176
  tea-set play, 183
  tests of, 279
    equipment, 288
  tower of cubes, of, 175
  writing, 183
Maturation, 127, 132
  central nervous system, of, 129
  criteria of, in neonates, 64
  definition, 7
  development depending on, 129
  species differences, 139
Mean age, 240, 252
Mental age, calculation of, 183
Mental handicap, 234
Mental retardation,
  brain growth in, 11
  echolalia in, 212
Merrill–Palmer scale of mental tests,
  175, 258
Michael Reed Picture Test, 156
Mimicry, 96
Miniature Toys Test, 164, 224, 286,
  287
Mobility,
  advantages of, 194
  cerebral palsy, in, 277
  deprivation of, 266
Moro reflex, 20, 38, 40
  clinical significance of, 61, 65
Mother,
  response to gaze, 158
Mother–child communication, 207
Mother–child emancipation, 278